Better Homes and Gardens®

SMART CHOICES IN ALTERNATIVE MEDICINE

Medical Reviewer
Samuel Benjamin, M.D.
Director, Center for Complementary and Alternative Medicine
State University of New York

Better Homes and Gardens® Books
Des Moines, Iowa

Better Homes and Gardens® Books
An imprint of Meredith® Books

Smart Choices in Alternative Medicine
Editor: Alice Feinstein
Associate Art Director: Lynda Haupert
Contributing Writers: Barbara Boughton, Jan Bresnick, Jack Forem, Mark Giuliucci, Phil Goldberg, Sara J. Henry, Lambeth Hochwald, Claire Kowalchik, Judith Lin, Diane Quagliani, Maureen P. Sangiorgio, Martha Schindler, Selene Yeager
Copy Chief: Catherine Hamrick
Copy and Production Editor: Terri Fredrickson
Contributing Copy Editor: Angela K. Renkoski
Contributing Proofreaders: Ed Malles, Debbie Morris Smith, Margaret Smith
Illustrator: Thomas Rosborough
Indexer: Sharon Duffy
Electronic Production Coordinator: Paula Forest
Editorial and Design Assistants: Kaye Chabot, Karen Schirm
Production Director: Douglas M. Johnston
Production Manager: Pam Kvitne
Assistant Prepress Manager: Marjorie J. Schenkelberg

Meredith® Books
Editor in Chief: James D. Blume
Design Director: Matt Strelecki
Managing Editor: Gregory H. Kayko

Director, Sales & Marketing, Retail: Michael A. Peterson
Director, Sales & Marketing, Special Markets: Rita McMullen
Director, Sales & Marketing, Home & Garden Center Channel: Ray Wolf
Director, Operations: George A. Susral

Vice President, General Manager: Jamie L. Martin

***Better Homes and Gardens®* Magazine**
Editor in Chief: Jean LemMon

Meredith Publishing Group
President, Publishing Group: Christopher M. Little
Vice President, Consumer Marketing & Development: Hal Oringer

Meredith Corporation
Chairman and Chief Executive Officer: William T. Kerr

Chairman of the Executive Committee: E. T. Meredith III

All of us at Better Homes and Gardens® Books are dedicated to providing you with information and ideas to ensure your family's health. We welcome your comments and suggestions. Write to us at: Better Homes and Gardens® Books, Health Editorial Department, 1716 Locust St., Des Moines, IA 50309-3023. Please visit our web site at bhg.com

If you would like to purchase copies of our books, check wherever quality books are sold.

First Edition. Printing Number and Year: 5 4 3 2 1 03 02 01 00 99
Library of Congress Catalog Card Number: 99-70561
ISBN: 0-696-20962-4

How to Use this Book

Interest in alternative medicine is exploding. Just this past year *The New York Times* reported that Americans make more visits to alternative health practitioners than they do to their primary care physicians. And, in 1997, they spent $21.2 billion on these visits. Clearly, this is more than a fad. It's a growing trend that shows every sign of being here to stay. And like every trend it has an upside and a downside.

You'll find the bright side of alternative medicine in this book—the therapies that have been tested by science and, in many cases, time-tested by generations of clinical use. The dark side of alternative medicine is that regulation is sporadic, varying from state to state. In this climate many alternative health practitioners and merchandisers make overly enthusiastic (or downright fraudulent) claims.

In short, there is wonderful healing potential in many forms of alternative medicine. And, at the same time, quality control continues to be a major issue.

The best advice for now is to rely on your primary care physician for diagnosis and treatment. When you choose alternative medicine, do everything you can to educate yourself about those therapies that really work. You can use this book to help you do just that, then discuss any alternative therapies you'd like to try with your physician. Doctors who are interested in alternative medicine frequently use the term "complementary" medicine, which simply means that they espouse the best that Western medicine has to offer and the best that alternative medicine has to offer. That's a good path for all of us to take.

A couple of precautions are in order. Pregnant women should be particularly vigilant about keeping their doctors informed about their alternative medicine choices. In particular, they should not be making decisions about herbs and dietary supplements on their own. It's also important to exercise caution when using alternative remedies for children—doses for herbs, for example, are much smaller. Please consult a pediatrician familiar with the therapy you're interested in trying.

Alice Feinstein
Executive Health Editor
Meredith® Books

NOTICE TO THE READER: This book is intended to provide you with information about alternative and complementary medicine. It is not intended to serve as a substitute for advice from your doctor. Every individual's health needs are unique. Diagnosis and treatment must be done through a health care professional. Please consult with a doctor for all your health care needs and let your doctor advise you about appropriate alternative therapies.

Contents

Foreword

Reading *Smart Choices in Alternative Medicine* will do more than just teach you, say, about acupuncture or herbs. As you finish the book you will notice that you have learned new criteria for how health care should be delivered, how you can integrate alternative therapies into your life, and how you can become your own best health advocate.

Better Homes and Gardens® Smart Choices in Alternative Medicine tells it like it is. It does not champion all of complementary and alternative medicine (CAM) because the fact is that some forms of alternative medicine just do not work. But safe alternatives do exist to many of the more dangerous and often ineffective medical therapies that our modern Western medicine (allopathic medicine) continue to use. These alternatives are especially important when it comes to treating chronic illness, an area where our allopathic medicine frequently falls short.

It's a good idea to educate yourself as much as possible about what CAM has to offer. Why? The development of alternative and complementary medicine has the potential to change the face of medicine as we know it. In fact, it's already doing so. For the sake of your own health care in the future, you need to know what CAM is all about, what really works and what doesn't, and how to use CAM therapies safely. And this book can help you do just that.

Americans in record numbers are already embracing CAM. In November 1998, the *Journal of the American Medical Association* published a study showing that Americans now pay more visits to CAM providers than they do to allopathic providers. And they spend more money out of pocket for CAM than they do for mainstream health care.

This same report also noted that nearly 42 percent of all Americans (by conservative estimate) are now using these healing methods. Use of herbs has almost quadrupled in just a decade, for example, while vitamin sales have increased by 180 percent.

America's support for CAM has been steadily increasing for quite some time. Nearly a decade ago, David Eisenberg, M.D., of Harvard/Beth Israel Hospital, published a study about CAM that sent shock waves of outright surprise not through the community of health care consumers who were seeking out these services in this country, but across the board rooms of austere teaching and hospital institutions. The study described a parallel system of alternative health care. This system was independent of the mainstream medical system, was not physician-centered, and was essentially unknown to most traditional health care professionals. But it was certainly known to much of the general public.

Perhaps more striking to doctors and researchers, however, was the realization that consumers were paying out-of-pocket for most of these therapies because insurance companies would not reimburse them for alternative techniques. How much were they paying? Nearly as much, the study said, as cash outlays for hospitalizations that same year.

Since then the American health care system has had two responses. On the one hand, it has acknowledged the need to study CAM and adapt those therapies that can contribute positively to patient care. On the other hand, it has attacked CAM's proponents, employing derisive language ("magic," "unscientific," "unfounded," "quackery," etc.) in the hope that this national movement can be staved off or maybe even reversed.

In the meantime, research into the effectiveness of CAM has quietly moved forward. Some doctors are now embracing these therapies and making them part of their own practices.

The time for change is clearly upon us, and none too soon. Allopathic medicine, certainly since the last world war, has become ever more entrenched in technology as the answer to our bodily and emotional needs. In the 1950s many predicted that infectious disease would be eradicated in a decade. Instead, we now live in the fear of "super germs"—created by our overuse of antibiotics and the subsequent microbial mutations that they helped create. Former President Richard Nixon in the 70s declared a "War on Cancer," allocating vast sums of money to find the technology to treat cancer successfully. Sadly, with few exceptions, we doctors are well aware that we have little to show relative to this extraordinary investment.

In fact, relative to the unprecedented investment we have made as a society in medical technology in general, the results have been precious little. Most advances in our health are related to societal change—smoking cessation, lower-fat diets, more exercise—not to the technology we funded with such abandon. Yet the costs continue to rise.

Take the case of coronary artery bypass surgery as an example. Bypass surgery is a technological marvel when it works. This surgery has been used for years as a treatment for angina (chest pain associated with blockage of the arteries feeding the heart). The assumption is that by diverting the blood supply in the affected arteries past these blockages patients would feel better and live longer than their counterparts who chose medications only. We now know that this assumption applies to only *a small percentage* of patients with this disease. For these people it works; for others it does not. Yet many such surgeries are still performed without clear indications that they will be helpful.

Meanwhile, Dr. Dean Ornish did careful research (covered in more detail elsewhere in this book) to demonstrate that diet, meditation, group work, and moderate exercise could, alone or in combination with medications, not only stop the progression of coronary artery disease but actually *reverse* it. All of these therapies fall into the realm of what allopathic medicine has viewed as alternatives. Dr. Ornish's research has shown that these methods do get the job done. Which would you personally rather face—bypass surgery or some serious alterations in your diet and lifestyle?

Yet Dr. Ornish's colleagues in our medical community by and large still resist his lifestyle-altering therapy—even though his approach is clearly supported by stringent research and his findings have been published in medical journals (in 1983 in the *Journal of the American Medical Association* and in 1990 in the British medical journal *The Lancet*).

I believe this failure to embrace Dr. Ornish's findings is because his methods are not technology-based. The other (and yet more important) reason, I believe, is that his methods rely on the patient and nonphysician personnel—shifting the emphasis of care from the doctor directly to a team that includes the patient.

What's so bad about medical technology? Nothing, when it's necessary and it gets the job done. But our allopathic system has steered a historical and financial course based on technology that has made it the most expensive system in the world, with per capita expenditures far exceeding those of any other country. In 1998 the national media gave wide coverage to a government report that by the year 2007 medical costs in this country will double, approaching $2.1 trillion. (That's *trillion*, not billion.) It's clearly time to give serious consideration to alternatives that are safe and effective.

To suggest that all of the mainstream health care providers in the U.S. oppose CAM or that the situation is hopeless would be inaccurate. A growing number of physicians and other health care professionals are eager to explore new ways of helping their patients. More than 75 American medical schools now offer some form of training in CAM. A growing number of clinical, training, and research centers offer CAM, including the State University of New York at Stony Brook, the University of Arizona, Stanford University, and Harvard. The University of California at Los Angeles (UCLA) offers a training program in acupuncture for physicians. Columbia University School of Medicine presents a week-long training program in herbal medicine for health professionals. In fact, an enormous demand for training in CAM comes from the medical community, and leading training institutions are collaborating to educate physicians, nurses, and others.

To support these efforts Congress has helped establish the Center for Complementary and Alternative Medicine at the National Institutes of Health. CAM has become a part of the mainstream, and its impact will be felt throughout organized medicine as it matures.

Out of this growing interest in CAM has been born a new paradigm—integrative medicine. It takes the best that allopathic medicine has to offer and integrates it with the best that alternative medicine has to offer. The key change, however, is the individual's power to take control. That's where you come in.

Better Homes and Gardens® Smart Choices in Alternative Medicine will be an important resource to you in the future, factually on the one hand and as a catalyst for thought on the other. This book is the portal to your own healing—facilitating your growth in mind, body, and spirit. I congratulate the authors for their work and welcome you as a fellow traveler in this exciting personal journey.

Samuel Benjamin, M.D.
Director
Center for Complementary and Alternative Medicine
State University of New York

chapter 1

acupuncture

PATHWAYS FOR RELIEF

The traditional theory is that you are helping the body heal itself and restoring it to balance. — *Ward Glenn Gypson, M.D.*

When Michael Fredericson, M.D., first saw Eva, she was in terrible pain with a condition known as "frozen shoulder." Unable to move her shoulder or carry trays of food in her job as a waitress, Eva had to stop working. Dr. Fredericson, who is both an acupuncturist and a physiatrist—an M.D. who specializes in treating physical complaints such as bad backs and sore necks—offered her a number of options, including physical therapy, a steroid injection, and acupuncture. Afraid of the side effects of steroids, she chose physical therapy and acupuncture.

"It was very dramatic," Dr. Fredericson says regarding the results. "After just one treatment, she felt well enough to go back to work. And after two to three months of both physical therapy and acupuncture, she had regained total motion in her shoulder. To get those kinds of results usually takes about a year."

Such success stories are part of the reason acupuncture is popular today. Over the past few years, it has garnered a reputation as one of the most effective forms of alternative therapy. And in November of 1998 the U. S. National Institutes of Health (NIH) Office of Alternative Medicine broke new ground for acupuncture when it released a positive consensus review of hundreds of acupuncture studies in the *Journal of the American Medical Association (JAMA)*. The scientists concluded that acupuncture does work in many instances, particularly for conditions such as chronic pain and nausea.

Yet even before the NIH statement, Americans were embracing this Oriental-style therapy with enthusiasm. In 1997, according to another 1998 study published in *JAMA*, Americans made more than 5 million visits to acupuncturists. In fact, since President Nixon's visit to China in 1972, there's been a rising tide of interest in acupuncture.

acupuncture helps heal

A National Institutes of Health (NIH) consensus panel reviewed thousands of studies for a research article published in the *Journal of the American Medical Association* in November 1998. The panel concluded that acupuncture was most effective for:

- Dental pain
- Nausea from pregnancy
- Nausea due to chemotherapy
- Postoperative nausea and vomiting

The review panel also found some scientific support—though sometimes only one positive research study—for using acupuncture to treat:

- Fibromyalgia (stiffness and pain felt deep within the muscles)
- Low back pain
- Menstrual cramps
- Tennis elbow (a type of tendinitis affecting the elbow)

Research evidence was less convincing, but still "promising" for using acupuncture for these conditions:

- Addiction
- Carpal tunnel syndrome
- Headache
- Osteoarthritis (a type of arthritis)
- Problems following stroke

Energy Medicine From China

Acupuncture is actually a French word that's a bit of a misnomer—it means "to stick with something sharp." A better translation from the Chinese for this brand of medical treatment is "energy medicine." And in fact, acupuncture, which has flourished in China since at least 400 B.C., is a complicated system of scientific thought based on revitalizing a type of energy called *qi* (pronounced *chee*). Traditional Chinese practitioners (and many modern-day proponents as well) maintain that this energy flows through the body in defined pathways, called meridians. Illness results when qi isn't flowing smoothly or when it gets stuck, the theory goes.

"In many ways, acupuncture doesn't make sense to Westerners," says Ed Weiss, M.D. But Dr. Weiss, an acupuncturist in Palo Alto, California, has found it to be surprisingly effective.

According to traditional Chinese theory, the body's 12 major meridians start in the chest, then travel to the hands and back to the head. From the head they flow to the feet and then back to the chest.

Each meridian links a number of areas of the body as well as various organs and their functions.

By activating some of the 2,000 acupuncture points on the body's meridians with thin needles, acupuncturists say they're stimulating qi and helping it to flow freely.

"The traditional theory is that you are helping the body heal itself and restoring it to balance," says Ward Glenn Gypson, M.D., an acupuncturist and associate clinical professor in the department of orthopedics at the University of California at San Francisco.

Much of the traditional language that surrounds the healing discipline of acupuncture tends to sound alien to Western ears. In acupuncture, the traditional philosophy maintains, the body can be likened to five elements: earth, metal, water, wood, and fire. Each of the elements is in turn linked to several meridians and to internal organs.

"These things are really metaphors for what's happening inside your body," explains Dr. Weiss. And when you carry the metaphors through diagnosis to treatment, explanations can get quite picturesque.

"A person who comes in with a sore neck often has a problem with 'wood and the liver,'" says Dr. Weiss, as an example. "He's very angry and frustrated. An interesting way to treat 'wood' could be to stimulate 'fire'—because 'fire' burns off excess 'wood.' Since the emotion that goes with 'fire' is laughter, you would try to get the person to laugh. Or you could treat points, such as at the base of the wrist, that calm the spirit, calm the heart, and so calm the 'wood.'"

Dr. Weiss adds, "The theory of acupuncture is actually very poetic."

What Exactly Does Acupuncture Do?

Western scientists have tried to come up with their own explanations for why acupuncture is effective, and they've had some success. Some studies have shown that acupuncture results in the release of body chemicals called opioid peptides that control pain. Placing acupuncture needles in the skin also seems to stimulate the immune system, alter blood flow, and cause the release of body chemicals, including hormones and neurotransmitters, resulting in a wide range of physiological effects. These effects include feelings of relaxation and decreased swelling and pain, according to Dr. Gypson.

Acupuncture also seems to stimulate the release of neurotransmitters that affect mood and appetite, according to Michael Smith, M.D., director of the acupuncture program at Lincoln Hospital in New York and author of a paper on acupuncture published in the *Encyclopedia Brittanica's 1998 Medical and Health Annual*.

As yet, Western science has developed no single theory to fully explain how or why acupuncture works, says Dr. Smith.

"But we do know that by supporting basic functions such as circulation, wound healing, and various immune and neurological functions, acupuncture promotes homeostasis—the balanced functioning of the whole person," he says.

The NIH study also found that there was considerable support in the scientific literature for the effectiveness of acupuncture in relieving nausea from chemotherapy, postoperative vomiting and pain, and dental pain. The study's authors also concluded that acupuncture may be helpful in problems such as addiction, headache, tennis elbow, low back pain, carpal tunnel syndrome, and asthma.

One problem that concerned the NIH consensus panel was the difficulty in producing high-quality double-blind placebo-controlled studies when testing acupuncture. In most scientific studies, a placebo or "dummy" treatment is given to one group—and then compared to the results from another group receiving the real treatment. But, particularly in studies on pain, people who receive placebo acupuncture treatment—that is, needles inserted at points that are not true acupuncture points—often experience some decrease in pain, though not as much as patients undergoing true acupuncture. Thus the use of such "sham acupuncture" treatments remains controversial, as do the results attained from such studies.

"There are also ethical problems in giving patients sham acupuncture treatments, because they're not getting the best treatment," says David Molony, acupuncturist, herbalist, and executive director of the American Association of Oriental Medicine.

Yet, despite this controversial issue, the NIH consensus panel concluded in the *JAMA* article that there was enough scientific support to endorse acupuncture as a promising therapy. And there's one very big plus: It is much more cost-effective and has fewer side effects than Western therapies used for the same conditions.

Banishing Pain

"Most any painful condition can be treated with acupuncture, some with more success than others," says Dr. Gypson, who reports good results in treating chronic pain. "Often I see patients who have tried everything and haven't been helped by Western medicine. But somehow acupuncture gives them relief."

A review study of research on acupuncture published in the *Archives of Internal Medicine* in November 1998 also found that the therapy was effective for back pain. Many studies on acupuncture are not of high quality, the researchers said, so they selected only studies of high quality for their analysis. Though most of the people treated in the studies had poor prognoses, those who received acupuncture fared better than those on a placebo.

Much Western research, such as the above study, has concentrated on acupuncture's ability to ease chronic pain. Yet some specialists in Oriental medicine say that such Western research doesn't really go far enough.

"Acupuncture is actually effective for a very wide range of conditions, not just for pain," Molony explains. "Conventional medical research is just not as accurate as thousands of years of observation and experience in Chinese medicine. And these firsthand clinical experiences tell us that acupuncture works for everything from chronic fatigue to infections."

Western physicians and researchers counter that anecdotal reports of clinical success are not enough to conclusively prove acupuncture's success as a wide-ranging therapy. Acupuncture must be validated in the highest quality placebo-controlled studies before it can be used for a range of conditions, they say.

Help with Addictions

Acupuncture treatment for addictions is one area where this therapy has become widely accepted, even though the NIH consensus panel could only conclude that this Eastern medicine may be helpful in such conditions. As well as helping smokers to quit, acupuncture is used widely to reduce the cravings of drug and alcohol addicts.

At Lincoln Hospital in New York, Dr. Smith has overseen the acupuncture program for 25 years. The program has been so successful that the acupuncture style developed there is now used in at least 1,000 settings around the world.

An inner-city hospital, where about 125 patients are treated with acupuncture each day, Lincoln is home to a multifaceted drug and alcohol treatment program. Patients hoping to beat their addictions are provided with acupuncture in groups. (Points on the ear are stimulated.)

"One way of looking at acupuncture is that it teaches the body to be more stable. Often patients report sleeping better and don't react as quickly when they're under pressure," says Dr. Smith.

He tells the story of one woman with a cocaine habit who fled to the hospital in fear of her husband, who was physically abusing her. After she and her husband both received acupuncture treatments, he found that he was less likely to fly off into a rage and resort to physical violence. And the woman was able to control her cravings for drugs more successfully.

"Patients report that they like acupuncture," says Dr. Smith. "It makes them feel good. And it's very useful early in drug treatment. It gets patients stable enough to participate in our other services, such as 12-step groups."

Dr. Smith calls acupuncture a "compassionate, convenient, and cost-effective foundation for addiction rehabilitation."

"Acupuncture," he adds, "relieves the drug abuser's fears about his life and the craving for drugs. Treatment can then shift from overcoming withdrawal symptoms toward taking concrete steps toward long-term social and emotional recovery."

How to Find the Best Acupuncturist

Knowing about the education and credentials of your acupuncturist can help you decide if he or she is right for you.

Most states require acupuncturists to be licensed, meaning that they have to pass a national exam. M.D.s, however, can offer

what about non-MD acupuncturists?

You may wonder about the difference between M.D. acupuncturists and licensed Oriental medicine acupuncturists (practitioners without an M.D.). And, in fact, there are some differences between the way these two groups approach acupuncture, although the distinction is not as clear as it used to be.

Besides doing acupuncture, many M.D.s may also have a practice in a Western specialty as well, such as orthopedics or family medicine.

Often they use acupuncture as an adjunct to Western therapies, often to relieve pain or physical conditions such as a stiff neck.

Acupuncturists who are not M.D.s but specialists in Oriental medicine may also practice other Eastern methods of healing, such as herbalism. They tend to use acupuncture much more widely, not just for painful conditions, but for the whole range of human illnesses.

"We look at Eastern medicine as a total system for healing the body, which involves both traditional Chinese herbs and acupuncture," says David Molony, executive director of the American Association of Oriental Medicine and author of *The Complete Guide to Chinese Herbal Medicine.*

There are some M.D.s, however, who practice herbal medicine and for all intents and purposes have given up their Western medical practice. Among them is Palo Alto physician Ed Weiss, M.D.: "I will prescribe Western drugs only when I have to. The reason is that I'm much more interested in the Chinese philosophy of medicine; it has a more holistic view of how the body works. And it seems more magical and is more fun for me and my patients than Western medicine."

acupuncture without taking such a test. They must have at least 200 hours of training and have an M.D. license from their state. An acupuncturist without an M.D. should also have attended a school accredited by the U.S. Department of Education for at least two years. In some states chiropractors can practice acupuncture. And in some states acupuncturists can only practice under an M.D. You should also check your acupuncturist by taking these steps:

- **Ask friends.** Look for an acupuncturist by asking your friends for the name of a good one. Ask your friends for as many details as they are willing to share. Basically, you want to know if the experiences were good ones.

- **Ask the acupuncturist about training.** Your acupuncturist should have at least two years of experience in acupuncture.
- **Notice if the first visit lasts at least a half hour.** It should include a lengthy discussion about your physical, psychological, and emotional symptoms.
- **Be wary of quick-cure promises.** Your acupuncturist cannot promise a cure on the first visit. He or she should provide a diagnosis only after taking a detailed history and performing an exam.

There are certainly different reasons for going to either an M.D. or an Oriental medicine acupuncturist. Generally, if you're used to Western medicine, you may feel more comfortable with an M.D. Likewise, if you're interested in combining acupuncture with other types of alternative healing such as naturopathy (many naturopaths also specialize in acupuncture) or herbalism, an Oriental medicine acupuncturist may be your best bet.

These days, many M.D.s trained in acupuncture are also incorporating other alternative therapies into their practices. M.D.s do, however, tend to charge more—up to $125 per office visit—but you often get reimbursed by insurance.

Lay acupuncturists can cost much less—the average is about $35 to $70 a session. You may be able to get reimbursed from insurance for care by a licensed acupuncturist, depending on the stipulations of your plan.

You can find an M.D. acupuncturist by calling the American Academy of Medical Acupuncture in Los Angeles at 213/937-5514. To get the names of lay acupuncturists in your area who also practice other types of Eastern medicine, call the American Association of Oriental Medicine at 888/500-7999 or visit their Web site at www.aaom.org.

Using Acupuncture

Your first visit to an acupuncturist will most likely begin with a long, detailed conversation, often lasting for a half hour or more. You'll talk about your symptoms as well as your psychological and emotional state. The acupuncturist may also delve into your family's history of illness, chronic illnesses that you've had in the past, and aspects of your personality.

Be prepared for some unusual questions. The acupuncturist may ask you what type of weather you function best in, your favorite colors, whether you like salty or sour foods, even detailed questions about what your urine looks like.

"What we're trying to understand is the patient's physical symptoms throughout his body as well as his personality as it relates to his health," explains Dr. Fredericson. "In Chinese medicine certain psychological types are prone to certain illnesses. By asking detailed questions we can often find out which meridian is the most involved in the patient's illness."

During the first visit, you'll most often have an acupuncture treatment for at least 20 minutes, sometimes more.

Just before the acupuncture treatment, the practitioner will take your pulse, a procedure far different in Chinese medicine than in Western treatments.

In Chinese medicine there are 12 pulses, six on each wrist. The acupuncturist will feel three superficial pulses and three deep pulses on each wrist. The deep pulses are taken by exerting greater pressure on the three superficial pulse sites—located at your wrist, 1 and 2 inches below your wrist on each hand.

Your acupuncturist may also tell you to stick out your tongue. He or she will check the color, the coating, teeth marks, even the shape of the tongue.

Both the pulse and the tongue are considered mirrors of the body in Chinese medicine, and by looking at them, a practitioner may be able to find which meridians are the most involved in your illness. Some acupuncturists use these diagnostic tools more heavily than others.

"I do take the pulse and I pay attention to it," says Dr. Weiss. "But I'm more interested in picking up other cues a person gives me about how they feel. I look at the way they dress, how they talk, and whether they seem to have low or high energy."

Acupuncture shouldn't be painful, though you'll be aware of the needles. Sometimes people say they're aware of the qi running through their bodies once the needles are inserted. Often people find that acupuncture makes them feel relaxed, even sleepy. In fact, acupuncturists report that some people seek out the therapy just because it makes them feel less anxious and stressed—not only during the acupuncture treatment, but after it as well.

Beyond Needles

Depending on your symptoms, your acupuncturist may try to energize the qi more fully by rotating several needles by hand or by applying a small machine to a few needles in order to stimulate them electrically, making them vibrate slightly.

The acupuncturist may also place suction cups over certain points on a meridian, with or without needles, to stimulate qi.

Another method is to use moxibustion—lighting a mugwort (a Chinese variety of sage) stick, which looks like a large incense stick. The moxa stick is then placed near the skin or a needle, providing a sensation of deep warmth. Sometimes, however, the acupuncturist will leave the needles entirely alone. The needles may be applied to the front and back sides of your body, your ears, hands, or legs.

Some acupuncturists also use acupressure, a type of massage meant to stimulate points on the body's meridians. Though generally considered less effective than acupuncture, acupressure has the capacity to alleviate symptoms and relieve tension when done by someone trained in Chinese medicine. Practioners use various techniques to energize the qi, such as shiatsu—a type of Japanese massage.

different styles, different needles

Different acupuncturists also use various styles of acupuncture and different sizes and numbers of needles. Most acupuncturists specialize in one style, while drawing on others occasionally. A practitioner who specializes in Japanese acupuncture will use needles that are so thin that they have to be guided into place with small plastic or metal tubes. Ancient Chinese acupuncture uses numerous small—but not hair-thin—needles at various points. Modern Chinese acupuncture—a pragmatic, less philosophical type of acupuncture—uses needles in only a few points.

There are also other styles of acupuncture from Vietnam, Germany, England, and France that have various philosophies and techniques.

Robbee Fian, a New York acupuncturist and president of the American Association of Oriental Medicine, has founded a style of shiatsu that is now used around the country. "Shiatsu is effective because it helps relax the body," she says. "And that often eases other health problems, because 85 to 90 percent of our illnesses come from stress."

Many acupuncturists also assign their patients acupressure massage to do at home. "It's a way of keeping the qi flowing in between visits," Fredericson says.

What to Expect

You should see some results from acupuncture within the first three to six visits. If you haven't, it may be time to seek out another practitioner or another type of therapy. Some patients recover fully after acupuncture treatment is complete, but others find it can only help ease their symptoms.

Acupuncturists say they often see patients improve after the first visit.

"Sometimes the improvement is sneaky," Dr. Weiss acknowledges. "The pain may not be better, but the patient feels better and is sleeping better. Or the pain is just as bad, but the patient can do twice as much activity before feeling pain."

Most people start out seeing an acupuncturist at least once a week, sometimes twice or more.

After a few months at most, you should be improved enough to schedule visits less often—say, once every two weeks or even once a month.

Many acupuncturists treat people with difficult chronic problems, and therapy can continue for many months or even years, though visits often become less frequent.

Other practitioners believe that acupuncture is a therapy that should be limited in nature.

"Normally I wouldn't see a patient for the same condition for more than six to ten treatments. By then acupuncture should have helped the patient significantly or aided a full recovery," says Dr. Fredericson.

Some patients may also return for a "tune-up" after their recovery. This happens often when they're under intense stress or if symptoms return.

"According to traditional Chinese medicine, you should return for acupuncture as the seasons change," Dr. Weiss says.

"What I tell people," he says, "is that it's important to get a treatment when your life changes in a big way—whether you're dealing with a new job, retirement, or going to a new school. A treatment can get you back into balance so you can deal successfully with anything that comes up."

Safety and Warnings

One of the advantages of acupuncture is that there are few side effects, especially when compared with Western medicine. Rarely, an acupuncture treatment can cause the condition to worsen temporarily. Or there may be some slight bleeding or bruising after the needles are taken out.

There have been a few reported cases of acupuncturists puncturing organs with the needles, but these cases are extremely rare.

Acupuncturists' needles are sterile and disposable today, so there's an extremely small danger of infection.

If you're on blood-thinning drugs such as Coumadin, you may have increased bleeding with acupuncture. But often this is not a significant problem, Dr. Gypson says. Always discuss your use of such medications with your acupuncturist.

You should keep your prescribing doctor informed that you are getting acupuncture.

Children younger than seven years and very ill patients should only be treated by acupuncturists who have considerable experience, says Dr. Weiss.

Pregnant women also should take care if they're seeking acupuncture. Acupuncture needles can bring on uterine contractions if they're placed in certain areas of the body, such as the abdomen. (Obviously, if you're pregnant it's important to let your acupuncturist know. You should also let your primary physician know that you are comtemplating acupuncture.)

Yet acupuncture can be effective in easing nausea during pregnancy.

"There are very few conditions that would prevent you from getting acupuncture. It's actually very safe," Dr. Gypson says. "Sometimes I run into a patient who's afraid of needles, but even these patients can be helped. We use electrical stimulation at points on the meridian instead of needles."

Dr. Gypson, who also treats patients with conventional Western therapies, maintains that acupuncture is not only safe, but can be a great addition to the other therapies he can offer patients.

"It gives them another choice," he says. "And they often benefit from using a blend of Western medicine—with its emphasis on physiology—and acupuncture, with a more holistic viewpoint of the body. Acupuncture often does help restore patients to harmony and balance."

Acupressure: Do-It-Yourself Relief

It sounds so simple. Instead of using a needle, acupuncture points can be stimulated, though not so deeply, by applying pressure with the fingers.

But guess what? Most acupuncturists *don't* advise trying acupressure at home, unless you have received specific instructions from an acupuncturist. The reason? Each person's illness and symptoms are highly individual, so each may need an acupressure exercise with a somewhat different twist.

"You have to know if the exercise fits your symptom," says acupuncturist Robbee Fian. "Is your headache in the front or the back of your head? And is the pain piercing or throbbing?"

So using acupressure that has not been prescribed by an acupuncturist is often ineffective. There are a few easy points, however, that are worth trying.

If you'd like to try a few simple acupressure techniques, try one or all of these next time you have a headache. Press each point firmly for a full 2 minutes.

Press your index finger to a point directly between your eyes.

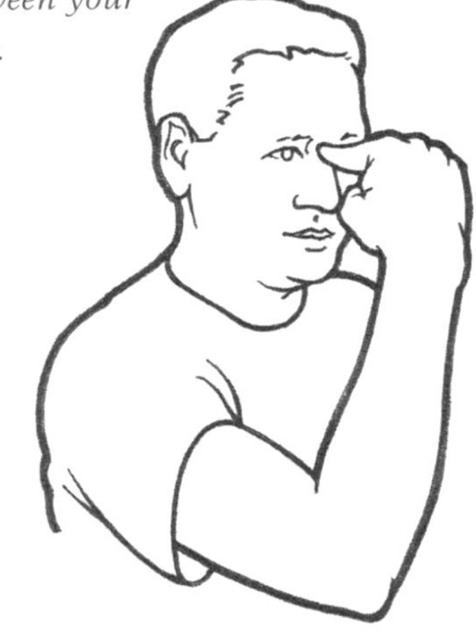

Press your index finger into the center of the top of your head, on line with your ears.

Press the thumb of your right hand into the web of flesh between the thumb and forefinger of the left hand. Switch hands and repeat. (Pregnant women should not do this one.)

resources

Books

Plain Talk About Acupuncture by Eleanor Mitchell (Whalehall, 1987)

This straightforward book is a classic in the field of acupuncture, one of the first Western books to explain acupuncture to a consumer audience. Since its first publication, it's been continually updated and is available in many bookstores.

Who Can Ride the Dragon by Robert Ken Rose and Yu Huan Zhang (Paradigm, 1999)

A thorough book about the link between Chinese culture and its medicine. The book delves into the origins of Chinese medicine and its symbols, which have often arisen from ancient Chinese religious myths. It also fully explains the practice of acupuncture and other Eastern medicines today. It's written in understandable prose by two practitioners of Chinese medicine from the People's Republic of China.

Understanding Acupuncture by Robert Felt and Stephen Birch (Churchill Livingstone, 1999)

An absorbing book that traces the evolution of acupuncture and Asian medicine from 168 B.C. The book combines a good explanation of acupuncture's history with scientific support for its use. It also offers practical tips about when acupuncture is a wise choice for treatment. The book is written by scholars, but is engaging enough to keep anyone's attention.

chapter 2

aromatherapy

MAKING SCENTS OF HEALING

> A bottle of lavender treats a million things, and it's not scary if used wisely.—
> *Shelli Rizzi, herbalist and aromatherapist*

You come home late, stressed out after a high-pressure day at the office. You reach for your trusty bottle of lavender essential oil, pour several drops into a steaming bath, and climb in. And, as always, you feel your stress level start to fall as soon you inhale those soothing vapors. Ah, aromatherapy works its magic once again.

It certainly smells good. That accounts for the "aroma" part of the word. But is it really therapy?

Aromatherapy, the practice of using essential oils—concentrated plant essences—to relieve stress, invigorate, heal, and promote wellness is an ancient one. The Bible is filled with references on the use of concentrated plant scents, such as frankincense and myrrh. Cleopatra was legendary for her use of rose and jasmine oil. And monks in the Middle Ages were among the first to distill plant essences and administer them for purposes of healing.

But it wasn't until the 1920s that the word aromatherapy was coined by a French chemist working in a perfume factory. It was this chemist, Rene-Maurice Gattefossé, who burned his hand and recovered from his burns by applying some lavender oil that happened to be nearby. He went on to classify a number of essential oils and their medicinal properties.

The Sweet Smell Of Money

Since Gattefossé's findings, aromatherapy—based on the premise that fragrance affects how you feel and that everyone has an emotional response to smell—has become more and more mainstream. Over the past decade, a plethora of aromatherapy products—from room sprays and candles to bath oils and lipsticks—has appeared on the market that claim some sort of therapeutic benefit.

In fact, in 1998, sales of aromatherapy products reached $520 million. The interest in aromatherapy is, of course, due to our

what are essential oils?

You open a bottle of essential oil. It's expensive, but seems worth it because it smells so darned wonderful. But what exactly *is* it?

Essential oils, so named because they are created from plants' essences, are complex chemical structures extracted from nearly 400 types of plants. To get these oils, manufacturers use various parts of the plants, including flowers, leaves, bark, roots, fruits, grasses, and resins. These plant parts become oils either by steam distillation, expression (mechanical pressing), by using carbon dioxide (a cold process), or by employing solvents.

Many essential oils don't feel particularly oily, not at all like olive oil or corn oil, for example. In fact, they can seem downright runny. Be assured, however, that they are true oils and will float on water and mix quite nicely with other oils.

Natural essential oils are ... well, essential to aromatherapy. Aromatherapy practitioners, naturopaths, and those who do therapeutic massage wouldn't think of using synthetic fragrances created in a laboratory. Commercial products you pick up at the cosmetics counter or at bath shops, however, often use synthetic fragrance oils.

What's the difference? To begin with, price. Natural essential oils are more expensive to produce because they require so many plants. It takes 16 pounds of fresh peppermint leaves, for example, to make an ounce of peppermint essential oil.

There's also a chemical difference. Aromatherapists maintain that the complex chemical structures of real plant essences lie at the mysterious heart of aromatherapy's ability to heal. Are they right? We don't know; the scientific jury is still out on this one.

If you enjoy candles, room fresheners, and bath oils that have a pleasant synthetic scent, go ahead and enjoy them. But do be aware that unless they are made with true essential oils, they may not really be aromatherapy in the strictest sense of the term.

growing desire to find natural ways to relieve aches and pains, to reduce stress, and to relax.

But there's a big difference between the beauty industry's romantic definition of aromatherapy and medical aromatherapy practiced by massage therapists and naturopaths.

What's labeled "aromatherapy" at the cosmetics counter is frequently created with synthetic oils and has very little science behind it. True aromatherapy is created with real plant essences and has some (but still not a whole lot) legitimate science behind it. Medical aromatherapy strictly focuses on the physiological affects of certain pure essential oils, such as lavender for reducing stress (and thus reducing blood pressure) or eucalyptus for easing sinus headaches. If you're going to spend your money to enjoy the wonderful fragrances of aromatherapy, you should at least know what you're getting.

The Healing Power Of Aromas

Despite centuries (millennia?) of history, the use of plant essences for aromatherapy is a mere youngster when it comes to scientific inquiry. In fact, of all the therapies in this book, aromatherapy may well be the one that has the least solid science behind it. But there is *some*, and what there is shows that there may well be something to this admittedly pleasant form of therapy.

At the Smell and Taste Treatment and Research Foundation in Chicago, neurological director Alan Hirsch, M.D., has spent his career focusing on what happens when we lose our sense of smell. He has also spent the majority of the last 15 years studying the scientific basis of aromatherapy. His brain-wave studies show that some scents (such as chamomile or rose) increase the alpha brain waves associated with relaxation, while other scents (such as rosemary or sage) boost the beta waves that make us more alert.

Dr. Hirsch's foundation currently has approximately 85 active studies under way. A number of the studies focus on things like the affects of aroma on anxiety and depression. Still, Dr. Hirsch feels that most of the claims made for aromatherapy remain untested scientifically.

Dr. Hirsch has remained intrigued with the many possibilities for the healing powers of plants, however. One of the areas he has studied is the effects of odors on obesity.

In one study of 105 people, he asked participants to inhale a scent when they felt like eating to see if the practice could help them lose weight. "We looked at why you feel full after you've eaten," he says. "It's not true that the stomach is full. The reason is that your brain interprets the amount you've eaten *and* the food you've smelled."

It seemed to Dr. Hirsch that if people's brains signaled a sense of fullness simply by smelling food, this process might be used as a tool for weight loss. So he set up a study that followed more than 3,000 people over the course of six months. The participants smelled green apple, banana, and peppermint on a regular basis throughout the day. And they lost, on average, five pounds a month.

Dr. Hirsch reports a direct correlation between sniffing and weight loss. "The more frequently they sniffed, the more weight they lost," he says. He's not quite ready, however, to recommend this as a weight-loss technique. "The smells could have acted as a displacement mechanism like a food diary," he says. "Maybe the odors satisfied their cravings. We have much more research to do on this topic."

Sniffing a bottle of essential oil whenever you're hungry is not likely to do any harm, however. It's certainly worth a try as a weight-loss technique.

Anxiety, Headaches, And Other Conditions

Dr. Hirsch has also done studies using the scent of green apples to treat migraine headaches. He's found that the scent does, in fact, reduce their duration and severity. He's also used the scents of cucumber and green apple for reducing claustrophobia. And he's found that mixed floral smells increase the speed of learning by 17 percent.

Aromatherapy may also play a part in sexual health, according to Dr. Hirsch. "We've done a number of studies on perfume and sexual arousal as well and found that the smell of lavender and pumpkin pie enhanced male arousal and that licorice and cucumber aroused females," he says.

Dr. Hirsch is, of course, not the only scientist looking at the healing powers of scent. In fact, a 1994 study at Case Western Reserve University School of Dentistry in Cleveland, Ohio, showed researchers that a floral fragrance reduced anxiety in dental patients. During the study, machines that aerosolize fragrant oils were used to dispense scent at a barely detectable level into an exam room. The 42 study subjects—all patients getting a root canal—were randomly subjected to either the floral scent, a spicy blend, or no scent. Patient anxiety levels were assessed before and after treatment. And 82 percent of the floral fragrance group had less anxiety than the spicy blend group or the control group that got no fragrance at all.

In Europe, aromatherapy is more widely accepted by the medical profession. Aromatherapy remedies for jet lag are offered on many Europe-based overseas flights. Aromatherapy is even taught in French medical schools.

Britain, however, is the international headquarters for aromatherapy, with many organizations based there. And among medical professionals there, aromatherapy is a widely accepted practice. At the Royal Liverpool University Hospital in England, for example, nurses use aromatherapy fragrances to relieve tension in patients before they undergo treatments.

aromatherapy helps heal

- Anxiety
- Colds and flu
- Headaches
- Muscle aches
- Obesity
- Stress

Specific Scents for Specific Problems

What about all those treatments for specific problems that aromatherapists offer? What about the books full of formulas—the ones that say sniff six drops of this for a cold and drizzle the oils of four specific plants in your bathwater to relieve stress? Is there anything to all this? Maybe. But the fact is that medical science has only just started to determine whether aromatherapy actually works, not to mention which scents might work to treat which conditions.

When you get advice from an aromatherapy practitioner, that advice is based not so much on science as on healing traditions that go back for centuries. The advice is based on the practice of other aromatherapists who have gone before and what their clients have told them, back through the years.

The advice is also based on nebulous things like tradition, intuition, and word-of-mouth anecdotes. That doesn't mean it's wrong. It *does* mean that the science behind it is simply not there. And you should be aware of that if you choose to use this kind of therapy.

If you follow certain precautions, aromatherapy is safe and pleasant to use. And you may well experience some of the healing benefits that practitioners claim for their products and therapies.

If you'd like to try aromatherapy, keep in mind that your practitioner will probably be schooled in other alternative medicine modalities, such as herbal medicine or massage therapy.

The goal of your session will likely be to help you find the scents that evoke positive emotions, in the hope that smelling, inhaling, or applying them topically through massage will help you feel less stressed and help relieve pain. (Aromatherapists, by the way, often make the claim that plant essences can penetrate your skin during massage and enter the bloodstream. There is no scientific validation for this claim whatsoever.)

And even though this process wasn't called aromatherapy in ancient times, essential oils have been known for thousands of years to lift the mood and affect virtually every system in the body, including circulation, nervous system, and digestion, says James Dillard, M.D., author of *Alternative Medicine for Dummies.*

Remember, too, that the word "aromatherapy" has a host of different meanings, says Avery Gilbert, Ph.D., a sensory psychologist in Montclair, New Jersey. "Aromatherapy can mean massage or it could mean one-on-one therapy where you listen to the patient and develop a blend of essential oils for him or her."

With these things in mind, here's what practitioners of aromatherapy have to say about their art.

Where aromatherapy stands out is its ability to help alleviate minor ailments, says Shelli Rizzi, an herbalist and aromatherapy practitioner in Redding, California.

how to find the best practitioner

There isn't a spa in this country that doesn't offer aromatherapy facials, massage, and other treatments. And aromatherapy is included in many wellness programs. But aromatherapy practitioners aren't licensed in the United States. Although certificate programs are offered at different institutes nationwide, there are currently no industry standards for aromatherapy practitioners. Anyone can hang up a shingle.

One way to check a practitioner's degree of commitment to alternative medicine is to see if he or she is trained in other areas, such as naturopathy, Chinese medicine, herbal medicine, or massage therapy, suggests Shelli Rizzi, an herbalist and aromatherapy practitioner in Redding, California.Look also at who they've studied with, she says.

Find out how long the person has studied and has been practicing, says Rizzi. "I'd be far more interested in whether he or she is an herbalist or an acupuncturist than if he or she has a certificate from an aromatherapy program, because those could last anywhere from one month to a year."

If you're working with a chiropractor, naturopath, herbalist, or physician who is interested in alternative medicines, ask for a referral. You can also ask your friends about their experiences with aromatherapy.

How easy it is to find a practitioner and how much you'll spend during your appointment depend on where you live. Most aromatherapy practitioners charge an hourly rate ranging from $40 to $80.

"There are some people who just do aromatherapy, but in this country aromatherapy has been hyped as a spa and beauty care practice," says Rizzi. "Most people go to an aromatherapy practitioner for stress relief or body care. If someone comes to me for stress relief, I look at their overall health. Then, I incorporate aromatherapy."

"The thing you can't escape is that everything has a mind/body connection," she says. "So if you've had a stomachache because you're stressed out, it's linked to your body and your mind. When you apply aromatherapy to that problem, it means you open a bottle of essential oils and trigger something in the mind.

You can take care of yourself and your family in simple ways. A bottle of lavender treats a million things, and it's not scary if used wisely."

"You can experience instant benefits," says Judith Jackson, a certified aromatherapist, licensed massage therapist, and author of *The Magic of Well Being.* Jackson's treatments and products are featured by leading spas nationwide. Practioners believe that some essential oils, like lavender, vetiver, and marjoram, have relaxing properties. "When someone comes to see me, I take a profile," says Jackson. "I get enough to find out what their problem is. As you progress with this as a therapist, you can tell right away what they need."

What to Expect

There are no licensing requirements for aromatherapy practitioners in the United States. In contrast, in Europe, where aromatherapy is more widely recognized, aromatherapy practitioners are licensed just like massage therapists.

Here, your experience will vary depending on whom you meet with.

At your first appointment, you'll probably discuss your diet and lifestyle. An aromatherapy practitioner will likely ask if you're taking medications, if you have a heart or lung problem, or whether you have allergies.

After getting a sense of the problems you're dealing with, your practitioner may offer you an essential oil blend. The practitioner may incorporate massage (using those essential oils) in his or her practice since many aromatherapists are licensed massage therapists as well.

For right now, aromatherapy has a way to go before it crosses into the arsenal of conventional medicine practices.

"We'll eventually see aromatherapy as a true medical intervention," says Dr. Hirsch. "The idea is that this could be part of treating disease."

So, along with your prescription for Imitrex for your migraines, for example, someday you might also get a vial of green apple smell. Or, along with Prozac for depression, you'll be given lavender.

"We're not there yet," says Dr. Hirsch. But by 2020, we'll be there."

Safety and Warnings

When it comes to using aromatherapy safely, there are a few things to keep in mind, says Mindy Green, director of educational services at the Herb Research Foundation in Boulder, Colorado.

- **Don't use undiluted essential oils.** Many essential oils can irritate, burn, or cause photosensitive reactions. A photosensitive reaction means that the oil makes the skin more sensitive to sunlight, making it easier to burn. Citrus oils are especially problematic in this regard. Be sure to read the label on the bottle and note whether the essential oil is already diluted, since many commercial products come that way.

To dilute it yourself, add about five or six drops of essential oil to 1 ounce of a carrier oil. Jojoba oil never goes rancid, making it a good choice. It is more expensive than safflower or almond oil, which are also good choices. Also, adding a few drops of vitamin E oil to the mix can help keep the mixture fresh.

- **Use only when appropriate.** Skip aromatherapy altogether if you're pregnant since some oils (like pennyroyal) can prompt miscarriage. If you have asthma, high blood pressure, epilepsy, open wounds, diabetes, rashes, or a neurological disorder, get approveal for the use of aromatherapy from your health-care provider.
- **Keep your aromatherapy practitioner informed.** Be sure to inform your practitioner if you're taking any prescription medications.
- **Do the skin test.** Before you use any essential oil for the first time, dab a little of the diluted oil on your inner arm or the nape of your neck. Wait for 12 hours to make sure there's no redness or itching. If you don't get any response to it, feel free to apply the oil more liberally. And remember, just because the books say an oil is generally mild, doesn't mean *you* won't have a reaction to it.
- **Watch for allergies.** "If you're sensitive to synthetic fragrances, you may be allergic to essential oils," says Green. "If you're allergic to chamomile tea, you might be allergic to chamomile essential oil."

If you're doing an aromatherapy bath at home, start with just two to five drops per tub. Certain oils, like peppermint, citruses, and lemongrass, may cause skin irritation so start with fewer drops. In addition, cinnamon, clove, nutmeg, or ginger can burn the skin. And, while the warm water adds to the therapeutic benefits of the oils, you'll still get irritated from the oils if you happend to be allergic.

- **Treat skin irritations.** If your skin does get irritated, apply vegetable oil directly on the outbreak. Check with your physician if the rash doesn't clear in 24 hours.
- **Never take an essential oil internally.** The most toxic are eucalyptus, hyssop, mugwort leaf, sage, tansy, thujone, and wormwood.

If you have an aromatherapy book that tells you to take the oils internally, discard the book. This is not something you should be doing on your own.

- **Err on the cautious side with children.** Although essential oils are safe for kids, geranium and some of the citrus essential oils are photosensitizing and can cause a serious sunburn when children are exposed to the sun. It's best to avoid using those oils on children.
- **Follow directions.** Read all label warnings on the essential oil packaging and use as directed.
- **Protect your eyes.** Keep essential oils away from your eyes because they can cause irritation.
- **Store for freshness.** Store your essential oils in a cool place or refrigerate the essential oils you buy. Keep in mind, though, that the shelf life for most oils is about two months.

Do-It-Yourself Aromatherapy

Essential oils are available at your local health food store and via mail order or the Internet. It's fun to experiment with different aromas but, before you buy, remember that essential oils are often quite costly because they're so expensive to produce. Buy in small quantities.

Keep in mind, too, that while essential oils may be natural, they're also powerful natural chemicals, says Jackson.

"Essential oils have a real power to affect your mood, your skin, your energy, and you have to use them in just the right dose," she says.

If you want to be the smartest at-home aromatherapy user, be sure to consult the myriad books on aromatherapy that can help guide you in terms of how much you use, how you store the oils, and that you use the right base.

There are a number of ways—besides just opening the bottle and sniffing—to enjoy your oils.

- **Sleep with it.** "You can drizzle some on a cotton ball and place it under your pillow," advises Jackson.
- **Diffuse it through your room.** A safe way to enjoy aromatherapy is to fragrance a room using an electric vaporizer. You can also buy a lightbulb ring that sits atop a lightbulb. It releases aroma as soon as the bulb heats up.
- **Get misty.** You can place water and an essential oil in a plastic spray bottle and mist a room, says Pamela Allardice, author of *The Art of Aromatherapy.*
- **Burn it.** During the winter, place rosemary or lavender on the wood in your fireplace for a relaxing evening at home.

Curing What Ails You

There are dozens of essential oils and hundreds of remedies to choose from. Aside from following an aromatherapy practitioner's advice, there are a number of things you can try on your own. Here are several of Jackson's favorites for various conditons:

- **Colds:** Inhale an infusion of eucalyptus oil in steaming water. To make an infusion, add 10 to 15 drops of eucalyptus in a bowl of steaming water. Close your eyes and inhale the mixture for two to three minutes for up to four times daily. Eucalyptus cools the body if you have a fever, dries mucous secretions, and shrinks swollen sinuses. Another way to clear your sinuses? Place a drop of eucalyptus oil on your pillow.
- **Headaches:** Apply a few drops of diluted lavender, peppermint, or rosemary oil to your temples. Massage them using deep strokes. Close your eyes and apply pressure to your forehead, jaw, and temples.
- **Indigestion and gas:** Massage either basil and chamomile or fennel and peppermint over your abdomen. (Again, place two drops of each essential oil into 1 ounce of carrier oil and massage as needed.)
- **Mouthwash:** Place one drop of peppermint or lemon essential oil in 1 half-cup of water. Gargle and rinse. (Do not swallow the oils.)
- **Muscle aches:** Prepare a dilution of two drops each of eucalyptus and rosemary or arnica and juniper in 1 ounce of carrier oil. Mix. Massage directly onto sore muscles.
- **Stress:** Mix 10 to 20 drops of lavender and rosemary in a full bath. Soak.

resources

There are several national organizations working to enhance the profession of aromatherapy. For more information on using essential oils or selecting an aromatherapy practitioner, contact the following organizations or read the following books. :

Organizations

American Alliance of Aromatherapy
P.O. Box 309
Depoe Bay, OR 97341
800/809-9850

National Association for Holistic Aromatherapy
P.O. Box 17622
Boulder, CO 80308–7622
800/566-6735

Pacific Institute of Aromatherapy
P.O. Box 6723
San Rafael, CA 94903
415/479-9121

Books

Aromatherapy A-Z by Connie and Alan Higley (Hay House, 1998)

Aromatherapy: A Complete Guide to the Healing Art by Kathi Keville and Mindy Green (The Crossing Press, 1995)

Scentual Touch: A Personal Guide to Aromatherapy by Judith Jackson (Henry Holt and Company, 1986)

The Art of Aromatherapy by Pamela Allardice (Crescent Books, 1994)

chapter 3

ayurveda

TRADITIONAL HEALING FROM INDIA

In order for us to regain health, we have to regain balance.
—*Christopher Clark, M.D.*

Want to understand what ayurveda is all about? Just look outside your window. This intricate system of health developed in India more than 5,000 years ago, yet its theories seem incredibly modern. Ayurveda (pronounced eye-your-VAY-dah*) is all about the importance of balance in nature. Think of how many natural disasters occur when Mother Nature's elements are off-kilter. Hurricanes, blizzards, and forest fires are only a few of the nasty consequences. Well, people are susceptible to a few natural disasters of their own when they don't live balanced lives. Only instead of calling them tornadoes and typhoons, we give them names like heart disease and cancer.*

"When people live excessively, drinking too much, smoking, eating the wrong foods, living with too much stress, and so forth, they develop what ayurveda calls imbalances," explains Christopher Clark, M.D., medical director at the Maharishi Ayur-Veda Health Center at the Raj Health Resort in Fairfield, Iowa. These imbalances can range from minor ailments such as dry skin and heartburn to major conditions like hypertension, obesity, and diabetes if they remain unchecked.

"In order for us to regain health," says Dr. Clark, "we have to regain balance. Even better, we should work every day to stay in balance so we never have to get sick to begin with. That's the real premise of ayurveda—optimal health."

It's in Your Constitution

So what does it mean to live in balance? For one, it means following some of the regular rhythms of nature, like going to bed at nightfall and waking with sunrise. But it also means eating, exercising, sleeping, and conducting our lives in a way that is in tune with our body's specific metabolic needs. Ayurveda teaches that though we are all human beings, we each have a unique physical constitution that dictates our personality, our physical makeup, and the lifestyle that suits us best.

"If you just look at how different you are from your friends and family, the fact that we each have different constitutional needs becomes pretty obvious," explains Hari Sharma, M.D., professor emeritus in the department of pathology at the College of Medicine and Public Health at Ohio State University in Columbus and author of *Contemporary Ayurveda.*

It's your unique constitution that explains why you may always need a sweater, while your husband is perfectly comfortable in a T-shirt; or why some folks seem to stay wafer thin no matter how much they eat, while others can't seem to lose an ounce no matter how much they diet. It's precisely why we don't all think, look, or act alike.

How did we become so different? The answer is at the heart of ayurveda. Ancient ayurvedic texts teach that the universe is comprised of five basic elements: space, air, fire, water, and earth. Those elements combine naturally into pairs that they call *doshas,* or universal forces. There are three doshas that comprise everything in the world around us, including ourselves. They are: *vata* (space and air), *pitta* (fire and water), and *kapha* (water and earth).

ayurveda helps heal

Though more research needs to be done, ayurvedic physicians promote ayurveda as a health system for preventing disease and increasing well being. It may also be beneficial in the treatment of non-acute, chronic conditions, including:

- Allergies
- Digestive disorders
- Headaches
- High blood pressure
- High cholesterol
- Respiratory ailments
- Skin conditions
- Stress

When you were born, the theory goes, the elements from your mother and your father combined to create your unique body type or constitution, known in ayurveda as your *prakruti.* As a result, each of us ends up having more of some elements than others, so we each have different characteristics. People with higher amounts of vata, for instance, will tend to be lighter and airier, while kapha people will be heavier and earthier.

Balancing the Elements

The trick to good health, according to ayurveda, is keeping the elements of your constitution in balance, which is not as easy as it sounds. Though your innate constitution, or prakruti, remains constant throughout your entire life, your body is highly susceptible to the forces around it, including the weather, the seasons, your lifestyle, what you eat on a daily basis, and how you exercise.

These outside elements build up to form your day-to-day constitution, which is called your *vikruti*. Ideally, your prakruti and your vikruti—your general body type and your day-to-day constitution—should match one another exactly. But in reality, that rarely happens, says Atsuko Rees, M.D., of the Maharishi Ayur-Veda Medical Center in Pacific Palisades, California.

"Just driving on the freeway can throw you out of balance," says Dr. Rees. "Add all the unhealthy aspects of modern culture like fast food, sleepless nights, tons of caffeine, alcohol, and nicotine, as well as stress and pollution, and it's practically impossible to live without imbalances. And it's those imbalances that are to blame for all the chronic conditions that we see today."

"Unlike Western medicine that teaches that if we aren't sick, we are healthy, ayurveda teaches that health is a continuum between optimum wellness and disease," explains Dr. Sharma. "Most people fall somewhere along the middle. They're not really sick, but they're not really well either. They're just living out of balance.

"The problem is that the longer you live this way, the more likely you are to suffer the cumulative effects of your imbalances and finally show symptoms. Some of these symptoms are minor, like headaches and constipation, but others can be major health threats, like heart disease, cancer, and diabetes. Ayurveda can correct these imbalances before they become a problem."

How much of a difference can living in balance actually make? Maybe a lot. Researchers at the Maharishi University of Management in Fairfield, Iowa, compared the health insurance expenditures of 693 people following the lifestyle recommendations of ayurveda with 4,148 similar people who didn't practice ayurveda. After 11 years, those who followed an ayurvedic health system had about 60 percent fewer health expenditures than those who did not.

What's more, when the researchers broke down these health insurance expenditures in categories according to disease, they found that the people practicing ayurveda were significantly healthier in 17 disease categories, including digestive problems, respiratory conditions, heart disease, and cancer.

The researchers credit the ayurvedic approach to health, which includes eating a largely plant-based diet, eliminating alcohol and tobacco, and practicing stress-reducing meditation, for the vast differences in health insurance expenditures.

"Once you truly know and understand yourself, it becomes easier to take responsibility for your health and avoid diseases of all kinds," says Vasant Lad, BAMS, MASc, director of The Ayurvedic Institute in Albuquerque, New Mexico, and author of *The Complete Book of Ayurvedic Home Remedies*. "That is where ayurveda is strongest. It empowers you to change your diet, lifestyle, and attitude in the ways that are best for you. It is the art of living and the art of balance." (Dr. Lad's degrees are from India and indicate several years of training in ayurvedic medical school.)

Understanding Your Dosha

The first step to maintaining a healthy balance, according to the ayurvedic tradition, is determining your dosha combination. Though all three doshas are present in all of us, most people are primarily a combination of two, with one being predominant. (To figure out your own dosha combination see "What's Your Dosha?" on page 27.)

As a rule of thumb, you are most likely to go out of balance in your primary dosha. The following is a guide to understanding the three doshas.

- **Vata (space and air).** A combination of space and air, vata is the most changeable of the doshas. The word vata itself comes from the Sanskrit (an ancient Indian language) word *vaayu*, meaning "that which moves things."

Vata people are vivacious, imaginative, and unpredictable. Physically, vatas tend to be either very tall or very short with thin, bony features; cool, dry skin; and fine hair. They also tend to be sensitive to cold. Though they have many new ideas, vata people often have a hard time following things through to completion. Of the three doshas, vata types also have the hardest time adhering to their appropriate lifestyle recommendations.

In the body, the vata force is responsible for all movement, including the movement of air in and out of the lungs, the flow of blood, and the flow of electrical impulses—including thought—through the body.

Because of their changeable nature, vatas have the hardest time staying in balance of any of the doshas. An excess of vata is believed to cause diseases of wind and dryness, such as intestinal gas, chapped lips, fatigue, rough skin, arthritic joints, constipation, and insomnia. When imbalanced, vata people also may become anxious and worrisome.

Generally, vatas should avoid things that aggravate the vata dosha. They should avoid light, dry, cold foods, for instance, while favoring warm, cooked foods and warming spices. They should also take special care to stay warm and moisturized in cold, dry climates or seasons. And they should try their best to maintain a steady eating and sleeping routine.

- **Pitta (fire and water).** It would be safe to say that most of the nation's CEOs are pitta people by ayurvedic standards. Made of fire and water, pittas are the steam engines of the world. They are intense, intelligent, fiery, and filled with drive. They correspond with our Type-A personality—always on the go, taking on new challenges, and commanding leadership roles in most situations.

They have strong metabolisms, which give them large appetites and thirst. They generally have well-muscled, medium builds. Because they're so warm, pittas tend to have ruddy complexions that flush easily. They're generally not well suited for very warm climates or seasons.

In the body, pitta is responsible for metabolism. It is the force that digests food, turns food into energy, and creates thought and intelligence.

what's your dosha?

The following are some of the dominant characteristics of the three doshas—vata, pitta, and kapha. Put a check by those characteristics that best describe you. The columns with the most checks are your primary doshas.

VATA	PITTA	KAPHA
• Dry, curly hair	• Thin, fine hair	• Dark, full hair
• Thin, bony physique	• Medium, muscled build	• Heavyset, curvy, strong
• Dry skin	• Ruddy, freckled complexion	• Oily, smooth skin
• Vivacious, imaginative	• Fiery, intense	• Steady, slow
• Dislikes cold	• Dislikes heat	• Dislikes damp cold
• Light sleeper	• Moderate, sound sleeper	• Heavy sleeper
• Intuitive	• Articulate	• Compassionate
• Easily fatigued	• Strong	• High stamina
• Quick to learn and forget	• Medium mental capacity	• Slow to learn, good memory
• Anxious under stress	• Irritated under stress	• Relaxed under stress

An overload of the pitta dosha can lead to, in ayurvedic terms, diseases associated with heat such as fever, infection, inflammation, skin rashes, diarrhea, ulcers, heartburn, and sore throats. Pitta people who are out of balance also are easily aggravated and tend to fly off the handle when angry.

Eating spicy, hot foods is not recommended for pitta people. Instead, people with dominant pitta doshas should seek out cooling foods and liquids, such as mint teas, sweet fruits, and cold salads. Pittas are also advised to avoid the blazing sun during the hot summer months.

- **Kapha (water and earth).** The thick, heavy combined forces of water and earth make the kapha dosha the slowest and most relaxed of the three. Slow moving, kapha people take a long time to process ideas, digest meals, and get moving in the morning. They have soft, lustrous skin and hair, and large eyes. They dislike cold, damp weather. And their physical build is strong, with solid musculature and broad, well-developed bodies, though they do tend to carry more weight than they should. Of the three doshas, kapha is the most stable.

Within the body, the kapha dosha is said to be responsible for the building processes of the body, from forming new cells to laying down fresh bone. It is the fluid in the joints, and it is the driving force behind mental processes like understanding, loyalty, and forgiveness.

When the earthy kapha dosha slides out of balance, the result is usually obesity, as well as general dullness, high cholesterol, sinus problems, fatigue, constipation, and excessive sleep. Usually steady and loyal, an imbalanced kapha also can become stubborn and lazy, often seeking emotional solace through food.

While kaphas naturally crave kapha-aggravating foods like cakes, ice cream, meat, and milk, they should try to avoid these cool, sweet, and often fatty foods. Instead, they should favor what ayurveda considers bitter or astringent foods like leafy greens, apples, and poultry.

Though all the talk of forces and doshas can sound rather mystical to Western ears, these explanations of dosha constitutions simply explain the differences among people we already see, says Dr. Clark. "It explains the vast mental and physical differences among people, like why some people remain cool under pressure, while others explode; why some folks love spicy foods, while others can't tolerate even mild peppers; and why different people are prone to different diseases."

You can also think of these ayurvedic definitions as more detailed descriptions of terms Western doctors already use to describe people, such as Type-A personalities, couch potatoes, endomorphs (large, heavy builds), ectomorphs (thin, lanky builds), and mesomorphs (lean, muscular builds).

"Ayurveda just has a different language for describing the same reality we all live within," says Nancy Lonsdorf, M.D., Ph.D., coauthor of *Woman's Best Medicine.* "We can say you have an excess of kapha, or we can say you have high cholesterol. The difference is that ayurveda works to treat the root of high cholesterol—the kapha imbalance—instead of just treating the symptom."

Daily Health Prescriptions

Along with living in accordance with your dominant dosha, ayurveda prescribes disease prevention through a series of daily, monthly, and yearly routines that rejuvenate the body and help keep you balanced. Though you can get benefits from any one of these things, ayurvedic physicians recommend that you adopt as many as possible to stave off the effects of aging and to live a longer, healthier life.

"The real power of ayurveda is that it is a complete, holistic health-care system," says Shri K. Mishra, M.D., professor of neurology at the University of Southern California in Los Angeles. "Ayurveda takes care of your mind, body, and spirit. It's not just tests and pills and surgery. But it is yoga, meditation, diet, herbs, cleansing, and a healthy lifestyle. It is also medicine for the people, meaning that everybody can help care for themselves."

Unfortunately, because ayurveda is as much a lifestyle as it is a medical system, there are few clinical studies that show the benefits of ayurveda as a whole for fighting disease. There are numerous studies, however, on some of ayurveda's individual lifestyle recommendations, such as meditation and yoga. The following are some of the lifestyle routines ayurvedic physicians recommend and how they can help keep you healthy.

Dosha Diets

The most important element of ayurveda is diet, says Dr. Lonsdorf. "If you are willing to change your diet to eat according to ayurvedic recommendations for your dosha, you can get about 50 percent improvement in your health."

For details on how to eat to balance your dosha, it's best to consult with an ayurvedic practitioner, who can customize dietary recommendations to your individual body type and medical status. Here are a few examples of the kinds of things you might hear.

In a nutshell, vata-dominant people should be eating foods that stabilize vata, including warm foods and beverages, as well as foods that are predominantly sweet, sour, or salty. Vata foods include items like sweet potatoes, peppers, beans, rice, nuts, and grapefruits.

Pitta people should emphasize cooling foods and drinks that are predominantly sweet, bitter, and astringent. Pitta foods include leafy greens, cranberries, wheat, and milk.

And kapha-dominant people should favor foods that are light, dry, and warm as well as those that taste primarily spicy, bitter, or astringent. Kapha foods include leafy greens, apples, and barley.

Daily Routines

"Like the wildlife around us, our bodies do better if we live in a regular routine along with nature—rising, sleeping, and eating at about the same time each day, rather than living in a hectic manner," says Dr. Sharma. The following is a basic ayurvedic routine.

- **Rise early.** Rising at or shortly after sunrise—definitely before 8 a.m.—is the best time to start the day and avoid sluggishness.
- **Eat the most at noon.** Breakfast should be eaten before 8 a.m., and it should be light. Dinner should also be a light meal and is best eaten before 6 p.m. for optimum digestion. Make lunch your largest meal of the day and try to eat as close to noon as possible to get the best digestion and maximum benefits from your food.
- **Walk in the morning.** Moderate exercise is recommended in the morning hours or in the midafternoon.
- **Brush and gargle.** Brushing your teeth, lightly scraping or brushing your tongue, and gargling with warm oil are all recommended to keep a clean, healthy mouth.
- **Give yourself a brief massage in the morning.** Using warmed oil, stimulate your circulation by massaging from your face to your feet in light, circular motions.
- **Bathe daily.** Bathe or shower in warm water using a mild soap.
- **Meditate.** Meditation should be part of your morning and evening routine for maximum stress reduction and optimal mental health.

- **Retire early.** To avoid a night of restless sleep and sluggishness come morning, try to get to bed by 10 p.m.

Meditation Heals the Heart

Ayurvedic physicians recommend taking time in the morning and evening to meditate. "This might be the single most important element to slowing the aging process," says Jay Glaser, M.D., of the Maharishi Ayur-Veda Health Center in Lancaster, Massachusetts.

Never meditated before? It's simple, says Dr. Glaser. "The goal is to reach a state of restful alertness, without any thoughts, emotions, or perceptions for 20 minutes at a time," he explains. It takes a little practice, but you can start by just sitting quietly and clearing your mind for five minutes and working your way up.

"Practicing meditation will vastly reduce your stress and improve your overall mental and physical health," he says.

Though researchers have suggested that meditation can be useful for combating everything from addiction to cancer, the best recent research results have been in the area of heart disease. And because meditation lowers stress, it is particularly useful for lowering high blood pressure.

When researchers from the Maharishi University of Management in Fairfield, Iowa, studied 111 African-American men and women, ages 55 to 85, with high blood pressure, they found that those participants who started practicing transcendental meditation experienced significant drops in both their systolic and diastolic blood pressures (both the high and low part of the blood pressure reading), while those who practiced other kinds of stress management techniques experienced no significant changes in their blood pressure.

Yoga, Herbs, and Purification

Ayurveda also advocates regular exercise. But ayurveda is not one of those "no pain, no gain" disciplines. In fact, ayurvedic physicians *prefer* light to moderate exercise rather than vigorous activity. The best daily exercise? Yoga.

"Yoga is wonderful for promoting balance, strength, flexibility, and improving mental health," says Dr. Glaser. "It's also much more gentle than you think. An ayurvedic physician can show you a few postures to get started." (For more details, see "Yoga" on page 297.)

For most people, a daily ayurvedic routine also includes taking some herbs. Ayurveda uses herbs like "tuning forks," explains Dr. Lonsdorf. "They are the helpers in our quest for harmony and balance."

Plus, many ayurvedic herbs are powerful antioxidants, says Dr. Sharma, so they are good for just about everybody. (Antioxidants, which include vitamins C and E, help neutralize free radicals. These are the naturally occurring molecules that damage the body's cells.)

Unlike Western herbs, which are generally sold individually, ayurvedic herbs come in combinations, sometimes containing as many as 15 herbs in one preparation.

Though we need more research to thoroughly understand how these herbs work, their antioxidant powers have been well documented. In one small study of 10

self-care

Back in ancient times, ayurvedic doctors were paid only while their patients were well. If you got sick, you stopped paying. Though times have changed, ayurveda is still widely regarded as a system for disease prevention. That means it requires a great deal of ongoing self-care. Remember, you should always seek consultation with an ayurvedic physician before trying to treat yourself at home.

Once you understand the fundamentals behind ayurveda, basic self-care for minor ailments is simple. Along with following the general daily care regimen that ayurveda recommends, such as meditation, dosha diets, exercise, and proper rest, most self-care remedies involve herbs.

"Because we live in a world where it's so difficult to stay in balance, even if you do the right thing, herbs are tremendously helpful to help your body handle the stresses of daily life," says Nancy Lonsdorf, M.D., Ph.D., coauthor of *Woman's Best Medicine.* Here are a few herbal prescriptions to try.

- **General balance:** To promote general wellness, try drinking herb and spice teas that balance your dominant dosha.
- **Vata-balancing teas:** cinnamon, clove, ginger
- **Pitta-balancing teas:** mint hibiscus
- **Kapha-balancing teas:** clove, ginger, chicory
- **Digestion:** Good digestion is absolutely vital to good health. To avoid indigestion, try taking herbal teas such as ginger, fennel, cinnamon, and cloves before or after meals.
- **Energy:** For listlessness and fatigue, try eating a few almonds or dates every day. Or take herbal preparations that include licorice, fennel, or peppermint.

There is a wide array of ayurvedic herbal preparations you can buy. When choosing ayurvedic herbs, a good bet to ensure quality is to purchase them from a reputable source, such as:

The Ayurvedic Institute
11311 Menaul, NE
Albuquerque, NM 87112
505/291-9698

Maharishi Ayur-Veda International
(www.maharishi.com)

Another safe bet is to buy ayurvedic herbs at a local natural foods store. "Just be sure to always read the labels," says Lakshmi Prakash, Ph.D., senior research scientist at Sabinsa Corporation in Piscataway, New Jersey. "The label should say that you are buying standardized extracts. I would not buy loose, bulk herbs in the United States."

how to find the best practitioner

In India, doctors of ayurveda receive a Bachelor of Ayurvedic Medicine and Surgery (BAMS) degree, which equals five and a half years of medical school there. No schools in the United States offer that degree, though doctors with BAMS can practice to a limited degree in this country. Unfortunately, there is no licensure for these practitioners in the United States, so they are hard to evaluate. Also, few insurance companies will pay for treatment from a non-M.D. ayurvedic practitioner.

One route is to find an ayurvedic physician who also holds a Western medical degree such as an M.D. or D.O. Deepak Chopra, M.D., former chief of staff at New England Memorial Hospital and the author of *Perfect Health, Quantum Healing, Unconditional Life,* and *Ageless Body, Timeless Mind,* is the most famous of these. That way not only will your visits be covered by most major medical insurance, but the doctor also will be able to prescribe general medical tests or medications if necessary.

You can also receive quality care from a non-M.D. BAMS (make sure they hold this degree from India), but you'll have to pay for it yourself. There are only a handful of ayurvedic clinics found in North America. For a list of practitioners nearest you, call the Maharishi Ayur-Veda Clinics System at 800/255-8332 or contact:

The Ayurvedic Institute
11311 Menaul, NE
Albuquerque, NM 87112
505/291-9698

men and women with high cholesterol, researchers at Ohio State University in Columbus found that when the volunteers took a commercial ayurvedic preparation of herbs called Maharishi Amrit Kalash, they had significantly less free-radical damage to their cholesterol than before they started taking the herbs. That means less hardening of the arteries down the road.

"Since free radicals play an important role in diseases like heart disease, cancer, and even aging itself, these herbal compositions can be very important for preserving health and preventing disease," says Dr. Sharma.

Just as your car needs a tune-up and oil change every so many miles, your body needs a cleanup and adjustment on a regular basis, according to ayurveda.

Ayurvedic physicians do this through a purification system known as *panchakarma*. Though the process is a bit different for everybody, panchakarma generally involves herbal massages, steam baths, warm oil treatments, and herbal enemas to loosen and rid the body of impurities.

"Panchakarma is a way to get rid of a lot of toxins in a short amount of time," says Dr. Rees. "In general, we encourage people to do panchakarma once or twice a year, but if someone has serious health conditions, we may do more intensive treatment."

By applying all of these lifestyle recommendations, you can reduce wear and tear on your physical body; keep your stress levels low; and live a much longer, healthier life than most people in this culture, says Dr. Lad. "It's never too late to start reducing the effects of stress on your body," he says, "because the more you reduce physical and mental stress, the less likely you are to suffer from diseases of all kinds."

"We are doing more research all the time," adds Dr. Glaser. "I've seen ayurveda treatments provide tremendous benefits for a wide array of about 40 or 50 chronic conditions including migraine headaches, asthma, depression, high blood pressure, irritable bowel syndrome, menopause complications, and arthritis."

"Ayurveda also has a great deal to offer in terms of complementary care," says Dr. Mishra. "If you have cancer, of course, you must see a Western physician to be diagnosed and receive treatment. But you also can work with an ayurvedic doctor to receive treatments that will help strengthen your immunity, reduce your stress, and help you feel better."

Seeking Ayurvedic Care

The first choice you'll need to make if you seek ayurvedic care is what kind of doctor to visit. In this country, there are classic Western M.D.s who also hold degrees as ayurvedic doctors, and there are BAMSs (Bachelor of Ayurvedic Medicine and Surgery) who were trained in India and are practicing in the United States.

If you visit a doctor who is an M.D. as well as an ayurvedic doctor, he or she will be able to use Western tools of diagnosis such as X-rays and MRIs, as well as prescribe medicine. If, on the other hand, you choose to seek treatment from a non-M.D. practitioner, you will need to keep your regular doctor abreast of what you are doing with your ayurvedic care provider.

"If you are very sick, then your first trip should be to your regular doctor," says Dr. Lad. "Then, after he or she prescribes drugs to treat your disease, we can work to bring you to optimal health and to prevent you from becoming sick again."

An initial visit with an ayurvedic physician can last up to two hours as the doctor takes a complete medical history, performs a thorough ayurvedic exam, and provides detailed treatment recommendations. Make sure you schedule plenty of time for your first visit.

Follow-up appointments are generally much shorter.

During a general physical exam, an ayurvedic doctor will begin by taking a good look at you. How white are your eyes? Is your tongue heavily coated? Is your skin clear?

Then, the doctor will ask you a series of questions, not only about your current state of health, but about your lifestyle and your emotional well-being. The doctor also will perform a physical test, pressing on your glands and abdomen to feel for abnormalities. Finally, he or she will conduct a "pulse diagnosis." This involves testing the strength of your pulse in different locations.

When the examination is complete, you can expect the doctor to explain your condition in both Western and ayurvedic terminology. "I will tell them, 'You have high blood pressure' or 'You have a cyst,'" says Dr. Glaser, "but I will also explain what that means in ayurvedic terms. I will tell them where their imbalances are and how they need to treat them. Sometimes that means prescribing medicines just as a Western doctor would. But it always involves ayurvedic treatments to get to the root of the problem."

When it's all over, you'll likely walk out of the door with about 10 ayurvedic treatment recommendations including dietary changes, exercise, mediation, and herbal supplements.

So you don't become overwhelmed, most ayurvedic physicians advise that you to ease into these adjustments. "You certainly can't do everything at once," says Dr. Rees. "So, we ask that you adopt these changes gradually, maybe starting with diet and working from there. As you begin to feel better and better, making the rest of the changes will be easier."

Be prepared to give ayurveda a little time to work, however. "Unlike superpotent modern medicines that can work overnight, but which also can have nasty side effects, ayurveda works more safely and more slowly," says Dr. Lonsdorf. "I tell people to give it two to four weeks. But about 90 percent of patients start noticing significant improvements after about 10 to 14 days."

Though costs vary depending upon where you live and the treatment you receive, expect to pay between $40 and $100 for an initial consultation.

resources

Organizations:

The Ayurvedic Institute
11311 Menaul NE
Albuquerque, New Mexico 87112
505/291-9698
FAX: 505/294-7572
www.ayurveda.com

Maharishi Ayur-Veda Clinics System
800/255-8332
www.maharishi.com

Books:

The Complete Book of Ayurvedic Home Remedies by Vasant Lad (Harmony Books, 1998)

The Book of Ayurveda by Judith H. Morrison and Robert Svoboda (Fireside, 1995)

Contemporary Ayurveda by Hari Sharma and Christopher Clark (Churchill Livingstone, 1997)

chapter 4

biofeedback

DO-IT-YOURSELF HEALING

... a mind–body communications technique, which for the first time allows man to communicate with his inner self.
Barbara Brown, Ph.D., a pioneer in biofeedback research

Not too long ago in a third-floor office suite in Los Angeles, a woman named Laurel sat in an easy chair with a wide band wrapped across her forehead and around her head. The band contained a number of tiny temperature detectors, which continuously monitored the blood flow to different parts of her head. (When more blood flows to an area, it warms up.)

In front of Laurel, on a computerized TV monitor, rising and falling bar graphs gave her visual feedback, telling her when she was successful in increasing the flow of blood to the target areas of her brain. A softly beeping tone gave her auditory feedback as well, rising in pitch when she was successful, falling lower when she was not.

Laurel is a patient of Hershel Toomim, Sc.D., cofounder of the Biofeedback Institute of Los Angeles, and the machine she used is his own invention. Dr. Toomim, now in his early eighties, has been working in biofeedback since the 1960s. Laurel, a "brilliant and artistic business woman," as Dr. Toomim describes her, suffered brain damage when she became poisoned as the result of inhaling toxic fumes at work.

"She was unable to read," says Dr. Toomim, "and in fact she could hardly even think; she'd forget before she got to the end of a sentence what she had intended to say. Sometimes she would forget to get dressed in the morning."

Laurel spent more than 20 sessions with what Dr. Toomim calls her "thinking cap" on, calmly directing her blood to flow to the damaged areas of her brain.

As Dr. Toomin explains it, by watching and listening to see when she was successful, she gradually learned to control the flow, sending nourishing and healing blood into the damaged areas. As a direct result of this therapy, Dr. Toomin believes, Laurel regained 95 percent of her brain capacity. She came through, ready and eager to resume her active and creative life.

Most biofeedback cases are not nearly so dramatic. But across the country, techniques like this, and others that monitor muscle tension, skin temperature, heart rate, and other bodily functions, are enabling thousands of people to relieve headaches, arthritis, and other types of pain, to sleep better, dissolve tension and anxiety, increase attention and concentration, manage their high blood pressure, and heal many other physical and emotional ills.

> **biofeedback helps heal**
>
> **Research continues to find new uses for biofeedback. Not everyone is a good candidate, but this therapy has proven helpful for many conditions:**
>
> - Alcoholism
> - Anxiety
> - Asthma
> - Attention deficit hyperactivity disorder (ADHD)
> - Depression
> - Headaches and migraines
> - High blood pressure
> - Irritable bowel syndrome (IBS) and other digestive disorders
> - Pain
> - Stroke, spinal cord damage, and other neuromuscular conditions
> - TMJ and other jaw problems
> - Urinary incontinence

What Is Biofeedback?

The term "biofeedback" was coined in the late 1960s. It refers to procedures by which people learn to modify their internal functioning and improve their health, using signals from their own bodies. Sensitive instruments act as a kind of "sixth sense," providing continuous information about the internal workings of the body.

With the use of biofeedback technology, our every response is instantly picked up and fed back to us, so we gradually learn to use our mind to influence our body. Barbara Brown, Ph.D., one of the pioneers of biofeedback research, described it as "a mind-body communications technique, which for the first time allows man to communicate with his inner self."

Prior to the 1960s, all sorts of complex "inside-the-skin" processes that we normally take for granted—such as circulation, blood pressure, heart rate, digestion, glandular activity, and breathing—were all considered involuntary, that is, outside the realm of conscious control and regulation. (All of these processes are regulated by the autonomic nervous system.)

Research Pioneers Faced Opposition

The first researchers who reported that these internal bodily functions could be controlled faced intense opposition from the scientific community. Since then, well over 3,000 articles and 100 books have documented the validity of those early studies.

The implications of being able to influence all these vital processes with just our mind and will are truly revolutionary. It means that just as we now think, "I will get up and walk across the room," and our body responds by engaging nerve impulses and muscles, so too we could say to our heart, "I want you to slow down" or to menstrual cramps or painful joints, "It's time to stop hurting." And they would respond!

We could gain tremendous control over our health and well-being. All we would need to learn is how to communicate to these subtle levels. Is this really possible? To a degree it is, and that's what biofeedback training is all about.

Feedback In Daily Life

Why should this concept seem strange? After all, we use various kinds of feedback all the time. While cooking, for example, we taste the pasta sauce to see if it needs more basil, oregano, or garlic. We add a little something and taste again.

When we drive, we use incoming visual signals to stay in our lane and not drive too fast for the traffic. We adjust our driving moment to moment according to the information (feedback) that we receive.

After the holidays, we may use feedback from the bathroom scale to assist us in self-regulating our weight downward.

In relationships, we observe the effects our words and actions have on our spouses, children, coworkers, and friends, and we act appropriately to maintain a harmonious flow of love and communication.

Peter Parks, Ph.D., a psychologist at the Menninger Foundation in Kansas, maintains that "people with difficulties in relationships often have not adequately developed their ability to pay attention to their impact on others." In other words, they don't respond to feedback and adjust their behaviors.

One of the simplest examples of feedback is the thermostat in your home. This device detects any change in temperature, then uses that information to trigger an adjustment by activating the furnace or air-conditioning system. This keeps room temperature at just the right level for your comfort.

Outside the usual range of awareness, our enormously intelligent bodies ceaselessly respond to internal and external information. Our bodies make countless adjustments every second to maintain health and balance.

In biofeedback training we consciously and intentionally do the same thing—though on a very small scale.

How Does Biofeedback Work?

During a biofeedback training session, sensitive electronic sensors, designed to detect very slight changes, are placed in a safe and painless way on your body. They may be positioned:

- **Over muscles,** where they can register slight variations in muscle tension
- **On the scalp,** where they pick up tiny changes in the brain's electrical activity

- **On the skin,** where they continuously monitor minute temperature changes

The signals are fed to a computer that amplifies the signals from the sensors and sends them on for display.

The types of displays vary. They may be in the form of:

- **A tone that changes in loudness or pitch**
- **A bar graph on a computer screen that rises or falls**
- **A light that flashes**

There are several other possible forms as well.

If you are attempting to relax tight muscles in your neck, for example, the monitor might display a light that becomes fainter as you relax, brighter as you become more tense. Or, you may hear a tone that becomes louder or beeps more often as your muscles tense.

The interesting part is that changing the display is entirely up to you.

Teaching Yourself To Relax: A Biofeedback Session

Let's say you want to relieve the tension in your neck and shoulders. And you've already been hooked up to the sensors. If you know how to meditate or practice some form of relaxation therapy, you might begin that procedure. Or, you might give yourself a quiet suggestion: "My neck and shoulders are warm and relaxed."

For many people, what works best is creative use of the imagination. Imagery, many experts say, is the most effective language for communicating with our bodies. When we imagine something (especially if several of the five senses are involved), the body responds as if what we are seeing and hearing internally is real, just as we may wake up from a bad dream sweating and with our heart pounding.

Thinking of tasting a lemon can cause saliva to flow (try it!). Images of anger or fear can increase our heart rate and muscle tension, while images of tender caresses can stimulate sexual arousal. Whether an event is real or imagined, the nervous system responds.

So, to relax those tense neck muscles, you can try visualizing light or sending healing energy to the tense muscles; that might work. Or, you may simply imagine a relaxing scene, like lounging on the beach, hearing the soothing rhythm of the waves, feeling the warm sun, and smelling the scent of salt water and suntan lotion on warm skin.

Machines Provide Information

Whatever strategy you try, feedback from the biofeedback instruments will immediately show you how you're doing, thus making learning faster. Based on what you see or hear, you may continue what you are doing or take another direction.

While mentally basking in the sun and relaxing, you may suddenly recall something stressful—the crowded drive over to the clinic or a problem at home or at work. Just from these thoughts, your muscles will tense up again, and the feedback will be right there to tell you.

It's a trial-and-error process of continual adjustment. Gradually, you will learn to

5 main types
of biofeedback

The effects of biofeedback are determined by measuring various bodily functions. Here are the five main types of biofeedback in use today:

EMG (electromyograph). Uses electrodes to measure minute electrical impulses in muscles. The most frequently used biofeedback instrument, the EMG can detect muscle tension in your face, jaw, shoulders, or in any muscle. Feedback from the EMG tells you if you are tensing your muscles or relaxing them. It is used to treat insomnia, anxiety, asthma, high blood pressure, and menstrual cramps, as well as muscle tension.

EEG (electroencephalograph). Often referred to as neurofeedback, EEG biofeedback measures brain waves—subtle patterns of electrical activity in the brain—through electrodes placed on the scalp. Brain waves have been classified into four main categories:

- **Beta** (normal waking consciousness, including concentration and focus)
- **Alpha** (associated with relaxation) Alpha training was popular during the 70s and 80s as a way to promote relaxation, but there is considerable disagreement among researchers as to its effectiveness.
- **Theta** (dreaming or daydreaming)
- **Delta** (deep sleep)

GSR (galvanic skin response). Measures the amount of resistance to the flow of a tiny electrical current on the palm of the hand. Moisture on the skin allows the current to flow easily. Tension makes the palms sweaty and lowers resistance. High resistance indicates relaxation. (This is the machine commonly used for the famous "lie detector" test.) GSR is often combined with EMG and temperature training.

Heart rate. Various devices (some as simple as wristwatch-type pulse monitors) measure the heart rate. Heart rate regulation is an important component of many biofeedback stress-reduction programs. Our hearts speed up during anxiety or "fight or flight" reactions and slow down during relaxation. A related type of biofeedback, which works with blood pressure, can help you see which of your thoughts and attitudes raise or lower your blood pressure and help you gain control of it.

Thermograph or ST (skin temperature). Uses sensors to measure very slight temperature gradations, usually in the fingers, hands, or feet. Tension and stress constrict blood vessels, while relaxation tends to increase blood flow and bring warmth to these areas.

the paradox of success: using your will to let go

One of the great secrets to success in biofeedback is effortlessness. Ordinary conscious activity revolves around the active use of will, and success depends to a great extent on how much effort we exert. If you say, "I will get up now and mow the lawn," you can do it; results will be proportionate to your efforts. But when working with bodily functions that are ordinarily involuntary and subconscious, like the beating of our hearts, willpower doesn't work. We need to develop and use what researchers have called "passive volition" or "doing without trying."

As Larry Dossey, M.D., says in his book, *Meaning and Medicine*, "One can only gain control and 'make it happen' by letting go."

We need to become calm, quiet, and settled. It is a subtle process of focusing our attention (by imagining, visualizing, or mentally suggesting the desired change) while remaining in a relaxed state.

regulate the amount of muscle tension, the speed of your heartbeat, the type of brain waves you are generating, the warmth in your fingers, or whatever it is you are trying to achieve. You are in control.

Best Uses for Biofeedback

Biofeedback is helpful in healing a wide variety of conditions, but it is particularly beneficial for stress-related disorders. Learning to relax and dissipate tension is part of virtually all biofeedback training. Research has substantiated its effectiveness in all of the following:

- **Anxiety.** Biofeedback helps both adults and children reduce anxiety symptoms, emotional as well as physical.

  Researchers at Ball State University in Muncie, Indiana, used a combination of EMG and thermal biofeedback to treat a group of 150 seventh and eighth graders who had been identified by their teachers as anxious. After receiving only six sessions of each type of biofeedback, the children showed a significant reduction in their anxiety levels.
- **Asthma.** In one study, people with asthma who were instructed in deep, diaphragmatic breathing were able to increase their air intake by 49 percent. When biofeedback training was added, they improved another 22 percent.
- **Attention Deficit Hyperactivity Disorder (ADHD).** Neurofeedback (EEG biofeedback) has helped hyperactive children and

children with ADHD improve their ability to concentrate, leading to better school performance and sometimes eliminating the need for medication.

- **Headaches and migraines.** One of the most successful and scientifically validated uses of biofeedback is relief and prevention of tension headaches and migraines. Tension headaches are usually treated with EMG (muscle) biofeedback, migraines with thermal biofeedback.

In dozens of studies, people who experience headaches report reduced pain, decreased frequency of headaches, the ability to stop a headache at its inception, and a greatly decreased use of medications.

- **High blood pressure (hypertension).** Many people have learned to regulate their blood pressure, lowering high readings to a healthy level. The most effective method appears to be thermal biofeedback, in which individuals learn to warm up their hands or feet using Autogenic Training or another relaxation technique (For more details on these techniques see "Relaxation Therapies" beginning on page 207.)

In one study of 77 people with high blood pressure, researchers found that most could lower their blood pressure significantly and either entirely eliminate medications or cut usage in half. Benefits remained strong nearly three years after their training.

- **Pain relief.** Biofeedback therapy has been very successful in treating chronic pain, including that from low-back pain, rheumatoid arthritis, menstrual cramps, and other conditions. It helps decrease stress chemistry and increases the effectiveness of the body's natural painkillers (endorphins and enkephalins). Biofeedback is often part of the treatment program in pain clinics across the country.

- **Stroke, spinal cord damage, and other neuromuscular conditions.** Muscle biofeedback (EMG) can be very helpful to people who have had a stroke or people with impaired mind-body coordination due to nerve damage.

This is especially true if biofeedback treatment is begun early enough (within three months). Quick treatment helps restore nerve cells that may not be allowing communication between the brain and the muscles.

- **TMJ and other jaw problems.** Painful conditions such as TMJ and bruxism (grinding the teeth) are generally due to too much muscle tension held in the jaw.

Using EMG biofeedback, individuals can learn to reduce the muscle tension and thus reduce the frequency and intensity of the pain. Most of the people who researchers studied required only about eight sessions to master the muscle relaxation.

- **Urinary incontinence.** This condition, which affects millions of Americans, especially older women, can be helped dramatically with EMG biofeedback, often in conjunction with learning Kegel exercises. (These are exercises that teach control over the muscles that allow urine to flow from the body.)

In addition to the above, other health problems that can be helped by biofeedback include depression, alcoholism, and various gastrointestinal disorders, such as irritable bowel syndrome (IBS).

Most people go into biofeedback seeking relief for one of these problems, whether a painful or debilitating physical condition or some kind of emotional or mental stress. But according to Kenneth Pelletier, Ph.D., M.D., clinical professor of medicine at Stanford University in California, "the treatment of specific symptoms is only one limited application of biofeedback potential."

An even greater value, he suggests, may lie in its contribution to preventive medicine, "its ability to introduce people to the concept of the relaxation response, which would help them reduce daily stress prior to developing disorders."

How to Find a Biofeedback Trainer

Because biofeedback is used to treat such a wide variety of conditions, it is important to find a therapist who specializes in what you need. Here are several ways to locate a trainer appropriate for you:

- **Ask the pros.** Get a referral from the Association for Applied Psychophysiology and Biofeedback (AAPB), the main professional organization for biofeedback practitioners.

  Contact them at 10200 West 44th Ave., Suite 304, Wheat Ridge, CO 80033; 303/422-8436; www.aapb.org.

  Or contact your state or local Biofeedback Society.
- **Use the phone directory.** Look under Biofeedback.
- **Go through your medical contacts.** Ask your doctor for a referral. Or, try hospitals, pain clinics, and university psychology or psychiatry departments.
- **Shop around.** It is important to feel comfortable with your biofeedback therapist or trainer and confident in his or her capabilities, so don't hesitate to investigate more than one before committing yourself to a program. If you have any doubts, get another referral.
- **Check credentials.** You should work with someone who has been certified by the Biofeedback Certification Institute of America, urges Steven C. Kassel, a marriage and family therapist and president of the Biofeedback Society of California.

Setting Up a Personal Program

When you visit a biofeedback lab or training center, you will usually begin with an introductory session that is often given free. This session will be both informative and diagnostic. You will learn about how biofeedback works, and you'll probably be given some tests and evaluations. The therapist will take a verbal health history and inquire about your current problem or concern in order to suggest a program for you. A thorough medical evaluation may be required.

If you decide to go ahead with the training, you and the therapist will set a schedule. Sessions typically last 45 minutes to an hour and are usually once a week. Your program may be as short as

eastern origins

a short history of biofeedback

Biofeedback instruments are a modern gift to understanding the mind-body connection and the possibilities of self-healing. But experiments with self-regulation have been going on for thousands of years.

The world views of India, China, and Tibet do not consider it impossible to use the mind to gain mastery over one's body, and stories of "supernormal" control by yogis and Zen masters who could slow their hearts or live for days inside a sealed box occasionally reached the West, but were generally dismissed as fables.

In 1973 Elmer and Alyce Green of the Menninger Foundation journeyed to India to study accomplished yogis and found that some did indeed have extraordinary abilities. The Greens, who were already engaged in biofeedback research on self-regulation, documented the abilities of Swami Rama, an Indian monk and teacher, to voluntarily alter his heart beat and body temperature. They watched him increase the temperature of one side of his hand while decreasing the temperature on the other side of the same hand! The warm side turned pink, the cooler side somewhat gray. The difference in temperature was 11 degrees.

Swami Rama admitted that it had taken him years to develop this control. With the help of biofeedback, trainees at the Menninger Foundation soon learned to warm their hands at will in as little as two weeks. Since then, researchers have verified the unusual mind-body coordination of some practitioners of both yoga and Buddhism.

Before the Greens, a few lone scientists in the late 1800s and early 1900s experimented with control of the so-called "involuntary" muscles, but most of the Western scientific community did not accept the notion that our will could have an impact on our bodies. It wasn't until the 1960s that biofeedback research began to blossom.

six weeks (this is common) or as long as 20 or even more, depending on the condition you're being treated for.

Costs vary, but average between $70 and $150 per session, partly depending on where you live (it's higher in big cities). Some insurance companies, including Prudential, Mutual of Omaha, and the Kaiser Permanente hospitals, offer access to biofeedback therapy with limited coverage. Sometimes costs can be billed under psychotherapy or major medical, and you may be fully or partially covered.

When you arrive for your first session, you will sit comfortably in a quiet room, get connected to the instruments, and have some instruction in how they work—and then begin your process of self-exploration and regulation.

Your Relationship With the Machine

"Some people are fascinated with the technology," says the Menninger Foundation's Dr. Parks, "and others would rather stay away from it. The important thing is to use it for a transformative purpose." The technology provides not only a way to "read" your body and learn more about how it functions but also an opportunity to master "the subtle internal movement of mind that changes the body in the desired manner," as one expert phrased it.

Once you have mastered what it takes to regulate your heart rate or your blood pressure, reduce your pain, or whatever you are learning to do, you will be able to do it at any time, anywhere—without the biofeedback equipment.

People do not become addicted to biofeedback machines or dependent on them. The equipment helps them learn some valuable new skills, but then they are self-sufficient and on their own, though they may choose to do some follow-up at a later time.

Biofeedback and Mind-Body Medicine

In its short history, biofeedback has made major contributions to our understanding of the relationship of mind and body and how they interact in sickness and in health. "Research into biofeedback is the first medically testable indication that emotion and mind can relieve illnesses as well as create them," notes biofeedback pioneer Dr. Brown. The view that the body is somehow separate from our thinking and feeling is rapidly disappearing.

This shift parallels new knowledge in physics, in which the old Newtonian model, which breaks reality down into isolated parts, is giving way to the deeper perception of quantum physics, which sees life as an interconnected, interacting web of energies and processes.

Nothing in life is truly isolated, not mind from body, nor the individual human being from the environment.

According to Harris Dienstfrey, author of *Where the Mind Meets the Body*, "It turns out that no system of the body is truly autonomous and closed off to the influence of the mind.... Somewhere in the mind is the capacity pure and simple to direct the body to do its bidding. The mind can consciously ask the body to change, and the body will comply."

What You Can Do At Home

"There's little need to use training equipment at home once you master a method of relaxation or self-regulation using the instruments in a clinical setting," says Kassel. If you do decide to use biofeedback instruments at home, "be well informed before selecting equipment," he adds.

Ask for suggestions from a professional. There are many sources of equipment, and levels of quality vary. Many machines are not as accurate and sensitive as the models used in a professional clinic setting. Check out warranties and be sure to get complete, clear instructions.

Just to get an idea of how biofeedback works, here are two inexpensive, safe, and simple methods you can experiment with on your own at home. You may find them quite effective. If you experience migraine headaches, mastering one of these simple approaches and using it when you feel a headache coming on may save you from a great deal of suffering.

Digital Thermometer

For this one, you'll need a simple indoor/outdoor thermometer with a digital readout.

- **Hold the thermometer.** Place it in your hands so your fingers are touching the temperature sensor.
- **Take a reading.** After a minute or so, note the temperature of your fingers as a baseline.
- **Watch your breath.** Then, preferably with eyes closed, follow your breathing. Pay careful attention to your breath as it goes in and out.
- **Or focus on your hands.** Simply turn your attention to your hands. You may notice a pulsation in your fingers or some feeling of warmth.
- **Stay focused.** Keep returning to your breathing, or to awareness of your hands, every time your attention drifts away. Do this for about 10 minutes.
- **Check the temperature.** You may notice that your hands feel warmer, and the temperature has risen a few degrees.
- **Keep trying.** Try this every day for a few days.

Here's another method to try:

- **Focus on your hands.** With eyes closed and the thermometer in your hands, think quietly to yourself, "My hands are heavy and warm."
- **Repeat your phrase.** After about 10 or 15 seconds, repeat again, "My hands are heavy and warm." Continue in this way for about 10 minutes and check the temperature.

Pulse Monitor

- **Purchase an inexpensive wristwatch-type pulse monitor.** (It looks like a wristwatch but tells your pulse rate instead of the time. Sporting goods stores carry these for runners who like to keep tabs on their pulse rates.)
- **Take a reading.** Sit down and after a few seconds note your heart rate.
- **Focus on your breath.** Then, with eyes closed, use the "watch-your-breath" exercise suggested on page 45.
- **Take another reading.** Check your pulse rate again. You may be surprised to find it several beats slower.

In general, working with a professional will be more beneficial than learning at home. They will not only have high quality equipment, but they are also trained to help you every step of the way.

Safety and Warnings

Biofeedback instruments can do you no harm. They simply provide information to you about what is going on within your body and brain. Nor can the techniques used by biofeedback therapists harm you. For the most part, they are simply relaxation techniques to help you reduce stress.

- **Work with trained professionals.** It's still a good idea, however, to work with someone certified by the Biofeedback Certification Institute of America, according to President Kassel. "There are some contraindications for biofeedback, some times when it either shouldn't be used, or used with caution," he says. "A certified practitioner will know how to guide you and help you make the right choices as you are learning to re-regulate body processes."
- **Monitor your medications.** There's one other thing to keep in mind. Your need for medication may change as you undergo biofeedback training. The relaxation procedures are often so effective they may have a positive side effect: For certain medical conditions, you may be able to reduce your medication doses.
- **Check with your doctor.** If you are currently under a physician's care for certain conditions, you'll have to consult with him or her before beginning a program involving biofeedback. Here are the conditons to be concerned about:
  - Diabetes
  - High blood pressure
  - Thyroid disorder
  - Serious depression

Explain what you are going to be doing, and ask him or her to monitor your progress.

healing a headache

One day in 1966 Elmer and Alyce Green, researchers at the Menninger Foundation, were monitoring a woman who was learning to warm her hands using biofeedback equipment. Suddenly her hand temperature increased 10 degrees in just two minutes. At the end of the session, they checked with her: "What happened a few minutes ago?" Her reply surprised them: "How did you know that my migraine headache went away?"

Hmm. If you can think your hands warm, does that mean headaches go away? It turned out to be a good question. And so began the studies that would establish biofeedback as an effective treatment for migraines.

It seems that intentionally increasing the flow of blood to the hands or feet diverts excess blood from the head, which many researchers believe is the main cause of migraines. Numerous studies show that both adults and children can learn to prevent an oncoming migraine just by warming their hands. (Simply warming your hands on a heater will not do the trick. This has to be mental. Try visualizing a bowl of soup in your hands.)

"Headaches are one of the conditions that best respond to biofeedback therapy," says Rob Kall, spokesperson for the Association for Applied Psychophysiology. "It's common for people to experience big improvements in three to four sessions, and to no longer have headache problems after eight to ten sessions." Relief for persistent headaches, however, may require up to 20 sessions.

Once people learn viable self-relaxation strategies to relieve their headaches without medication, the ability remains. In one study, 63 people with chronic, frequent headaches received six to twenty sessions of biofeedback training, resulting in a 93 percent decrease in office visits to doctors, a 90 percent reduction in medications, and a 75 percent drop in emergency room visits over five years. A larger study, reported in the journal *Headache Quarterly,* followed 395 people for four years after they received biofeedback training. Sixty-eight percent experienced decreases in headache duration and frequency, and 56 percent were able to decrease or limit their use of medications.

A study of children who had both tension and migraine headaches found that they were able to reduce their number of headaches by 70 percent and their use of medications by 87 percent. These children only needed an average of seven training sessions.

It sounds like biofeedback is certainly worth a try if you've been plagued by persistent headaches that haven't responded to treatment.

resources

Here are the best sources for information and referrals about biofeedback and trained practitioners:

Organizations

Association for Applied Psychophysiology and Biofeedback
10200 W. 44th Ave., Suite 304
Wheat Ridge, CO 80033
303/422-8436
www.aapb.org

The Biofeedback Certification Institute of America (at the above address) provides a directory of certified practitioners, including their background and experience. Call 303/420-2902.

Center for Applied Psychophysiology
Menninger Clinic
P.O. Box 829
Topeka, KS 66601–0829
785/350-5000
www.menninger.edu

The Menninger Foundation is one of the oldest and most respected centers in the world conducting research and offering treatments using biofeedback in their clinic.

Books

New Mind, New Body by Barbara Brown, Ph.D. (Harper & Row, 1974)

Mind as Healer, Mind as Slayer by Kenneth Pelletier (Dell, 1977)

Timeless Healing by Herbert Benson, M.D. (Scribner, 1996)

The Fine Arts of Relaxation, Concentration and Meditation by Joel Levey (Wisdom Publications, 1987)

chapter 5

bodywork

HANDS-ON HEALING

If you teach an individual to be aware of his physical organism and then to use it as it was meant to be used, you can often change his entire attitude to life. —*Aldous Huxley*

The field of bodywork was one of the most accessible new approaches to health that emerged out of the 60s. "Before then," one woman recalls, "I don't think I knew anyone who went for a massage or saw a bodywork practitioner. Now, according to the New England Journal of Medicine, *massage therapy is the third most sought-after alternative medical treatment in the country (after relaxation techniques and chiropractic). Tens of thousands of licensed bodyworkers provide more than 75 million treatments a year.*

Multi-faceted Benefits

Proponents—increasingly backed by scientific research—say that massage and other forms of bodywork can bring relief from everyday aches and pains and help dispel a wide variety of ailments. These disciplines can help renew your energy and vitality, relieve tension and anxiety, and alleviate common complaints such as headaches, stiffness, menstrual cramps, neck pain, and eyestrain.

Rather than being cures in themselves, these methods appear to help your body heal itself by facilitating circulation and dissolving stress.

Various types of bodywork may also help strengthen the immune system, making you more resistant to disease. Some proponents go further and claim that these techniques may enliven the body's inner intelligence—its natural tendency to be healthy and whole.

What does medical science say about all these claims?

Research does indicate that massage increases the flow of oxygen and nutrients to every cell in the body. During a massage the body's own natural painkillers (endorphins) are released into the bloodstream, helping to subdue pain.

Mental calm increases, along with a feeling of emotional well-being.

But most people don't get a massage because they've read scientific studies about it. The tremendous popularity of bodywork is due mostly to personal recommendations. "People who walk into a massage session stressed and anxious and walk out an hour or so later relaxed and radiant are the best advertisement," one enthusiastic client said.

What Is Bodywork?

It just means rubbing here and pressing there, right? It's not quite that simple. There are so many different types of bodywork that a single definition is all but impossible.

In this chapter "bodywork" is used as a catchall term to include conventional massage (lying passively on a table while a massage therapist kneads your muscles) as well as nonmassage methods of working with the body. Some involve dancelike movement, others use pressure on points on the body to redistribute energy flow. To simplify, we'll break bodywork down into four broad categories:

- **Massage** is systematic, hands-on manipulation—rubbing, kneading, pressing—of muscles and soft tissues. Common types are Swedish, deep tissue, and sports massage. These methods are based mainly on a Western view of the body as consisting of its structural components—muscles, bones, tissues, and organs.
- **Asian** bodywork systems are based on the principle that the body (like all living things) has a vital energy or life force circulating through it that must be kept free-flowing and dynamic for health to be maintained. These systems include both pressure point techniques, such as acupressure and shiatsu, and movement methods, such as tai chi and qigong.
- **Movement re-education or somatic education methods** aim to consciously re-educate the body toward more healthy and natural posture and movement. Though they work with both structure and energy, the main focus of these methods is on function—how the body moves and performs its many activities.

The Alexander Technique, the Feldenkrais Method, and Tragerwork are among the most popular and effective of these systems.

- **Energetic systems** (just like the Asian methods above) are based on the principle that a vital energy runs through and around the body. But most of the systems in this category that we'll look at were developed in recent decades in the West. Members of this family include Therapeutic Touch, polarity, and reflexology.

Why Bodywork Works

"Massage increases the circulation of blood and lymph," says Walter Dominguez, a massage therapist in Los Angeles. "The increased blood flow brings more oxygen and nutrients to the cells, and the improved flow of lymph helps to carry away toxins and waste products. The result is healthier cells and tissues."

Research indicates that the oxygen content of the blood may increase as much as 10 to 15 percent after a massage. Practitioners say the rhythmic pressure and stimulation given to the body during massage sessions harmonize the nervous system and send more blood to the internal organs, thus tuning up the entire body.

"It's almost impossible to have a good massage and not feel deep relaxation and a reduction of anxiety and stress," says Dominguez. "And we all know how closely related stress and illness are. I keep reading that at least 75 to 80 percent of diseases are stress related. So reducing stress almost automatically translates into better overall health."

Other forms of bodywork have similar effects. The Alexander Technique, for example, which focuses primarily on retraining the body to stand, sit, and move naturally and without tension, has been shown to improve breathing; modify the stress response; improve posture, balance, and coordination; increase range of motion; and relieve pain.

Many experts believe "touch therapy" is the oldest of the healing arts, an ability as ancient and natural as life itself. When something on your body hurts or feels stiff, you instinctively rub, press, or hold it. When someone close to you feels physical or emotional pain, you spontaneously reach out to hold or touch in order to convey your sympathy and support.

Research has shown that animals gently petted or cuddled grow faster, have stronger immune systems, and are less fearful than animals who don't receive that physical attention. Similar results have been found from touching human infants.

One reason touch therapies are so effective is that they use the great sensitivity of our skin. A 1-inch square section of skin contains thousands of tiny nerve endings. No wonder it feels so good to be touched, and being touched can have such a powerful effect on our health, vitality, and well-being.

A Short History of Bodywork

In one form or another, massage and bodywork have been part of the human experience for millennia. In the Western medical tradition, the use of touch for healing goes back at least as far as Hippocrates (fifth century B.C.), the Greek physician often referred to as "the father of Western medicine."

Homer, author of *The Illiad* and *The Odyssey*, describes the rejuvenative powers of oil rubdowns for exhausted warriors. Historians say the Roman emperor Julius Caesar received a daily massage and Pliny, the Roman naturalist, found massage helpful in soothing his asthma.

Massage seems to have faded from favor for centuries beginning in the Middle Ages, but it made a comeback in the early 19th century when a Swede named Per Henrik Ling, influenced by what he learned on a trip to China, developed the method of kneading, pressing, and tapping that is now known as Swedish massage. His system found its way across Europe and to the United States. In 1894 a group of English women founded the Society of Trained

Masseuses, most likely the first professional association of massage practitioners.

Massage was commonly used during World War I to treat soldiers but didn't become truly widespread until the 1960s.

That's when a wave of natural and holistic healing systems and techniques swept across America in response to a growing understanding of the relationship between mind and body and a renewed acceptance and appreciation of our bodies and their needs.

In the East, where the traditional systems of healing have continued unbroken for literally thousands of years, medical texts such as *The Yellow Emperor's Classic of Internal Medicine* in China and the *Charaka Samhita* and *Sushruta Samhita* of Indian ayurvedic medicine describe various types of massage and pressure point therapies, and how and when to use them. These techniques are still widely practiced in Asian nations and have become common in the West as well.

In recent decades, scientific research has begun to validate the effectiveness of these methods of healing. Progressive businesses in several countries offer massage to their employees as a preventive measure. Fortunate executives may treat themselves to a brief neck and shoulder "chair massage" to relieve muscle tension at their desks.

Massage: More Than a Rubdown

Massage therapists press, rub, knead, squeeze, and otherwise stroke the muscles and soft tissues of the body. Massage may be vigorous and use quick strokes, or it may be quiet, slow, and gentle. It can be light or deep and penetrating.

You may think it looks easy and uncomplicated, but professionals work long and hard to master anatomy and learn a repertoire of strokes, and understand when and where to apply them. The basic strokes of Swedish massage, the most common type practiced in the United States, have fancy French names:

- **Effleurage (stroking)** consists of sliding the hands evenly over the body surface in long, gliding strokes. It is relaxing and soothing.
- **Petrissage (kneading)** is like kneading bread. The massseur (male) or masseuse (female) uses a rhythmic motion to grasp and lift muscles away from the bones, pressing and squeezing, sometimes lightly, sometimes more firmly.
- **Tapotement (percussion)** is a quick, light patting or tapping stroke that is stimulating and helps relieve muscle cramps and spasms. It can be performed with the outside edge of the hand (hacking), the fingertips (tapping), cupped palms (cupping), or loose fists (beating).
- **Friction,** performed with the palm or fingers, consists of small circular movements in which the hand rests on the skin (it does not slide over the surface) and moves the superficial tissue over the deeper tissues. Friction is said to warm and soften the muscles and fascia (the connective tissue beneath the skin that separates it from muscles and organs) and increase circulation.
- **Vibration** is similar to friction in that the therapist's hands stay pressed against the

what if you're shy?

Are you shy about your body? Would you be reluctant to lie on a massage table with all your clothes off, even if a person of the same sex were giving the massage?

Here are a few things you should know: First of all, a professional bodyworker will never ask you to remove more clothing than you are completely comfortable removing.

Second, for most types of bodywork other than massage, wearing loose clothing is normal. Taking your clothes off is neither needed nor appropriate. So, if removing your clothing is not an acceptable option for you, explore one of the other modalities that are described in this chapter.

Third, when you go for a massage, the therapist will leave the room or send you to another space (perhaps a bathroom) where you can remove your clothes. A large bath towel or a sheet will be provided for you to wrap yourself in before you lie down on the table, and you will remain covered during the entire session, except for the area being worked on at any one time.

For a full body massage, removal of all clothing is standard procedure. This is partly so that all areas of the body can be easily worked (the buttocks, for example, contain large muscles that hold a lot of tension) and partly because the oil used in the massage will stain any clothing you have on.

If you are uncomfortable with full nudity, leave your underwear on, but be prepared to find oil stains. Keep in mind that an experienced bodyworker has seen just about everything there is to see in terms of the variety of weights, shapes, sizes, and colors of bodies.

skin without gliding over it. A vibrating motion is set up by shaking the hands or fingers rapidly and rhythmically. The masseur or masseuse may also lift the muscle away from the bone before vibrating it.

Your Massage Session

If you've never had a massage, you're probably curious about more than the kinds of strokes a massage therapist is likely to use. Here's a quick snapshot of a typical visit.

Your massage therapist may work in a fitness center, health club, or gym; in a spa or resort; or in a chiropractor's office or holistic health clinic along with other alternative practitioners. More and more, massage therapists are employed to help patients in hospitals and nursing homes.

Many practitioners will make house calls, bringing along a portable folding massage table that sets up in seconds. But a large number of practitioners are quiet entrepreneurs who simply work from a room in their own homes. The massage therapist we'll describe is one of those who works from a home office.

Before you lie down on the table for your massage, the massage therapist will probably ask you a number of questions about your health history or have you fill out a detailed questionnaire. Be honest in your answers. The therapist may identify certain reasons why massage is not the best thing for you. He or she also wants to know whether you are looking for some specific results, such as relief from a stiff neck or lower back pain, or just general relaxation and stress reduction.

The massage therapist will then leave the room so you can undress. You'll put your clothes in the space provided, climb up on the padded table, cover yourself with the sheet or large bath towel that is waiting for you (some therapists use both), and lie down. You have just completed almost everything you will have to do for the next hour! (Later, you may be asked something as arduous as, "Please roll over on your side.")

When your massage therapist returns, he or she may put on some soft music. If you don't like it, feel free to ask for something more to your liking. Or, you may wish to have no music playing at all. Similarly, you may feel like talking, or you may wish to keep silent and just go with the sensations of the massage. As a trained professional, your therapist will be responsive to your preferences.

Your massage therapist will then uncover a part of your body, perhaps your arms and shoulders or your legs, and begin to gently rub on a little massage oil as he or she strokes and kneads the muscles. As the massage progresses, the therapist will uncover only the parts of your body being worked on, allowing you to keep warm and comfortable under your covering.

When you are lying on your back, your massage therapist may place a rolled towel or small pillow under your knees or beneath your head. Always speak up if you are uncomfortable with anything the therapist does—perhaps a stroke is too strong, or the pillow's in the wrong place—or if there is anything you need.

Most of the time, you will feel relaxed—*very* relaxed. But sometimes that deep relaxation can release more than muscle tension.

Some held-back emotions might rise to the surface, or you may find yourself getting a little weepy. Don't worry; your massage therapist is used to this. He or she knows it is one possible result of a successful massage.

When the massage is finished (a typical session lasts an hour and costs between $35 and $75), the therapist will leave the room for a few minutes, allowing you some privacy to lie quietly and enjoy the feelings of pleasure and warmth that are flowing through you. Some people doze off during this time; some may snooze blissfully for a few minutes during the actual massage.

When you are ready, you can stand up and wipe off any excess oil (you can use the towel that has been covering you) and get dressed. Or, before you leave, a shower may be available, or a warm bath using therapeutic oils. Then you're off to the rest of the day feeling deeply relaxed and refreshed.

bodywork helps heal

Elliot Greene, past president of the American Massage Therapy Association, says "headaches, insomnia, digestive disorders including constipation and spastic colon, arthritis, asthma, carpal tunnel syndrome, sinusitis, and minor aches and pains are some of the problems that can respond to massage therapy." Indeed, a wide range of ills can be profitably treated by the various bodywork modalities. The conditions most extensively researched and/or widely reported by satisfied clients include the following:

- **Anxiety.** From young children to the elderly, massage techniques have been found to help reduce anxiety by inducing relaxation.
- **Arthritis.** Bodyworkers say that people with arthritis often experience relief because improved circulation to the joints reduces inflammation and pain. Directly massaging the hands help relieve symptoms.
- **Headaches.** Most headaches other than migraines are caused by muscle tension, primarily in the neck and shoulders. A back rub, whether of the homegrown variety or on a professional's massage table, greatly relieves this tension and is highly effective for headache relief.
- **High blood pressure.** A few studies now confirm that a particular procedure called "slow stroke back massage" can moderate high blood pressure.
- **Pain.** Bodywork can be effective in relieving many kinds of severe pain.
- **Pent-up feelings.** The relaxation and release of deep-lying tensions in the body during a massage may result in some crying or other emotional release. Massage therapists are familiar with this phenomenon and will let you cry in peace or talk with you about it if you feel like talking.
- **Posture and movement.** The relaxing effects of massage, and the more dynamic approaches such as the Alexander Technique and Feldenkrais Method, help free the body from habitual poor posture and painful movements.
- **Premature infants.** Gentle massage helps preterm infants gain weight and achieve better growth.
- **Sore muscles.** Athletes of all abilities know the benefit of a good rubdown after physical exertion to soothe tired muscles and prevent pain the next day.
- **Stress and tension.** The relaxation and release of tension from a good massage are legendary and hardly need scientific corroboration. Proponents maintain that massage can help a number of known stress-related conditions, such as insomnia, asthma, and digestive disorders. So, it makes good sense that the relaxation produced by bodywork would be beneficial.

Variations On a Theme

Several contemporary massage methods are based on Swedish massage.

• **Deep tissue massage** works to loosen tight muscles and release deep-lying tensions far below the surface of the body, often in the back or shoulders where many layers of muscle may cover the source of tension or pain. The strokes used are slow and powerful. Therapists may use their body weight and even their elbows to get to areas that need releasing. This kind of deep work frequently brings pent-up emotions and memories of traumatic events to the surface to be released.

• **Sports massage** is essentially Swedish massage adapted for athletes, with some deep tissue work as needed. Massage before an event or activity acts as a warm-up, loosening muscles and getting circulation going. Afterward, it soothes tired muscles and helps remove waste products, thus helping to prevent pain later. Sports massage is also effective in relieving sore muscles and treating injuries such as sprains and strains. Some experts believe sports massage can help athletes rise to peak performance and to enter "the zone" in which mind and body function effortlessly and at their best.

• **Trigger point therapy,** a more targeted type of bodywork that focuses on individual muscles, is an effective and often remarkable method of pain relief. The therapist uses firm pressure with fingers, knuckles, or elbows to press for only a few seconds on small, hard, painful knots of tension deep in the muscles. These trigger points may be "referring" pain to other parts of the body as well, which may suddenly feel better when the point is pressed. (Bonnie Prudden, fitness expert and founder of the school of trigger point massage known as Bonnie Prudden Myotherapy, began her work when a friend pressed on one painful spot in her neck, instantaneously relieving a stiff neck.)

• **Rolfing** was created by the biochemist Ida P. Rolf, Ph.D. One of the most intensive methods of deep tissue bodywork, Rolfing manipulates the body's muscles and the fascia (connective tissue surrounding the muscles) in a series of 10 sessions.

The goal is a substantial straightening and realigning of the body from head to toe that is aimed at improved posture and movement, increased energy, and overall emotional and physical health. Rolfing sessions can be somewhat painful and are a bit more pricey than many other types of bodywork, ranging from $75 to $100 an hou—even higher for an experienced Rolfer in a metropolitan area.

Though not much scientific evidence exists for the effectiveness of the above bodywork systems, there is abundant anecdotal evidence pointing to their value and safety.

Movement Re-Education Systems

Some bodywork systems involve what's known as "somatic education"—a conscious retraining of the body away from stress-formed patterns of posture and movement and toward a free-moving, graceful, natural way of being in the world.

These methods emphasize the importance of consciousness or mindfulness, a moment-to-moment awareness of how you are holding your body, how you are moving, how you are feeling. In the words of Aldous Huxley, a student of the Alexander Technique, "If you teach an individual to be aware of his physical organism and then to use it as it was meant to be used, you can often change his entire attitude to life."

This seems to be the case with thousands of individuals who have used the following practices. Although these methods may include some table work that resembles massage, they differ in that they call upon the client or student to learn new patterns of awareness and movement, let go of self-limiting patterns, and learn to use the body in a more balanced, efficient, and comfortable way.

The Alexander Technique

As a young Shakespearean actor touring in Australia in the last years of the 19th century, Frederick Matthias Alexander often became hoarse and sometimes lost his voice on stage. Unable to find successful medical treatment, he began a careful process of self-observation in an attempt to find the cause of his problem.

By watching his movements in mirrors, Alexander discovered that he was generating his own disability. An unconscious, habitual tendency to move his head backward and down created tension in his neck and throat, which then affected his voice. By carefully reversing this movement, he solved his problem and at the same time laid the foundations for one of the most successful schools of bodywork.

Way ahead of his time, Alexander anticipated the mind-body movement of the 1980s and 90s with his emphasis on conscious awareness as a vital part of healing. He repeatedly used the term "psycho-physical" to indicate, as he said, "the impossibility of separating 'physical' and 'mental' operations in our conception of the human organism."

"The correct way to refer to the Alexander Technique is 'psycho-physical re-education' or mind-body learning," says Michael Frederick, a longtime Alexander teacher in Ojai, California. "That's what Alexander himself called it."

The Alexander Technique has certainly had its share of endorsements from everyone from popular entertainers to M.D.s.

"As my Alexander teacher taught me to sit in a state of lumbosacral poise, I gradually eliminated my chronic low back pain," says John H. M. Austin, M.D., professor of radiology and chief of the division of radiology at Columbia-Presbyterian Medical Center in New York City. "The Technique is true education. When compared with the physical and financial cost of back surgery, a course of instruction is very inexpensive."

Over the course of the past century, many famous people have used and endorsed the Alexander Technique, including the playwright George Bernard Shaw, the philosopher and educator John

Dewey, and performing artists such as Julie Andrews, William Hurt, Jeremy Irons, James Earl Jones, Paul McCartney, Paul Newman, Joanne Woodward, Robin Williams, and members of the New York Philharmonic Orchestra.

The technique is taught at the world-famous Juilliard School of Music in New York City and the UCLA School of Theater, Film, and Television. When Nikolaas Tinbergen of Oxford University was awarded the Nobel Prize for Medicine in 1973, he devoted half of his acceptance speech to praising the work of Alexander.

So how does the Alexander Technique manage to make enthusiasts of so many famous people?

Alexander's central finding was what he called "the primary control," the relationship between head, neck, and spine, Frederick says. That relationship can be either compressed or free and natural. "In a natural state," he says, "the head balances lightly on top of the spine, the torso expands, and breathing is easy." By contrast, "bad" posture habits tend to produce a collapsed way of sitting and standing, shallow and inefficient breathing, and the tight shoulder, back, and neck muscles so common today.

In a session with an Alexander instructor, you work one on one to become more aware of your body, to recognize ingrained habits of posture and movement. "As you sit there, do you notice some tension in a shoulder or in your lower back?" asks Frederick. "Are you leaning on one hip more than the other?" Little by little, without criticism, you learn about yourself.

Armed with this knowledge and the teacher's guidance (through verbal instruction and an occasional gentle touch to help you grasp a new way of sitting, standing, or moving), you learn to release areas of tension. "It's a process of seeing how you set up interfering patterns of movement," says Frederick, "and then taking them away, letting them go. It's like the creation of a beautiful sculpture. The work of art is what's left when the unnecessary marble has been cut away. When you let go of tension, what you have left is right balance, a more healthy and comfortable way of being."

Sessions are typically 45 minutes to an hour, are done fully clothed, and take place partly on a massage table (where your teacher carefully moves your head or limbs to help you relax) and partly in activity and movement. Costs run from $45 to $70 per session.

Alexander teachers generally suggest a series of 30 to 40 sessions over three to six months, in order to overcome long-standing habits and truly re-educate the body.

The training of an Alexander teacher is one of the most rigorous programs in the bodywork field. For certification by North American Society of Teachers of the Alexander Technique (NASTAT), individuals have to complete 1,600 hours over a minimum of three years. NASTAT has trained about 600 of the 2,500 Alexander teachers worldwide.

Applying the Alexander Technique

One of the unique aspects of the Alexander Technique is that the teacher helps you understand and become more

the alexander technique

basic movement

The basic movement at the heart of the Alexander system is extremely simple. When doing it, keep in mind that this is a subtle movement, not aerobics, and it requires no effort or strain.

- **Get comfortable.** Begin by sitting or standing comfortably.
- **Focus on your body.** Be aware of how your head, neck, and torso feel, and the quality of their relationship. If you find yourself slumping, don't try to reverse or correct it by standing up stiffly. Just observe.
- **Release your neck.** Now, very gently and delicately, free your neck and allow your head to release up and away from your shoulders. The forward/upward movement will be very slight, almost imperceptible. You are not tucking your chin into your neck, nor stretching your neck. "Up" means upward from your shoulders, not up toward the ceiling. If you are lying down, up is in a horizontal direction.

  Let your body lengthen and your torso expand gently outward as your head releases upward from your shoulders. There is no "right" posture here, just a natural relationship of your head, neck, and torso, a coming back into proper balance.
- **Note how you feel.** You may feel a lightness and rightness, an openness or easiness of breath or movement.

You may use this basic movement at any time—sitting, standing, walking, exercising, even lying down.

comfortable with activities of importance to you. Suppose, for example, that you put in many hours in front of a computer. You may spend a lot of time and money purchasing just the right, ergonomically correct chair and table, but once you sit down, you may negate these efforts by slumping or slouching.

Here are some Alexander Technique tips from Frederick to help you avoid back strain, carpal tunnel syndrome, headaches, and other occupational hazards:

- **Be aware.** Note the space between you and the computer.
- **Focus on how you sit.** Keep both feet on the floor in front of you. Sit evenly on your two "sitting bones," not rolling back onto your tailbone.
- **Use support if you need to.** If you find yourself repeatedly collapsing in a slouch, support the lumbar region of your back (that's where the curve is) with a pillow so you can maintain an upright posture without strain.
- **Pay attention.** Keep coming back to an internal awareness of the relationship of

your head, neck, and torso, and repeat the "basic movement" described on page 59.

- **Stay loose.** Don't try to be rigid or hold a particular posture, but gently and in a simple way, have a sense of internal length.

If sitting all day is not an issue, you may instead work on enhancing your onstage movements as an actor or speaker, your moves on the basketball court, your posture while playing a musical instrument, your skills at comfortably lifting little children, or any other movement or posture that concerns you.

The teacher will help you observe yourself so you can see and feel the source of your difficulty, then will guide you in learning to sit, stand, and move with balance, poise, and comfort.

The Feldenkrais Method

Like the Alexander Technique, the Feldenkrais Method is primarily an educational system. According to pioneering health educator Andrew Weil, M.D., the Feldenkrais Method is based on the premise that we have all forgotten how to move with the natural ease of a baby.

Our bodies have become rigid and set in bad habits of movement, which adversely affect our physical and emotional health. Through this method, we can unlearn those habits and "rediscover the free, effortless sense of movement we had in the first few years of life," says Dr. Weil.

A remarkable man, Moshe Feldenkrais, Ph.D., (1904–1984) left home at age 13, earned degrees in mechanical and electrical engineering and a doctorate in physics, and was one of the first Europeans with a black belt in judo. Like Alexander, Feldenkrais developed his healing system because of a personal health problem. When doctors told him in 1940 that a knee injury was so severe he would never walk again unless he had surgery, he set about to prove them wrong.

Feldenkrais taught himself to walk (partly by observing young children's natural movements) and soon was teaching others what he had taught himself. The Feldenkrais Method has two phases, both designed to eliminate habitual patterns of movement that are limiting, inefficient, or painful.

The first, Awareness Through Movement, consists of classes in which groups of students perform some of the hundreds of simple exercises developed by Feldenkrais to facilitate natural movement. These slow-moving exercises involve common everyday moves like bending, turning, and leaning. Lessons last 30 to 60 minutes, at a typical cost of only $6 to $15 per person (classes may have from two to twenty participants).

Instructions are purely verbal, and there is no massage or physical contact. "These precisely structured movement explorations involve thinking, sensing, moving, and imagining," says the class description provided by the Feldenkrais Guild. In private Functional Integration lessons, the second Feldenkrais format, the teacher offers some gentle hands-on guidance in movements tailored to individual needs.

Fully clothed, the student lies on a padded table or sits, stands, or moves, practicing self-observation and responding

the magic of the method

If you would like a taste of the Feldenkrais Method, try this sample Awareness Through Movement lesson:

- **Get comfortable.** Sit comfortably on the edge of a chair, with your hands resting in your lap.
- **Slowly and gently turn your head to the right.** Turn only as far as you can without strain or pain. Notice a point on the wall where your head stops—the farthest point you can comfortably see. Return to the center.
- **Turn gently and slowly to the left.** Again, only so far as you can move without pain or strain, and again note the farthest point you can see when movement stops. Return to the center.
- **Support your head.** Now, raise your hands together in front of your face and cradle your head in your open hands, with your chin resting on the heels of the hands.

  Your fingertips will be somewhere around your eyes. In this position, your elbows will rest on your chest.
- **Turn again.** Keeping the elbows as if glued to your chest and with your hands still cradling your head, gently turn to the right as far as you comfortably can, then back to the center. Because of your arm position, your whole upper body turns along with your head. Make the same turn to your left and return to center.
- **Turn without support.** Now, drop your hands back into your lap, then repeat the head turns that you did at the beginning of this exercise. Turn first to the right then to the left.
- **Notice the change from the first time you tried it.** Without any effort on your part, this simple exercise has expanded your range of motion.

to the practitioner's tactile communications. At least four private sessions are recommended. A typical session could cost anywhere from $40 to $100, depending on your location and the experience of the teacher.

Esalen Institute cofounder Michael Murphy says Feldenkrais work, just like the Alexander Technique, "can produce a feeling of freedom, lightness, and balance accompanied by new spontaneity and pleasure." This corresponds well to Feldenkrais' stated goal: "to make the impossible possible, the possible easy, and the easy elegant."

Though not a great deal of hard scientific verification is yet available, there is an abundance of anecdotal evidence from the more than 1,000 teachers in the United States and their satisfied students, including former basketball star Julius Erving, the late author and editor Norman Cousins, former Israeli prime minister David Ben-Gurion, actress Whoopi Goldberg, and classical musicians Yo Yo Ma and Yehudi Menuhin.

To become certified, Feldenkrais practitioners must complete 800 to 1,000 hours of training over a period of three to four years. To find a trainer certified by the Feldenkrais Guild of North America, see the Resources section at the end of the chapter.

"I have long been intrigued by this subtle form of retraining the nervous system," says Dr. Weil, who adds he has found it "much more useful than standard physical therapy" for patients whose range of movement has been restricted by injury, cerebral palsy, stroke, fibromyalgia, or chronic pain.

"I also believe that the Feldenkrais Method can help older people achieve greater range of motion and flexibility," he says, "and help all of us feel more comfortable in our bodies."

The Trager Approach

Tragerwork, like both the Alexander and Feldenkrais systems, aims at helping you relax and let go of any long-standing energy blockages and patterns of tension in your posture and movements. But the method developed by Milton Trager, M.D., is quite different.

The main principle of Tragerwork is applied while you lie down, preferably on a massage table. No clothes have to come off, and no predetermined techniques or massage strokes are used. Rather, the Trager practitioner is taught to intuitively sense tensions in your body and respond to them.

By moving your head, limbs, and trunk in a gentle, almost playful way—rhythmically shaking, vibrating, rocking, gently rubbing, even bouncing—the practitioner frees tight muscles and locked joints and gives your body a taste of what it feels like to be relaxed and loose. The experience is pleasurable and, though relaxing, is also enlivening. Sessions typically cost from $75 to $95.

The other aspect of Tragerwork is known as Mentastics (mental gymnastics). These easy, dancelike exercise movements help you replicate, through your own movements, the pleasurable feelings the therapist helped you experience on the table and increase your awareness of light, free, effortless movement.

Asian Bodywork Systems

The basic concepts governing Asian bodywork have been explained in "Acupuncture," which begins on page 1. Primary among these principles is the idea that bodies are not just structures (bones, muscles, organs, etc.) but also energy systems.

"Our modern world has been dominated for several centuries by a mechanistic, materialistic view of life, which views the body as a kind of machine," says Steve Shimer, licensed acupuncturist and coauthor of *Healing with Pressure Point*

Therapy. "This view is becoming obsolete. Breakthroughs in science are revealing a world very similar to the one described by the ancient healers, a world of energy, relationships, and interdependence in a field of Unity."

What this means is that our bodies are not "frozen sculptures," as Deepak Chopra, M.D., phrased it. Rather, the human organism is dynamic and ever changing, ever renewing itself, alive with energy. According to this understanding, the energy (known as *chi* or *qi* in Chinese medicine, *prana* in ayurveda) flows through the body along energy channels known as meridians. When the energy flow becomes blocked or goes out of balance, the door opens for disorder and disease. When the flow of life energy is balanced, the body's natural defenses remain strong and health is maintained.

The central purpose of the Asian schools of bodywork is to maintain balance or restore it if it is disrupted.

Think of the meridians as the streets crisscrossing your city. Sometimes traffic flows smoothly, and it's a pleasure to drive around town. Other times, however, accidents, stormy weather, or plain old rush-hour traffic congest the streets and bring traffic to a crawl. Similarly, stressful living, heavy food, physical injury, lack of exercise, or any one of hundreds of lifestyle factors can cause slowdowns and blockages of the energy in our bodies and impede our progress through life.

These energy therapies offer a way to get traffic moving again.

Acupressure

Acupressure is a Chinese system of pressing on specific points on the body thought to be centers of energy (qi), located along the meridians or energy channels. From these points, the qi can be stimulated, pacified, or released if it is blocked, using finger pressure that is either light or firm, steady or intermittent, depending on the condition to be treated.

Proponents of acupressure assert that it can be effective in the treatment of almost any condition, and it (or its counterpart, acupuncture) is integral to Chinese medicine, a complete system of healing.

It is said to be especially effective for pain relief, especially of headaches, muscle cramps, spasms, sinus pain, arthritis, and menstrual cramps, as well as for overall stress reduction.

Shiatsu

The word "shiatsu" means thumb or finger pressure, but if you visit a shiatsu practitioner for a treatment, you may find that the therapist uses his or her palms, knuckles, elbows, fists, and even feet.

The Japanese version of acupressure, shiatsu was probably brought to Japan by Buddhist monks in the sixth century. According to acupuncturist Shimer, "The principles of energy, meridians, and points are essentially the same in shiatsu as in acupressure but with different names."

In Japan, the life energy is called ki (pronounced *key*) instead of qi (pronounced *chee*). The points, known a tsubos

can you feel the energy?

This exercise is most easily done if you stand up, feet about shoulder width apart. Rub your palms together briskly for about a minute. Hold your arms out in front of you, elbows bent, hands facing each other, but at a 45-degree angle (not perpendicular to the floor), palms slightly down. Hold for a few seconds, then drop one arm part way down. Put your hand back even with the other hand. Drop it down. Put it back. Do you feel a difference? You can also try moving your hands closer, then farther apart, then closer again. Many people can feel a subtle current of energy, a warmth, or even a tingling, when the hands are facing each other or are closer together. The energy dissipates when one hand drops down or the hands move far away from each other.

(pronouned *soo-bows)*, are seen as vortexes of energy, places where the energy gathers. They are sometimes compared to volcanoes, where energy from within the earth's core rises to the surface.

"These are the points at which energy is particularly active and can be most easily influenced for release or balance," says Shimer. The main difference between the two, Shimer explains, is that in shiatsu, pressure is generally applied more vigorously than in acupressure. Shiatsu practitioners use their thumbs whenever possible in order to apply firmer, stronger, rhythmic pressure. "Also, some shiatsu practitioners place more emphasis on meridians than pressure points. Their rationale is that if you learn the location of the meridians, you will have a sense for the flow of the energy in the body and will instinctively feel the position of the points," says Shimer. Acupressure and shiatsu practitioners are found in increasing numbers throughout the United States and are becoming ever more popular as research verifies their effectiveness, and insurance companies and HMOs become more receptive to alternative and complementary treatments. You may find them at holistic health clinics, affiliated with chiropractic offices or massage therapists, or in private practice.

Marma Therapy

Marma therapy is a science of touch little known in the West until the last 10 to 20 years. It is part of ayurveda, the ancient Indian system of natural medicine. (See page 23 for more details on ayurveda.)

Like its Chinese and Japanese counterparts, marma therapy stimulates sensitive, vital points on the body that govern the flow of life energy (known in ayurveda as *prana*) and the functioning of organ systems. The traditional texts describe numerous channels that resemble the meridians of acupressure and list 107 major points. According to Sushruta, one of the ancient ayurvedic sages, these pressure points are areas of high concentration of life energy.

The classical texts state that the three most important marma points are at the crown of the head, the heart (in the center of the chest), and the pelvic area. The way to enliven the marma points is through touch, which is considered the most powerful of the five senses when it comes to healing. Practitioners also use therapeutic marma oils, applying specific oils at specific points to treat specific symptoms.

In ayurvedic terms, the marmas are said to be the junction points linking our consciousness with our body. Marma therapy, the theory goes, thus enlivens the connection of mind and body, matter and consciousness. (The texts say that the body is pervaded by consciousness or life energy "as the sky is pervaded by the sun's rays.") Practitioners maintain that this heightened awareness triggers a spontaneous natural healing response.

It's not yet easy to find an expert in marma therapy, but it is a growing field in the West. Consult a center that offers ayurvedic medicine for referrals.

Tai Chi and Qigong

If you travel to China and look out your window early in the morning, you may be captivated by visions of men and women of all ages performing slow, graceful, rhythmic exercises. They are practicing tai chi or qigong, ancient martial arts techniques that combine movement with breathing and mental awareness to energize and balance the body's qi or life force.

Even more than the related Western movement re-education techniques considered earlier in this chapter (such as the Alexander and Feldenkrais methods), these Asian practices offer a kind of meditation in motion that integrates mind, body, and spirit for health and balance. Many books and videos teach these exercises, but it is always better to learn from an experienced teacher. Classes are available throughout the country in colleges, community centers, and holistic health centers. (For more details on the health benefits of these disciplines, see *Tai Chi and Qigong* beginning on page 243.)

Western Energetic Systems

Acupressure and ayurvedic marma therapy are believed to be at least 5,000 years old. By contrast, various forms of Western energetic bodywork (sometimes called "bioenergetics") have been around no more than 100 years. Yet, they are proving themselves to be quite effective.

These methods are based on the view that our bodies, like the rest of nature, appear as solid structures on the surface but are vibrating with energy on deeper levels. Ultimately, all matter is energy; this is one of the accepted truths of modern physics. One of the increasingly accepted truths of modern medicine is that human beings, too, are dynamic and complex energy fields interacting with the energies of the environment.

Though you can't see this energy, it is there. Perhaps, like many practitioners of these therapies do, you can feel it. Try the simple exercise described in "Can You Feel the Energy?" on page 64.

Polarity Therapy

"I was teaching school in the Midwest," recalls Gloria Kamler, director of the Santa Monica Center for Integrated Therapy in California. "And one winter I took a class in Polarity Therapy, just to get out of the house. I actually felt energy in my hands right away, and when I practiced on people, their stiff necks went away, their digestion got better.... It was great, but a little strange.

"But then, one day, I realized—I saw with great clarity—that this was working because essentially we are all spiritual beings. There is a life force inside us, an energy or consciousness, which vibrates into physical form and actually weaves the fabric of our bodies. Dr. Randolph Stone, founder of Polarity, wrote that 'Energy is the real substance behind the appearance of matter and form.' I saw that I was helping to activate those subtle energy currents, which are more basic than tissues, muscles, and organs."

Polarity Therapy practitioners work with this fundamental energy through massage, foot massage (reflexology), breathing exercises, and a series of stretches and exercises that work to move and balance the body's energy. Polarity practitioners are certified by the American Polarity Therapy Association.

Research on Polarity is still scant but enthusiasts feel it can help balance the emotions, increase energy and vitality, and defuse stress.

Craniosacral Therapy

Quite unlike any of the deep tissue or vigorous massage methods, this subtle healing art involves very gentle pressure and manipulation of the craniosacral system, which includes the skull, vertebrae, and the sacrum (the bone at the base of the spine). This system contains the cerebrospinal fluid, which bathes and supports the brain and spinal cord.

"Health is an expression of life's inherent, ordering intelligence," says Scott Zamurut, a Craniosacral and Polarity Therapist in Boulder, Colorado. "It manifests primarily as slow rhythmic pulsations of energy up and down the spinal axis of the body," he says. It is this pulse that craniosacral therapists learn to feel.

When this system is even slightly misaligned, Zamurut says, "the organizing intelligence is hindered and health suffers." The therapist uses very light pressure—no more than the weight of a nickel—to make minute adjustments in the craniosacral system.

"This is very slow, very delicate, very meditative work," says Zamurut, "that allows the intelligence of the system to heal from within."

The therapy is so gentle that it is considered suitable even for babies, children, and delicate elderly. "It's helpful for pain relief, including jaw problems like TMJ, and for head injuries, sinus problems, and headaches," says Zamurut, "and these are the conditions that frequently bring people to us. But the therapy can be beneficial for many other conditions." Craniosacral sessions last from 45 minutes to an hour; costs are in the upper level of the price range for a good massage (which costs $35 to $75).

Reflexology

A close relative of acupressure and shiatsu, reflexology works with the body's energy by stimulating pressure points on the feet (and secondarily on hands and ears). In this system, the feet are seen as miniatures of the entire body, so by giving your feet a thorough workout, you can invigorate and/or relax your entire body.

Reflexology treatments rely on "reflex zones," somewhat more generalized areas than the very specific points and meridians central to shiatsu and acupressure. Ten zones are said to run vertically from the top of your head down to the soles of your feet. Practitioners maintain that every organ, gland, or bodily structure is located within one of these zones and has a related reflex area on the bottom of your foot. By pressing on these specific places on your feet (using a variety of techniques), practitioners maintain they can influence the energy and health of the organ systems of your body.

Reflexology was born in the 19th century when a Connecticut physician named William Fitzgerald discovered that he could do minor surgeries by using pressure on points on his patients' hands to prevent pain. Eventually he identified the reflex zones and called his work "zone therapy."

Eunice Ingham, an American physical therapist, later discovered that the feet were more highly responsive than the hands. She charted the reflex zones on the feet, creating the first maps showing exactly where to press.

Her nephew, Dwight C. Byers, continued her pioneering work. He is director of the International Institute of Reflexology in St. Petersburg, Florida, author of *Better Health with Foot Reflexology*, and teacher of some of the most prominent and successful reflexologists working today.

There are more than 25,000 trained and certified reflexology practitioners throughout the world. Although not a great deal of research has been conducted on reflexology, beneficiaries of this therapy find it extremely relaxing and helpful for a number of conditions, from headaches to PMS. "Most of us find that just a simple foot rub feels so soothing," says Byers. "Working with reflex zones takes it to a whole new level."

Safety and Warnings

Can something that feels so good and has so many potential benefits ever be harmful? You bet. Like everything in this world, bodywork is a mixed blessing.

If any of the following circumstances apply to you, check with your doctor before getting a massage or starting bodywork:

- Blood clot
- Cancer
- Circulatory problems
- Heart disease
- Infectious disease
- Pregnancy
- Swelling (edema)

resources

Organizations

American Massage Therapy Association
820 Davis St., Suite 100
Evanston, IL 60201
847/864-0123
www.amtamassage.org

Associated Bodywork and Massage Professionals
28677 Buffalo Park Rd.
Evergreen, CO 80439
800/458-2267
www.abmp.com

National Certification Board for Therapeutic Massage and Bodywork
8201 Greensboro Dr., No. 300
McLean, VA 22102
703/610-9015
www.ncbtmb.com

North American Society of Teachers of the Alexander Technique
310 Hennepin Ave. S., Suite 10
Minneapolis, MN 55408
800/473-0620
www.alexandertech.com
Info and teacher referral service

Feldenkrais Guild
P.O. Box 489
Albany, OR 97321
800/775-2118 or 541/926-0981
www.feldenkrais.com

Books

Bodywork: What Type of Massage to Get, and How to Make the Most of It by Claire Thomas (William Morrow, 1995)

Hands on Healing (Rodale Press, 1989)
Explores various modalities of bodwork.

The Massage Book by George Downing (Random House, 1972)
Considered a classic work on massage.

Massage for Common Ailments by Sara Thomas (Fireside, 1989)

The Book of Massage by Lucinda Lidell (Fireside, 1984)
Contains extensive instructions and illustrations on shiatsu and reflexology as well as massage.

Acupressure's Potent Points by Michael Reed Gach (Bantam, 1990)
Profusely illustrated, user-friendly book by the director of the Acupressure Institute.

The Alexander Technique by Wildred Barlow (Alfred A. Knopf, 1991)
From the founder of the Alexander Institute.

Better Health with Foot Reflexology by Dwight C. Byers (Ingham, 1996)
From the director of the International Institute of Reflexology.

chapter 6

chinese medicine
ORIENTAL WISDOM

> The doctor's job is to diagnose imbalances and devise a treatment program that restores harmony.
> *Steven L. Benedict, O.M.D., Chinese medicine practitioner*

Virtually every month for 14 years, Nancy had suffered severe menstrual cramps. All her doctor could do was prescribe medication to reduce the pain. Even then she would usually miss a day or two of work during her period because she was barely able to get out of bed. Then she heard that acupuncture was good for pain relief. Because acupuncture was covered by her health insurance, Nancy decided to check it out. She got more than she bargained for. The practitioner Nancy saw, Los Angeles acupuncturist Felice Dunas, Ph.D., had Nancy fill out a wide-ranging questionnaire, asked her a battery of questions that had nothing to do with cramps, felt the pulses on both wrists rather intently, and asked to look at her tongue.

To Nancy's surprise, Dr. Dunas said that her other problems—digestive upsets and mood swings—were related to her menstrual pain since, in Chinese medicine, every sign and symptom is a clue to a person's overall condition. Dr. Dunas could not guarantee immediate relief. In fact, she said, the best time to treat Nancy's cramps was when she was *not* having them.

Dr. Dunas recommended a series of weekly acupuncture treatments plus a combination of Chinese herbs to take daily. She taught Nancy self-massage for her legs, which she said would affect her lower abdomen, and advised her to eliminate cold food and drink and to brew ginger tea each day. She urged her to get more exercise, but

what the letters mean

You're used to seeing M.D. after someone's name. But when you get into alternative forms of therapy, other kinds of letters show up:

- O.M.D. or D.O.M. — Doctor of Oriental Medicine
- L.Ac. — Licensed Acupuncturist
- C.A. — Certified Acupuncturist

not while wearing shorts, because she needed to keep her legs warm. All of this, she said, would correct the imbalances that were causing Nancy's symptoms.

Nancy followed Dr. Dunas's advice. All of it. And a month later, her cramps were about 10 percent milder, and her bloating was visibly reduced. The following month her pain was further diminished, and the cramps lasted three days instead of five. That pattern continued until, after five months, her discomfort was so mild she did not miss a minute of work. Plus, her digestive problems were virtually gone, and her mood was even-keeled.

A "Complete Medicine"

Since the early 1970s, when Richard Nixon made his historic trip to China and Americans discovered acupuncture, Chinese medicine has been known mostly as a system of pain relief. "What needs to be understood," says Richard Hammerschlag, Ph.D., president of Yo San University of Traditional Chinese Medicine in Santa Monica, California, "is that it is a complete medicine whose way of looking at the body is different from Western medicine. They're two different metaphors for explaining how the body works, and both of them have a lot of advantages."

First codified at least 2,500 years ago, Chinese medicine (sometimes called Oriental medicine) could be called the granddaddy of holistic health. In olden days, the village physician in China was paid to keep the people well. He did this through regular physical exams and by paying attention to his patients' environment, emotional states, diets, and lifestyle. When people got sick, the doctor was expected to treat them at no additional cost. While the economics have certainly changed, the basic philosophy has not. Modern practitioners of Chinese medicine still emphasize prevention and view their patients as integrated systems of body, mind, and emotions.

Chinese medicine sees the body as an electrical system, explains Joel Penner, O.M.D., L.Ac., a professor at Emperor's College in Santa Monica, California, and author of a textbook called *Zang Fu Syndromes: Differential Diagnosis and Treatment*. "The electrical system moves what we might call life force or vital energy throughout the body," he says. "Health and well-being depend on the quality and distribution of that energy."

In Chinese that life force is called *qi* (sometimes written as chi, and pronounced *chee*). Qi is said to run through a latticework of subtle channels in the body. The existence of these channels, called meridians, has yet to be proved scientifically. When qi is strong and coursing smoothly through the system, the theory goes, our physiology functions harmoniously as nature intended. When qi is weak or its distribution is impeded, causing a deficiency or excess in specific areas, organs break down and systems go awry, leading to the symptoms of disease.

It's All About Energy

The techniques employed by practitioners of Chinese medicine are all designed to strengthen qi and get it flowing properly. "The basic understanding is that health represents a balance of energies in the body," says Steven L. Benedict, L.Ac., O.M.D., a private practitioner of Chinese medicine in Brentwood, California. "The doctor's job is to diagnose imbalances and devise a treatment program that restores harmony."

The most familiar method that Chinese medicine uses, of course, is acupuncture, in which fine needles are inserted into specific points on the body to regulate the flow of qi. Some practitioners supplement acupuncture treatments with heat. While heat-producing machines or heating pads might be employed, the traditional technique is moxibustion. An herb called mugwort or moxa is placed on top of the acupuncture needles or made into cones and set directly on the skin. (They're removed before the skin can burn.) Then they're burned like cubes of incense to heat the area.

Other hands-on treatments include acupressure, which uses touch instead of needles to stimulate meridian points, and various forms of manipulation and massage. Massage techniques might include *tui na*, a traditional therapy, which has been described as a combination of acupressure and chiropractic. "Tui na mobilizes qi and promotes blood circulation by manual contact with skin, muscle, nerve, and bone," explains Harriet Beinfield, L.Ac., coauthor of *Between Heaven and Earth: A Guide to Chinese Medicine*. The technique is used mainly on infants and the elderly.

A Tapestry of Treatments

The most widely used modality, aside from acupuncture, is Chinese herbology. Practitioners prescribe herbs in various combinations based on time-tested formulas to fit each individual's needs for prevention and treatment.

The Chinese have developed a sophisticated pharmacopoeia, classifying barks, roots, flowers, and seeds according to their qualities and properties. Some herbs are used to redistribute qi, some to concentrate it, some to purge the body of toxins, and some to tonify or strengthen specific organs or the body as a whole.

Some practitioners, especially those trained in China, put together packages of raw herbs for patients to cook at home. Because this is time consuming and many brews are unpleasant to taste, most people prefer to take their herbs in pill form. Manufacturers have obliged with a host of patent medicines that are available at many health food stores and herbal emporiums, especially in the Chinatown sections of major cities.

Some practitioners, however, insist that cooking the herbs, while laborious, has advantages. "Herbs are easily assimilated in this form, producing rapid results," maintains Beinfield.

Dietary and lifestyle adjustments are also central to Chinese medicine. Recommendations are generally based on each individual's diagnosis, not on uniform standards. And the advice can be quite different from what we in the West are used to. With diet, for example, many practitioners do recommend vitamins and other Western supplements; however, they consider not just the nutritional components of food but also its energetic influence on the flow of qi. They also factor in the effects of certain qualities such as heat and cold on the individual's condition.

Exercise recommendations are also geared to the individual. Sometimes individuals who are on a workout regimen are advised to change their routine because it is not appropriate for their energy balance. "We might recommend that they do that exercise at a different time, or do a different type of exercise instead, to generate greater harmony in their body," says Dr. Benedict.

In addition to the usual aerobic exercises, practitioners might urge certain individuals to hike in nature or walk barefoot on the earth—activities that can help balance the person's energy patterns.

Traditional Chinese movement and breathing practices such as tai chi and qigong might also be recommended. These slow, gentle exercises are said to enhance flexibility, strengthen the joints, and promote the efficient movement of energy through the body.

In some instances, lifestyle suggestions can even get sexy. "Chinese medicine holds that the proper use of sexual energy can bolster the immune system, strengthen internal organs, and enhance overall well-being," says Dr. Dunas, author of *Passion Play: Ancient Secrets for a Lifetime of Health and Happiness Through Sensational Sex*. Not only can Chinese medicine treat sexual dysfunction and enhance an individual's capacity for pleasure, she says, but the use of certain lovemaking techniques can revitalize the system and direct healing qi to where it's needed.

Three Billion Chinese Can't Be Wrong

Chinese medicine has been used effectively for thousands of years—not just on humans but on animals, notes Dr. Hammerschlag. So its effects can't be just psychological. And it has been studied rigorously in its homeland. Still, Chinese medicine has faced an uphill battle for acceptance in the West, where the demands for scientific proof are strenuous and research opportunities have been limited by lack of resources.

That has changed in recent years, as science has begun to catch up with the millions of citizens who have sought various forms of Chinese medical treatment.

In 1997, the National Institutes of Health (NIH) published a consensus paper delineating five areas in which acupuncture was found to be effective. Those areas are pain (both acute and chronic), respiratory problems, addiction control, gastrointestinal distress, and rehabilitation from neurological damage. The report also concluded that acupuncture "may be useful as an adjunct treatment or an acceptable alternative" for headache, asthma, and a number of other conditions. (For more details, see "Acupuncture" on page 1.)

But that's just acupuncture. Almost all the rigorous research in the West has focused exclusively on that one component of Chinese medicine.

"This is a major problem because it's rare to get treated with acupuncture alone," says Dr. Hammerschlag. "If studies on acupuncture find statistically significant benefits, it seems likely that the results would be even better if they studied Chinese medicine as a whole."

A limited number of scientific studies have been done on individual Chinese herbs. In 1987, for example, researchers looked at people with nasopharyngeal cancer in China. All the people in the study received radiation therapy, but half were also given a traditional Chinese herbal formula. That group did significantly better than those who had radiation only. Other findings suggest that certain Chinese herbs may have value in preventing and treating illness. A number of studies indicate, for example, that astragalus has a wide range of immune-enhancing effects and may be effective as an adjunct in cancer therapy.

Another Chinese herb, ligusticum, seems to enhance the immune system and act as an anti-inflammatory agent. And schizandrae has proven beneficial in the treatment of hepatitis.

Other studies indicate that various Chinese herbs may be useful in the treatment of liver disorders, irritable bowel syndrome, epilepsy, and cancer.

While such studies are encouraging for proponents of Chinese herbs, they do not accurately reflect the nature of the medical system as a whole. The problem with clinical trials on individual herbs, says Dr. Hammerschlag, is that practitioners seldom prescribe that way. Rather, they combine herbs known to complement each

give yourself an earful

In Chinese medicine, the ears are considered a microsystem of the whole body. And massaging the ears is thought to stimulate the flow of qi through the entire system, which is a good way to relax and revitalize.

Try an ear massage when you need to beat stress. Just create a calm environment (dim the lights, play quiet music) and slowly rub your ears between your thumb and forefinger. Take your time—10 to 15 minutes is recommended—and massage every part of your ears. A drop of oil on each finger can make it extra soothing.

other's effects and neutralize one another's potential side effects.

In addition, unlike Western pharmacology, the Chinese system does not prescribe uniform treatment for every illness. It might make sense, for example, to test whether a new drug relieves migraine headaches. But in Chinese medicine a migraine isn't just a migraine. It's viewed as a symptom of an underlying imbalance. Five people with the same headache symptoms can receive five different diagnoses and five different treatments.

A practitioner of Chinese medicine would treat the individual's imbalance, not just the headache, and he or she is likely to employ more than one type of treatment. So, it's difficult, if not impossible, to test whether in actual practice a specific herb is effective in treating migraines.

With interest in Chinese medicine growing among both physicians and the general population, it's only a matter of time before research on the system as a whole comes to light. When a more complete body of data materializes, we'll know exactly how to best use this ancient science. Until then, consumers can derive a certain amount of confidence from a few thousand years of clinical results and keep their family physicians informed of any treatments they receive from Chinese medicine practitioners.

chinese medicine helps heal

- Arthritis
- Cancer
- Cardiovascular disease
- Chronic fatigue
- Gastrointestinal disorders
- Liver problems
- Nausea
- Pain
- Respiratory conditions

An Ounce of Prevention, Pounds of Cures

"Chinese medicine is a complete system of internal medicine," says Dr. Benedict. "It treats respiratory conditions, gastrointestinal disorders, circulatory problems, liver problems, and so forth." In other words, you can turn to a practitioner of Chinese medicine for just about anything that ails you.

Aside from pain control, its most conspicuous success has been in the treatment of chronic conditions, particularly degenerative illnesses such as chronic fatigue, cardiovascular disease, and arthritis. "It doesn't just mask the symptoms or alleviate pain," stresses Dr. Penner, "it can actually return the person to normalcy."

There are limitations, however, and practitioners have been trained to recognize them. If you require surgery, you'll be referred to the proper Western specialist, although in many cases an East-West partnership might be just the thing.

"If a person is going in for an operation, it would be wonderful to treat them with Chinese medicine beforehand to boost their immune system and help them withstand the trauma of surgery," says Dr. Dunas. "And after the operation, Chinese medicine is wonderful for postoperative pain relief and postoperative nausea."

Of all the things Chinese medicine does well, though, preventive care is its forte. "The diagnostic procedures can detect changes in the body weeks or months before they become symptoms," notes Dr. Hammerschlag. "They can pick up an underlying imbalance in your system so it can be corrected before it becomes a major problem."

Practitioners claim that in many cases, including heart disease and cancer, their methods detect signs of trouble before high-tech procedures can spot them.

Good practitioners, however, also know their diagnostic limitations. They will send out for blood tests, urinalysis, Xrays, and other Western specialties whenever such tests are needed. Once a disease is manifesting itself, Western medicine does a better job of diagnosis.

Using Chinese Medicine

On your first visit to a practitioner you may be in for some surprises. "Like Western doctors, they will start out taking a history," says Steven L. Rosenblatt, M.D., Ph.D., L.Ac., a family physician and acupuncturist in Los Angeles. But they won't just ask about symptoms, he notes. "They'll be interested in your diet, your emotional state, how you sleep at night, your work, and other lifestyle information."

This is typically done through some combination of questionnaire and personal interview. Your practitioner may very well take a lot more time getting to know you than the average Western physician.

Then comes the diagnostic work, which is really different from the Western style. Your practitioner will probably examine the pulses on both your wrists—not to count the beats as M.D.s do, but to feel for subtleties of blood movement in six different locations.

"They're not only looking for speed," explains Dr. Penner, "they're looking for the quality of the pulse, like whether blood is coursing through strongly or weakly and whether it's thin or thick."

In Chinese medicine, each pulse position is correlated with specific organs, so the diagnosis also provides clues to what's going on in various parts of the body.

Your practitioner might also ask you to stick your tongue out. Instead of pressing on it with a wooden stick, however, he or she will look it over carefully. "The tongue indicates what's going on in the body," says Dr. Dunas. "We look at its thickness, its color, its coating, and various markings, all of which tell us about the patient's condition and the distribution of energy in the body."

Actually, your practitioner probably started to diagnose you the minute you entered the office. "A good doctor of Oriental medicine can determine quite a bit from the sound of a person's voice, various facial characteristics, and the feel of the skin when you shake hands," says Dr. Benedict.

Some practitioners will also touch (palpate) certain areas of your body and, when appropriate, take your blood pressure or order lab tests.

Diagnosis with a Difference

Be prepared to hear some new terminology when your practitioner explains your diagnosis. He or she might say, for example, that you have a "qi deficiency" or "qi stagnation" in a certain area of your body, meaning that vital energy is lacking or congested. You'll probably also hear the words yin and yang, a reference to the opposite qualities (feminine-masculine, cold-hot, wet-dry, dark-light, etc.) whose complementary interaction is said to govern all natural phenomena, including our bodies. Hence, you might have a "yin deficiency" or be told that your "yang energy is weak."

Nature metaphors permeate the jargon as well, so don't be surprised to hear terms like "damp," "fire," and "wind." And bear in mind that in Chinese medicine the heart, liver, kidney, lungs, and spleen are not just organs in the Western sense but systems or networks with a wide range of influence. "Each organ network refers to a complete set of functions, physiological and psychological, rather than a specific and discrete physical structure," explains Beinfield.

Dr. Penner offers an example of how that might work: "If we see someone with back and knee pain, whose feet and hands are hot; has ringing in the ears; a flush in the cheeks; a reddish tongue; and a thin, rapid pulse, we would probably conclude that he has a kidney yin deficiency."

Once the diagnosis is made, your practitioner will recommend a combination of treatment modalities to treat your condition and prevent future problems. Because Chinese medicine is considered an art as well as a science, if you go to several practitioners, you're likely to encounter a variety of treatment styles. But they'll all be built on the ancient foundation of common principles.

What to Expect

With acute conditions such as pain or injury, you might see results from Chinese medicine within minutes. With chronic disorders, though, healing usually occurs gradually, because treatment is designed to restore balance and strength to the entire system, not just alleviate symptoms.

"As a rule of thumb," says Dr. Penner, "strengthening deficiencies takes a month of treatment for every year the condition has existed." Thus, if you've had a problem for 10 years, you might see some improvement quickly, but it can take a year or so of herbs, acupuncture, and whatever else is prescribed before complete normalcy is restored.

More than ever, insurance companies are allowing visits to licensed practitioners of Chinese medicine. But the number of visits allowed and the conditions they agree to cover tend to be limited.

Be prepared to pay out of pocket. How much? It depends. The cost varies widely, depending on your location and your health-

finding a practitioner

Thirty-six states plus the District of Columbia now have regulations that license acupuncturists. Anyone with a state license and a degree from an accredited school has been trained in both acupuncture and all aspects of Chnese medicine.

Licensed practitioners generally have the initials L.Ac. (Licensed Acupuncturist) after their names, although in some states the designation is C.A. (Certified Acupuncturist). Many also have been certified by the National Certification Commission for Acupuncture and Oriental Medicine (NCCAOM). Many have also earned an O.M.D. (Oriental Medical Doctor) or D.O.M. (Doctor of Oriental Medicine) degree. If you're in a state without licensing procedures, make sure your practitoner has either been licensed in another state or certified by the NCCAOM. This assures that they've met basic standards of competency. You may find pracititoners in your area by contacting any of the national organizations listed on page 78.

care needs. You can expect to pay more for an initial evaluation than subsequent visits, with the price of the latter depending on the type of treatments provided.

Safety and Warnings

If you're worried about aftereffects from acupuncture, or catching AIDS or other infectious diseases from the needles, rest easy. Needling seldom causes anything more than a temporary ache, and even that occurs infrequently. And, assures Dr. Rosenblatt, "All the needles used these days are prepackaged, sterilized, and disposable. They are not reused."

- **Watch for herb-drug interactions.** As for herbs, the Chinese have learned over the course of thousands of years which ones to give in which combinations to reduce the risk of side effects to virtually nil.

  Some herbs might interact unfavorably with certain Western medications. So make sure that you keep both your regular physician and your practitioner of Chinese medicine fully informed about all the treatments you are receiving.
- **Make sure your treatment is customized.** As with any medical system, you stand a greater chance of adverse side effects if you self-medicate. It's inadvisable to take the herbs prescribed for your friend even if you have a similar condition.
- **Get advice from qualified people only.** Taking advice from the proprietor of a

resources

Books

The two books most often recommended as comprehensive introductions to Chinese medicine are:

Between Heaven and Earth: A Guide to Chinese Medicine by Harriet Beinfield, L.Ac., and Efrem Korngold, L.Ac., O.M.D. (Warner, 1996)

The Web That Has No Weaver: Understanding Chinese Medicine by Ted J. Kaptchuk (15th anniversary edition scheduled to be published November 1999)

Organizations

For information about licensing requirements, or to locate a qualified practitioner in your area, contact any of the following organizations:

American Association of Oriental Medicine
433 Front St.
Catasauqua, PA 18032
610/266-1433 or 888/500-7999
www.aaom.org

National Acupuncture and Oriental Medicine Alliance
4637 Starr Rd., SE
Olalla, WA 98359
253/851-6896
www.acupuncturealliance.org

National Certification Commission for Acupuncture and Oriental Medicine
11 Canal Center Plaza, Suite 300
Alexandria, VA 22314
703/548-9004
www.nccaom.org

Accreditation Commission for Acupuncture and Oriental Medicine
1010 Wayne Ave., Suite 1270
Silver Spring, MD 20910
301/608-9680

health food store or an apothecary in Chinatown can also be risky. "It can be detrimental to take something that is not appropriate for your condition," Dr. Penner points out. "If the person at the counter is not trained in Chinese medicine, they might not know what they are doing.

"A lot of people are taking ginseng, for example, but some can actually do themselves a lot of harm by taking it."

Bottom line: Have a licensed practitioner prescribe an herbal formula that's right for you.

chapter 7

chiropractic

GETTING ADJUSTED

Every year there are more visits to chiropractors' offices than to medical doctors' offices. Sometimes it makes you wonder who's the real alternative medicine. —*Jerome McAndrews, D.C.*

Five million years ago, man's ancient ancestor Australopithecus stood up on his stubby hind legs and started walking for the first time. Five minutes later came another milestone in human history: the world's first backache. While standing erect gives us great advantages over other animals, it comes at a price. More than eight out of 10 Americans will suffer from lower back pain at some point in their lives. In fact, in any given year about one-half of the population will endure at least one episode of back discomfort.

The Great National Pain

While most backaches resolve themselves within a few weeks, some can linger longer or never really disappear. This can lead to lost time at work, constant pain, and a frustrating loss of mobility. Between disability costs and doctor bills, the nation spends more than $20 billion every year to deal with back pain and related injuries.

Chiropractors believe that their unique back-adjustment techniques can help solve this huge problem. While chiropractic won't work for everyone, studies have shown that this therapy often eases back and neck pain significantly. There's also a little evidence that chiropractors can be useful with other ailments, including headaches, ear problems, and menstrual or abdominal pain.

Conscientious chiropractors will not claim to be able to cure such problems, but they do believe that fixing irregularities in the back will improve the overall health of patients. And they feel that their methods may help prevent future diseases by strengthening the body's ability to fight off invading germs, viruses, and other pests.

Chiropractic medicine has grown phenomenally as people look for alternative ways to handle their health. Now, nearly one in three people with serious lower back pain seeks help from a chiropractor. In

1990, visits to chiropractors' offices topped 160 million. In light of statistics like these, it's a little hard to call chiropractic care "alternative" medicine at all.

"I think we've come much further than that," says Jerome McAndrews, D.C. (Doctor of Chiropractic), a chiropractor and spokesman for the American Chiropractic Association. "Every year, there are more visits to chiropractors' offices than to medical doctors' offices. Sometimes it makes you wonder who's the real alternative medicine. Simply put, we're good at the back like nobody else is. And that's why we've become so accepted by the public."

chiropractic helps heal

The evidence is clear that chiropractic treatments can ease:

- Back pain
- Neck pain

And it really doesn't matter whether the pain is caused by a chronic condition or by trauma from a car accident, fall, or injury at work.

As for other conditions, the picture is much murkier. In fact, chiropractors make no claims that they can cure anything directly. They believe that adjusting the spine can offer long-term health benefits by allowing the nervous system to function more freely.

However, during the course of practice, chiropractors have found that treatments have sometimes helped with a number of conditions, including:

- Asthma
- Carpal tunnel syndrome
- Ear problems (otitis media, tinnitus)
- High blood pressure
- Headaches (including tension, migraine, and neck-related headaches)
- Jaw pain
- Menstrual pain
- Osteoarthritis
- Rheumatoid arthritis (only in early stages; treating people with advanced conditions is not recommended)

Chiropractic's Origins

While many alternative therapies trace their roots back thousands of years, chiropractic is a relative newcomer. On September 18, 1895, an Iowa man named Daniel David Palmer "adjusted" the neck bones of Harvey Lilliard, a deaf janitor from Davenport. Although the event has been shrouded in mystery and controversy ever since, Palmer claimed to have restored Lilliard's hearing with this one simple maneuver—and created chiropractic medicine at the same time.

Palmer's theories drew heavily on two healing arts that were popular in his day. The first was bonesetting. Bonesetters believed that manipulating or wrenching bones in different parts of the body could free up their motion and ease pain. Palmer also borrowed from magnetic healers, who believed that blockages in the body's energy flow caused disease.

Palmer's idea went like this: The nervous system carries healing and restorative energy, which Palmer called "innate intelligence." He believed that this energy kept the body functioning at optimal levels.

Since the vast majority of nerve impulses in the body travel through the spinal cord, Palmer felt that doctors should focus on this area when looking for the causes of disease. And since the spinal cord is housed in the spine, Palmer believed that out-of-place vertebrae in the spine could block the flow of innate intelligence.

Palmer called these spinal misalignments "subluxations" and contended that they were often the root cause of disease. Fixing subluxations was the key to his healing process.

He did this by using his hands to perform a series of high-speed adjustments to the spine. Properly done, the adjustments moved the vertebrae back into their normal positions.

Spinal Keys to Health

Today, most chiropractors don't adhere to Palmer's theory of innate intelligence. But they do believe that freeing nerves to send proper information to the body can do wonders for back pain—and help prevent other health problems from arising later.

The human spinal cord has 31 pairs of connecting nerves that relay messages from the brain to muscles, organs, and other body parts. These nerves also send information back to the brain. Nerve impulses control a great number of body functions—everything from conscious actions like moving your fingertips to involuntary actions like increasing your heartbeat.

Chiropractors believe that subluxations in the spine can interfere with the body's ability to send and receive these messages. This lack of communication can be at the core of many problems, although it's almost impossible to predict exactly what a subluxation can cause.

"That's why good chiropractors will never say that they treat specific diseases," says Robert Dubin, D.C., a chiropractor in private practice in Petaluma, California.

Many chiropractors have added new techniques to their healing arsenals as well, from modern treatments like ultrasound to time-honored procedures like massage. They've also changed the way they look at subluxations.

To Palmer, a subluxation was simply a misaligned vertebra that needed to be put back in place. Today, most chiropractors include loss of motion in a part of the spine as a subluxation, too. A joint that doesn't move in the manner it's supposed to, they believe, can cause just as much trouble as one that's out of alignment.

"Think of your body like a mobile hanging from the ceiling," Dr. McAndrews says. "In the beginning, everything is in balance, and the whole mobile looks good. But what happens when something gets out of balance? The whole thing tilts and starts hanging funny. One thing has to compensate to balance out the other—and pretty soon you've got problems where you never did before."

The Case for Chiropractic

The medical establishment and chiropractors have battled for decades over the effectiveness of chiropractic treatment. Until the 1970s, in fact, the American Medical Association held that chiropractors were "quacks" and refused to allow any of its members to consult with chiropractors. That changed in 1976 when a federal court found the AMA guilty of conspiring against chiropractors and of violating antitrust laws.

Since then, the medical establishment and chiropractors have held an uneasy truce, according to Scott Haldeman, M.D., Ph.D., D.C., clinical professor of neurology at the University of California-Irvine and an adjunct professor at Los Angeles Chiropractic College. This has allowed both sides to conduct scientific research to see how well, if at all, chiropractic treatment works.

"Until the late 1970s, there was just no good science out there about chiropractic," Dr. Haldeman says. "We had isolated stories from chiropractors, but nothing we could really substantiate." That has changed significantly, he says.

Numerous studies now show that chiropractic care is indeed effective in treating back pain. In fact, the federal Agency for Health Care Policy and Research ruled in 1994 that spinal manipulation can alleviate low back pain.

Dr. Haldeman, a member of that government panel, says the evidence is "very convincing" that chiropractic helps people with acute back pain. He also says there's a "growing database" of studies showing that it also helps with chronic back pain cases, although it's not clear whether the relief from the pain is permanent or short-term.

A 1998 study reviewed 15 major clinical trials on chiropractic and back pain. Nine of these trials showed "significant benefits" from chiropractic care, while four showed no benefit. The other two were inconclusive.

At the same time, a review of six neck-pain studies found that two showed chiropractic helped relieve pain. Two showed that chiropractic manipulation was better than conventional treatment. One showed that adding chiropractic care to regular care improved results. And one showed no benefit.

The authors of an analysis published in the *British Medical Journal* in 1996 found that "there is early evidence to support the use of manual treatments in combination with other treatments for short-term (neck) pain relief."

But chiropractic's usefulness with other health problems remains less clear. The evidence about chiropractic and headache relief is "just starting to develop," Dr. Haldeman says.

Of the few studies out there, one shows that manipulation helped with migraine headaches and one indicates that it may help with tension headaches. However, a 1998 Danish study of 75 people found that, over a 19-week period, chiropractic treatment did not help people with tension headaches any more than a fake laser treatment. Both treatments were combined with massage; interestingly, the massage itself may have helped people in both groups.

As for other conditions, it's just too early to tell. "All we have is anecdotal evidence about conditions like menstrual pain, hypertension, and earaches," Dr. Haldeman says. "It's going to take more than that before anyone can say that chiropractic helps in these cases." However, the authors of two more recent studies that looked at people with asthma said that chiropractic care failed to improve the condition.

No matter what the studies show, it's clear that people who use chiropractors are remarkably satisfied with their care. In fact, a survey of more than 700 members of a health maintenance organization in Washington State found that 66 percent of the people who saw chiropractors for their low back pain were "very satisfied" with their care—compared to only 22 percent of people who got conventional treatment.

Finding a Chiropractor

Unlike some alternative or complementary therapies, it's pretty easy to locate a chiropractor. In the United States alone, about 50,000 chiropractors are now practicing—an average of 1,000 per state. That number is expected to double over the next decade. But it's not a good idea to just dive into the Yellow Pages and choose a practitioner at random.

"It's just like finding any other service provider," Dr. McAndrews says. "You want to find someone that you like, who works well with you, and is qualified to offer the kind of options you need."

All 50 states require that chiropractors be licensed. Although the exact requirements vary from state to state, all chiropractors must earn an advanced degree from an accredited college of chiropractic (this usually takes four years) then pass a licensing exam.

Here are several tips to help you locate a good chiropractor.

- **Ask for proof of training.** Don't be afraid to ask the chiropractor for credentials; if he or she won't show them to you, leave immediately.
- **Ask about professional affiliations.** Chiropractors have the option of joining professional organizations like the American Chiropractic Association. These groups offer additional training, support, and treatment guidelines for chiropractors. Dr. McAndrews strongly recommends choosing a caregiver who belongs to at least one of these groups. "It shows that they've made a commitment to better themselves, and I think that's very important," he says.
- **Look into insurance.** If you are fortunate enough to have insurance coverage that includes chiropractic care, make sure the chiropractor you choose accepts your plan. This can save you lots of money in the long run.
- **Talk to more than one.** Once you've narrowed the field to several qualified chiropractors, ask them for a consultation.

keeping it straight

Most chiropractors describe themselves as "mixers." And it's not because they're fun at parties. It's because they're willing to mix in other healing methods—from nutrition to acupuncture—to meet their patient's needs. It is precisely this "mixing" that so may M.D.s object to. Yet there's a small number of practitioners called "straights" who will never hand you an aspirin, prescribe a massage, or put your joints in an ultrasound unit. "Straights believe only in adjusting the spine and letting the body do the rest," says David Koch, D.C., a chiropractor and president of Sherman College of Straight Chiropractic in Spartanburg, South Carolina.

Straight chiropractors believe that fixing subluxations (a chiropractic term for misalignments) in the spine may free the body's nervous system to ease back pain and other problems. There's no need to use other methods, straights believe, since subluxations are often the root cause of ill health.

Within the straight movement is another offshoot whose members call themselves "super-straights." Super-straight chiropractors believe that keeping the spine free of subluxations won't necessarily cure a particular disease but will allow a great enhancement in everyday life.

"I don't think adjustments will automatically fix headaches or cancer or anything else," Dr. Koch says. "It's not our objective to remove pain or cure conditions."

Still, a well-oiled spine can help the body and mind reach its full potential, according to Dr. Koch. "Maybe you can run a mile faster or digest food better. Or maybe it will enhance your daughter's ability to score over 1,400 on her SATs," he says. In other words, super-straights maintain, a spine that's kept in good working order with periodic checkups and adjustments can unlock the body's potential to be the best it can be.

None of this is proven yet, although Dr. Koch says many quality-of-life studies are under way. The bottom line for consumers: Decide whether straights or mixers sound right for you—and be sure to ask your chiropractor where he or she stands.

Sit down with each chiropractor and talk about your specific problems.

- **Get the specifics.** Ask if he or she has experience dealing with your needs. Have each one explain a typical course of treatment for someone like you—but understand that the actual procedures vary from patient to patient. Also ask if they offer complementary services like massage as part of their treatment package.
- **Go with your feelings.** Most of all, try to get a feel for how you'd work with the chiropractor. This is extremely important, since chiropractic care involves more than just taking medication and waiting for it to work. "It's a very personal process," says James Rynicki, D.C., a chiropractor in private practice in La Mesa, California. "A chiropractor will be giving you hands-on treatment, so you have to feel comfortable in his presence."

In addition, you'll probably be getting advice on exercise, stretching, and other health-related issues like nutrition. If you don't feel good during this first meeting, Dr. Rynicki says, you might have trouble following your program later.

What to Expect

Once you've chosen a chiropractor who suits you, it's time for the initial examination.

Expect to answer lots of questions on your first trip to the chiropractor. Most doctors will want you to fill out a detailed medical history. This will include questions about whether you have health problems like high blood pressure, high cholesterol levels, cardiovascular disease, arthritis, or other conditions that can affect the way you receive treatment.

"We want to know as much about you as any doctor would," says Jonathan N. Colter, D.C., a chiropractor in private practice in Huntersville, North Carolina. "That's the only way we can tailor a program that meets your needs and is safe." In some cases, a chiropractor will want to consult with your physician to share information about medications and other treatments you've received in the past.

The chiropractor also will talk to you at length about the specific problems you're having. For example: Do you have headaches? If so, how often, and for how long? Do you have trouble sleeping? Does your back hurt after certain activities? If you have pain in your back, how have you been treating it? Have you seen other doctors or chiropractors about your condition before?

Remember to be patient. The more information the chiropractor has, the better off you'll be once the treatment begins.

The Physical Exam

After all this information gathering, it's time for the physical exam. Depending on your specific needs, a chiropractor can choose from a wide array of tests. Here are some of the most common:

- **Walking.** "It's vital to see how a person carries himself," Dr. Rynicki says. "The body is not static; it's always moving. So how you walk tells a lot about how you feel." Expect the chiropractor to ask you to walk toward and away from him several times. This allows the chiropractor to judge how you're doing. And don't be surprised if some chiropractors, like Dr. Rynicki, sneak a peak at your stride as you head in from the parking lot and through the office door.

- **Weight-bearing test.** You'll be asked to stand with your left foot on one scale and your right foot on another. This will measure how much weight you carry on each side of your body. Most people distribute their weight evenly on both legs, within 5 pounds or so. If you're carrying 85 pounds on one leg and 65 on the other, it's often a sign that your skeletal system is out of kilter.
- **Spine Analysis Machine (SAM).** This is a simple visual test of your posture. The chiropractor will ask you to back up to a metal-framed device that has colored strings attached to it horizontally and vertically. You'll be asked to stand as you normally would while the doctor adjusts the strings to match how you're standing.

For instance, the right side of one horizontal string will be lined up with the top of your right shoulder, while the left side of the same string will be lined up with the top of your left shoulder. The chiropractor will then adjust other strings for your hips, center line, neck, head, and other body parts.

When the test is complete, you and your chiropractor will have a true picture of how you stand. This will measure how much you have started to compensate to deal with back pain, sore necks, and other problems. You may be surprised to see how much higher one shoulder rides than the other or how much lower you hold one hip compared to the other. With this information, the chiropractor can begin to construct a treatment plan that can straighten out these imbalances—and get your body hanging properly again.

- **Reflexes.** This is the old knee-jerk test that we're all used to taking. The chiropractor will lightly rap one of your joints with a rubber hammer to see how it reacts. If your reflexes aren't responding well, Dr. Colter says, it could be a sign that your nervous system is having trouble sending the proper signals.
- **Range of motion.** You'll be asked to move your neck and back as far as possible in each direction while standing. These measurements will show the chiropractor how much movement you have in your spine and where there's room for improvement.
- **Palpation.** This is the true meat-and-potatoes test of chiropractic treatment. While you sit, stand, and lie on a table, the doctor will palpate, or feel, the muscles and bones in your back and neck.

Chiropractors have undergone extensive training in anatomy, so they can often tell when something's amiss in your spine by touching the right spots. They'll also check for unusual muscle activity, like spasms or imbalance, that are a dead giveaway for underlying skeletal problems.

- **Xrays.** In many cases, a chiropractor will want to look under your skin to get a clearer picture of your spine. For this, he or she will need to take Xrays. "There's simply no tool that can give us a better idea of what's going on with your back," Dr. Rynicki says.

Chiropractors have been criticized for taking too many Xrays—and sometimes rightfully so. "There have been occasions where doctors have overused the tool," Dr.

back care basics

Chiropractic isn't a do-it-yourself kind of therapy. Without the right tools and techniques—not to mention the flexibility of a ballet dancer—trying to do a chiropractic adjustment on yourself might end up causing more harm than good. Of course, you can always help prevent back problems in the first place. Here are a few spine-friendly tips to help you avoid emergency trips to your chiropractor:

• **In bed.** Don't snooze on your stomach. This puts strain on your neck, no matter how you turn it. Instead, try sleeping on your side. Just make sure you adjust your pillow so that your neck is supported and in line with the rest of your spine. If you'd rather sleep on your back, that's fine. Simply place a rolled-up towel or small pillow under your neck to give it proper support.

• **At work.** For office workers, a good chair is key. The American Chiropractic Association says there should be 2 inches between the front edge of the seat and the back of your knees. Sit with your feet flat on the floor, with your knees at a 90-degree angle. If you can't sit that way, use an angled foot rest.

And don't forget to get up and walk around a few times per hour. Too many people lock into a position and stay there, which puts great strain on the neck and back.

If you do lifting as part of your job, be sure to do it the right way. Bend at the knees, not at the waist. And hold the object you're lifting close to your body to reduce strain on your back.

• **At play.** Always warm up properly. Do a few minutes of calisthenics, walking, or jogging before beginning any physical activity. This warms up all your muscles and gets blood flowing.

If you already have back problems, talk to your chiropractor or physician about the right stretches to meet your individual needs. These can vary greatly, depending on the condition of your spine.

• **Doing chores.** If you're standing at the workbench or in front of the kitchen sink, try lifting one foot higher than the other. Place it on the shelf under the sink or on a sturdy box. This eases the pressure on your lower back and can halt backaches before they start. (Those old-time saloons that had a foot rail had the right idea, at least in terms of helpful support for the back.)

• **On the go.** Men, don't put your wallet in your back pocket. Sitting on it can throw your posture out of whack. Put it in your front pocket or give it to your wife to carry in her handbag. Just make sure she carries that purse with the strap across her body. Constantly hanging a purse or bag off just one shoulder is another posture-killer.

• **Watching television.** Make sure you watch TV head-on. Turning your head to the side for long periods of time can cause a real pain in the neck. And never use the arm of the chair or sofa to prop up your neck. The angle is too steep. Instead, support your head with a pillow that keeps your neck in its normal position.

getting adjusted

A chiropractic spinal adjustment involves a lot more than just getting your neck cracked. Modern chiropractic has at its disposal a number of techniques. Here are some of the most common:

- **Diversified.** This is simple, hands-on adjusting, using high-speed movements that move the spine temporarily past its normal range of motion. "This is the one that most people think of when they think of chiropractors," says James Rynicki, D.C., a chiropractor in private practice in La Mesa, California. "It's the original back-cracking."
- **Thompson.** This technique uses a special spring-loaded table with segments that quickly drop to adjust the spine with the patient's own weight. Dr. Rynicki says it's especially useful for larger patients.
- **Activator.** An activator is a hand-held, spring-loaded gadget that the chiropractor can use to adjust individual vertebra. It was adapted from an old dentist's tool used to pull teeth. The activator can move faster than the human hand, allowing for better velocity with less force on your joints.
- **Flexion-distraction.** This is another table, one that moves the hips and legs in all directions. It's a great way to gently manipulate the spine and promote more flexibility.
- **Myofascial release.** This technique uses trigger points to help release muscle spasms that often accompany back pain. Done properly, Dr. Rynicki says, it can be tremendously helpful to patients who have acute pain.
- **Sacro-Occipital Technique (SOT).** Instead of high-speed, high-force adjustments, this technique relies on a series of pads and wedges. When placed in the right places, the wedges can gently move the skeletal system into proper alignment.

Dubin says. "But that doesn't mean Xrays in general are bad. They give us a tremendous amount of information that we can't get in other ways."

It's fairly common to have a baseline set of Xrays taken at the beginning of a treatment program, Dr. Colter says. If you've had Xrays of your spine taken recently, the chiropractor can sometimes use those instead of taking another set and exposing you needlessly to radiation. It's also fairly typical to have another set taken after a year or so to see if things have changed. But there's no need to take them any more often than that. If your chiropractor insists on taking them every month or two, Dr. Dubin says it's probably best to find another chiropractor.

Your first office visit can take anywhere from 45 minutes to a couple of hours, depending on how much information the chiropractor needs to collect.

Follow-Up Consultation

Once the tests are done, you'll be asked to schedule another appointment within a day or two. This brief delay gives the chiropractor time to analyze the results of the tests and create a treatment program tailored just for you.

When you come back for the second visit, the chiropractor will present you with a report of findings, detailing the discoveries and specific program you'll need to follow. There's usually no charge for this follow-up visit.

After that, it's up to you. If the report sounds logical and the treatments sound right, you can get things started, often on the same day as the second visit. If you have any doubts or questions, or if you want to consult your physician, family, or other sources about the course of treatment, by all means wait.

"Don't ever feel pressured," Dr. Dubin says. "Chiropractic care is something that you should want to do, not something you feel compelled to do."

There's really no typical course of treatment in chiropractic care, given the variety of problems that may need fixing. But it's common for a chiropractor to ask for two or three office visits per week for a period of a few weeks.

If this sounds like a lot, remember that a chiropractor is not just treating pain. He or she is trying to solve the underlying cause of the problem. "That takes a little time," Dr. Colter says. "Many times, your body has been compensating for quite a while. It may actually resist you putting things back in order at first. So we just have to keep reminding it about how things are supposed to be."

If you're suffering from a recent injury—perhaps from a fall or a car accident—a short-term treatment program may be all you need.

The chiropractor will try to put things back in working order as quickly as possible, and you'll be on your way.

But if you have a long-term problem—degenerating disks, bone spurs, old trauma from previous injuries—things could take a while. After the initial period, where the chiropractor treats you two or three times a week, you may need to return on a weekly basis for a period of months.

It takes time for chiropractic adjustments, stretching, and other therapies to take hold permanently, Dr. Rynicki says. "If it didn't happen overnight, it's not always realistic to expect it to go away overnight."

Having said that, Dr. Dubin warns that you should never sign up for a long-term group of office visits that require you to pay in advance.

"In truth, we never know exactly how many visits a person is going to need," he says. "I've had people walk in here for one visit and had their problem fixed immediately—but I've also had people come in here for months of visits before we see major results." You should always have the right to stop treatment at any time, with no strings attached.

The Treatments

Chiropractors have dozens and dozens of techniques available to them. But they all have one thing in common: None of them should hurt. If you feel a significant amount of pain, tell the chiropractor to stop immediately.

In addition to all the techniques for adjusting the spine, many chiropractors use other tools to help relieve their patients' pain.

These may include different types of massage, ultrasound therapy on different joints, heat and cold therapy, and even other alternative methods like acupressure or acupuncture.

"Many of us try to use things that treat your body in a holistic way," Dr. Dubin says. "Chiropractic may be the core of the treatment, but other techniques can add greatly to the process."

Most chiropractors recommend periodic checkups for preventive care. "This is different than traditional medicine, where you usually only go when you're sick," Dr. Rynicki says. "I think that going to a chiropractor once or twice a year can do wonders in keeping your body fit and healthy. "It's a lot like going to the dentist. Even if there's nothing wrong right now, it's still a good idea. The idea is to prevent problems before they start."

Safety and Warnings

There are a number of things to be aware of if you're contemplating chiropractic treatment.

- **Make sure you're a good candidate.** Sometimes, chiropractic care is not in the cards. People with certain health conditions may be at risk of further injury. Dr. Rynicki says these conditions include degenerative spinal disks that have already begun to fuse, advanced rheumatoid arthritis, certain previous surgeries or bone fractures, advanced osteoporosis, high blood pressure, diseases of the circulatory system, and some forms of cancer.
- **Get acquainted before you get intimate.** In most cases, don't expect to just walk in, lie down, and have your back cracked. Your chiropractor should take the time to get to know you first. "A responsible chiropractor will never work on you without first analyzing your needs thoroughly," says Dr. Colter. "If someone wants to do that, run, don't walk, out of the office as fast as your aching back will allow."
- **Avoid excess Xrays.** Your chiropractor will want a set of Xrays at the beginning of your treatment. It's also probably a good idea to take a another set after a year or so to check how things are going. Do not allow a chiropractor to Xray your back every month. If your chiropractor insists, find another chiropractor.
- **Never say ouch.** Chiropractic treatment should never hurt. If you experience any pain whatsoever, let your chiropractor know immediately.

chapter 8

food
FUEL FOR HEALING

You are what you eat. —*Dr. Henry Lindlahr*

Recognizing the powerful link between what we eat and our health is nothing new. Nearly 2,500 years ago, Hippocrates, the celebrated Greek physician and father of medicine, used food as an essential part of his formulary to treat what ailed his patients. During the 20th century, sophisticated scientific research has proved the validity of Hippocrates' ancient observations. What we eat can indeed make or break our personal health prognosis.

Early in this century, nutrition discoveries centered on preventing diseases such as scurvy and rickets, rampant conditions caused by vitamin deficiencies. A few decades ago, researchers began to investigate how consuming too much of some nutrients such as fat and sodium contributes to chronic conditions such as heart disease and cancer.

As this century ends and the next begins, the focus has shifted again. Now, nutrition scientists are working rapidly to enhance our knowledge about eating to optimize our health today, stave off disease tomorrow, and stay vital for years longer than our ancestors.

This chapter guides you through the latest findings on eating for optimum health. As these exciting discoveries unfold, one fact is certain: Eating well is not an "alternative" route to wellness but an integral part of everyone's picture of good health.

Nevertheless, it wasn't too many years ago that using diet as an adjunct to medical treatment *was* considered alternative. People who worried too much about things like whole wheat bread and getting enough vitamins were affectionately known as "health nuts." Although these days most doctors' training still doesn't include much about nutrition, most do recognize the importance of diet as part of preventing disease and getting well.

It's important to consider food in a book like this, however, as there are still any number of way-out recommendations mixed into the vast realm of alternative health. Some "alternative" diet recommendations are fine, while others are downright dangerous. And when you're healing, it's vitally important to know the difference.

The Power of a Plant-Based Eating Plan

Despite all the diets, health foods, and supplements popular today, the fact is, no one diet, food, vitamin, or mineral can guarantee good health. In fact, the only condition diet can outright cure is malnutrition. But the latest scientific research does offer compelling evidence that a particular pattern of eating contributes mightily to good health and disease prevention.

In a nutshell, this eating pattern is one that's abundant in plant foods such as grains, beans, peas, lentils, vegetables, and fruits; low in fat (especially saturated fat) from meat, dairy products, and fatty extras such as butter, margarine, and oils; and with the right amount of calories to maintain a healthful weight.

Eating a plant-based diet offers impressive health benefits. Research shows that this eating pattern helps prevent heart disease, cancer, high blood pressure, stroke, diabetes, birth defects, cataracts, and obesity. No wonder diet recommendations from numerous health authorities such as the Dietary Guidelines for Americans, the American Heart Association, the American Cancer Society, the American Diabetes Association, and the American Dietetic Association reflect this eating pattern.

make your vegetables mixed

Enjoy some of your veggies raw and some lightly cooked. Some vitamins are lost during cooking, but some phytochemicals are better absorbed from vegetables that are lightly cooked.

Strive for Five

The best advice calls for eating at least five daily servings of vegetables and fruits, preferably more.

Sure, you know fruits and vegetables are good for you. But did you know just how good? Diets rich in fruits and vegetables are linked with reduced risk for heart disease and high blood pressure and are especially potent cancer fighters. In fact, according to a 1997 landmark report from the American Institute for Cancer Research, overall cancer rates could fall by as much as 20 percent if people made only one simple change—eat five or more servings of vegetables and fruits each day. Yet, fewer than 1 in 4 American adults meet the five-a-day minimum.

What gives produce its health-protective punch? Research is still sorting out the specifics, but it suggests it's a complex interplay between the wealth of vitamins, minerals, fiber, and the hundreds of disease-fighting phytochemicals found in plant foods, rather than any one substance acting alone. That's why eating a wide and colorful array of fruits and vegetables is smart for basic good nutrition and also to receive the most health-enhancing benefits.

Here Are Some Standouts from the Produce Stand:

Cabbage and its cruciferous cousins fight colon and rectal cancers. *Best picks:*
- Arugula
- Bok choy
- Broccoli
- Brussels sprouts
- Cabbage
- Cauliflower
- Collards
- Kale
- Kohlrabi
- Mustard greens
- Radishes
- Rutabaga
- Turnip
- Turnip greens
- Watercress

Citrus fruits fight cancer and protect vision. Citrus fruits are loaded with powerful antioxidants (carotenoids and vitamin C) and a host of other phytochemicals that help protect against some cancers and stave off age-related macular degeneration, the leading cause of blindness in people more than 65. *Best picks:*
- Grapefruit (choose pink to get the most carotenoids)
- Lemons
- Limes
- Oranges
- Tangerines

Colorful fruits and vegetables boost the immune system and fight heart disease. Carotenoids such as beta carotene and lycopene give red, orange, yellow, and dark green vegetables and fruits their vivid colors. They are also powerful antioxidants that help boost the immune system, fight cancer and heart disease, and protect against macular degeneration of the eye. *Best picks:*
- Apricots
- Broccoli
- Cantaloupe
- Carrots
- Kale
- Mangoes
- Pink grapefruit
- Pumpkin and other orange winter squash
- Red and yellow sweet peppers
- Spinach
- Sweet potatoes
- Tomatoes
- Turnip greens

Beans and certain fruits and vegetables prevent birth defects. The folic acid in leafy greens, dried beans, and citrus fruits and juices helps prevent birth defects. As a bonus, this substance also helps fight heart disease and may prevent colon cancer. *Best picks:*
- Asparagus
- Broccoli
- Kidney beans
- Lentils
- Oranges and orange juice
- Spinach

Plus many enriched grain and cereal products also are fortified with folic acid.

plant chemistry lesson

it's good for you

It's a little daunting to read about nutrition these days. There are so many components of food that your body needs, so many new words to take in. Here are a couple of words that should be in your vocabulary.

Phytochemicals are chemicals found in plant foods that may prevent cancer and heart disease, boost the immune system, and slow the aging process. Plants contain hundreds of different phytochemicals.

Antioxidants are types of phytochemicals that help fight diseases such as cancer and heart disease and keep the immune system healthy by protecting body cells from damaging free radicals. Free radicals are natural by-products formed when body cells burn oxygen for energy. Antioxidants work to stop cell damage by deactivating free radicals. The best-known antioxidants are vitamins C and E, and the carotenoids, beta carotene and lycopene.

Eat More Whole Grains

Breads, cereals, muffins, pasta, and pizza crust are only a few foods made from grains such as wheat, rice, rye, oats, corn, barley, millet, and triticale, and their close relatives amaranth, quinoa, wild rice, and buckwheat. With whole grains, the bran and germ are intact, not processed away, as with refined grains such as white flour and white rice.

Whole grains are naturally low in fat and high in energy-giving complex carbohydrates, and provide fiber, B-vitamins, vitamin E, and trace minerals such as zinc and copper. But that's not all. Like fruits and vegetables, whole grains contain a host of phytochemicals that reduce the risk of cardiovascular disease and cancer. The active phytochemicals are concentrated in the bran and the germ, another reason to choose whole grains over refined versions.

To make sure you're getting the whole grain, choose breads that list a whole grain flour as the first ingredient and cereals labeled whole grain wheat, whole grain oats, or another type of whole grain. Experiment with unusual choices such as bulgur, quinoa, triticale, millet, wheat berries, and amaranth.

Whole grains also provide two types of disease-fighting fiber:

Insoluble fiber helps digestion and may play a role in preventing colon and rectal cancer. This is the kind of fiber that moves through the digestive tract without dissolving, so it helps your digestive tract run smoothly. *Best picks:*

- Baked products, such as muffins, made with whole wheat flour or wheat bran
- Bran cereals
- Brown rice
- Vegetables and fruits with edible skins or seeds, such as potatoes kiwi
- Whole wheat bread

Soluble fiber lowers cholesterol and helps prevent heart disease and control diabetes. This kind of fiber dissolves to a gummy texture as it's digested. When included as part of a low-fat diet, soluble fiber may reduce risk of heart disease by lowering blood cholesterol levels. It also helps control blood sugar in people with diabetes. *Best picks:*

- Apples
- Carrots
- Dried beans, peas, and lentils
- Oat- and psyllium-based breakfast cereals
- Oat bran
- Oatmeal

The National Cancer Institute recommends that we consume 20 to 35 grams of fiber each day, which includes a mix of insoluble and soluble types. Check the Nutrition Facts food label on the foods you eat to make sure you get the recommended amount. To avoid digestive discomfort, increase your fiber intake gradually and drink plenty of fluids.

Trim the Fat

Your body needs some dietary fat for important functions such as absorbing the fat-soluble vitamins A, D, E, and K, and supplying essential fatty acids. Children need these fatty acids and vitamins in order to grow properly, and adults need them for healthy skin. But dietary fat becomes a health hazard when we eat too much, especially too much of the saturated kind.

Eating too much saturated fat increases risk for heart disease by raising blood cholesterol levels. In fact, saturated fat drives up cholesterol levels more than any other type of fat. Meat, milk, and milk products such as cheese, butter, and ice cream are the main sources of saturated fat for most Americans. Saturated fat is also found in coconut, palm, and palm kernel oils (check for these on the ingredients lists of the foods you buy) and in smaller amounts in poultry, fish, and shellfish.

High-fat diets also are linked with increased risk of cancers of the colon, rectum, prostate, and endometrium (the lining of the uterus). Eating too much red meat—beef, lamb, pork, and products made from these meats—may increase risk for several types of cancer, most notably colon and prostate cancers.

Here's how to trim extra fat from your diet and choose the healthiest types for the fats you do eat:

- **Put more plant proteins on your plate.** You don't have to completely eschew meat to be healthy, but opting more often for protein-rich plant foods boosts your intake of fiber and phytochemicals, and displaces some of the saturated fat and cholesterol found in meat. Choose more meals based around dry beans, peas, and lentils, soy-based foods such as tofu and tempeh, and nuts and seeds.

Fish is a healthful choice as well. Eating fatty fish such as tuna, salmon, mackerel, lake trout, and swordfish once or twice each week may reduce the risk of heart disease. Experts believe these fish are protective because they're rich in omega-3 fatty acids (also known as linolenic acid), a type of polyunsaturated fat believed to cut the risk for heart attack. Like all fish, they're low in saturated fat, too.

When you eat meat, choose lean cuts such as those with the words "round" or "loin" in their names. Eat poultry without skin. Use cooking methods that add little or no fat such as baking, broiling, grilling, steaming, and poaching. Stretch smaller meat portions by using them in grain- and veggie-loaded dishes such as pasta, stir-fries, chili, stews, soups, and main-dish salads.

- **Look for low-fat dairy products.** Dairy products such as milk, cheese, and yogurt are famous for being chock-full of easily absorbable calcium, a key mineral needed for strong bones and to avoid osteoporosis. They're also an excellent source of protein, vitamin D (which your body needs to absorb calcium), vitamin A, phosphorus, and potassium.

Every day medical research is uncovering more benefits from dairy-rich diets: A diet high in fruits, vegetables, and low-fat dairy products helps reduce blood pressure. (Learn more about diet and high blood pressure in the "Good Nutrition Q&A" section on page 100.) And eating plenty of low-fat dairy products may reduce the risk of colon cancer.

So what's not to love about dairy foods? Basically it's the fat, saturated fat, and cholesterol found in full-fat versions. Fortunately, the dairy case is filled with fat-trimmed options. They're just as nutritious as full-fat versions and taste great, too. Look for reduced-fat, low-fat, and fat-free milk, yogurt, ice cream, and frozen yogurt.

For strong bones and to ward off osteoporosis, the National Academy of Sciences (NAS) recently upped daily calcium recommendations to 1,000 milligrams for adults ages 19 to 50 and 1,200 milligrams after age 50. As a point of reference, a cup of milk or 1½ ounces of natural cheese contains 300 milligrams; a cup of plain nonfat yogurt contains 450 milligrams. Calcium-fortified juices and many fruits and vegetables also provide calcium.

If you don't or can't get enough calcium through foods, making up the shortfall with a calcium supplement is wise.

Choose Oils and Fats Wisely

For heart health, make most of the fat in your diet the unsaturated or monosaturated kind. The difference between saturated and unsaturated fat falls into the realm of chemistry.

But all you really need to know is that saturated fat comes from animals and tends to be hard at room temperature. Think butter and lard. And monounstaturated and polyunsaturated fats are liquid at room temperature. Think salad oils.

Monounsaturated fat can help lower blood cholesterol when you substitute it for the saturated fat in your diet. Monos are especially heart-healthy because they work by lowering "bad" LDL cholesterol without lowering the protective "good" HDL cholesterol. Some research shows that monos may even help raise good

the daily
plant-based eating plan

This plan provides a framework for eating a plant-based diet that will support your healing no matter what kind of health challenge you are facing. Choose fruits, vegetables, and grains in their whole, unrefined form most often. Select lean meats and low-fat dairy products. And eat only small amounts of "extras" such as fats, oils, and sweets.

Vegetables. 3–5 servings. *A serving is:*
1 cup of raw leafy vegetables
½ cup of other vegetables, cooked or chopped raw
¾ cup of vegetable juice

Fruits. 2–4 servings. *A serving is:*
1 medium apple, banana, or orange
½ cup of chopped, cooked, or canned fruit
¾ cup of fruit juice

Grains. 6–11 servings. Choose whole grain varieties for at least three of your daily servings. *A serving is:*
1 slice of bread
1 ounce of ready-to-eat cereal
½ cup of cooked pasta, cereal, rice, or other grain

Protein-rich foods. 5–7 ounces.
Count each of these as 1 ounce:
½ cup of cooked dried beans, peas, or lentils
⅓ cup of nuts
2 tablespoons of peanut butter
¼ cup of seeds
½ cup of tofu
1 egg (limit to four yolks per week)
(A card-deck-size serving of cooked lean meat, poultry, or fish is about 3 ounces.)

Low-fat dairy products. 2–3 servings. *A serving is:*
1 cup of milk or yogurt
1½ ounces of natural cheese
1 cup frozen yogurt
1½ cups ice cream

Added fats and oils. Limit vegetable oil, butter, margarine, and salad dressing to 5 to 8 teaspoons each day. Choose monounsaturated oils such as olive or canola oils most often.

Desserts, sweets, soft drinks, and sugar. Include only small amounts if you can afford the calories.

cholesterol. Olive, canola, and peanut oils are high in monounsaturated fats.

Polyunsaturated fats are found in corn, soybean, sesame, sunflower, and safflower oils. Like monounsaturated fats, polys can help lower blood cholesterol when substituted for saturated fat. But, polys seem to work by lowering both the bad and good types of cholesterol. Some research suggests that consuming too much polyunsaturated

supplements for good insurance

Most nutritionists these days advise getting your nutrition mainly from food, with maybe a multivitamin supplement added for insurance. Is this really enough?

A number of doctors feel strongly that it is not. "One can easily say there is no hard data, but moderate dietary supplementation does no harm and may do good," says Samuel Benjamin, M.D., director of the Center for Alternative and Complementary Medicine at the State University of New York at Stony Brook.

Dr. Benjamin says he endorses a daily supplement regime that closely parallels the one that Andrew Weil, M.D., makes in his book 8 Weeks to Optimum Health. Here's what Dr. Benjamin recommends:

Vitamin C*	1,000 to 2,000 milligrams 2 to 3 times a day for a total of 2,000 to 6,000 milligrams a day
Mixed carotenes	25,000 IU
Vitamin E (mixed tocopherols)**	400 to 800 IU
Selenium	200 to 300 micrograms

These amounts are considerably above the Daily Values. It's a good idea to discuss dietary supplements with your physician, especially if you're contemplating doses above the Daily Values.

** This is a high dose of vitamin C and is inappropriate for people with certain conditions, such as kidney stones and ulcer disease. You should not take this much vitamin C without first discussing it with your doctor.*

*** The 400 milligrams for people under 40 and the 800 milligrams are for people over 40.*

fat can promote cancer. So, when choosing an oil, tip the balance toward monounsaturated types.

Margarines contain trans fatty acids, which are formed when polyunsaturated oils are hydrogenated (hardened) to give margarine its shape. The trans fatty acids in margarine tend to raise blood cholesterol, though not as much as the saturated fats found in butter or lard. If you do use margarine, choose a tub or squeeze variety. These softer forms contain fewer trans fatty acids than stick margarines. Trans fatty acid-free spreads are also available.

Even if most of the fats and oils you eat are the more healthful unsaturated types, it's still important to keep tabs on the total amount of fat you eat to cut risk of cancer and heart disease. All types of fat are calorie-rich, so eating too much can promote weight gain.

The American Heart Association (AHA) recommends consuming less than 30 percent of total daily calories from fat, with less than a third of that total coming from saturated fat. If you eat 2,000 calories a day, this amounts to less than 65 grams of total fat and less than 20 grams of saturated fat.

But don't worry about counting every fat gram you eat. Here's an easier rule of thumb from the AHA: Limit the amount of fats and oils you use in cooking and baking, and as spreads and salad dressings to 5 to 8 teaspoons each day, and select lean and lower-fat options for most of your other food choices.

Dean Ornish, M.D., has done research that found that eating far less fat on a daily basis—a mere 10 percent of calories from fat—combined with meditation and group support not only prevents but even reverses heart disease. See "Vegetarianism" on page 261 for more details on this approach.

Foods as Therapy

There has been a tremendous amount of research over the past few decades on the ability of the right kind of diets to fight disease. Researchers have looked at hundreds of foods and dozens of diseases. There's been a good deal of research, for example, showing that getting enough calcium helps prevent osteoporis (brittle bones) in later life. Much research on the health benefits of plant foods, however, has focused on their potential for cancer prevention. Here's how the National Cancer Institute ranks the cancer-protection activity of several foods and herbs:

- **Highest levels:** Garlic, soybeans, cabbage, ginger, licorice, carrots, celery, cilantro, parsley, and parsnips
- **Modest levels:** Onions, flax, citrus, turmeric, broccoli, cauliflower, tomatoes, peppers, brown rice, and whole wheat
- **Lower but measurable levels:** Oats, barley, mint, rosemary, thyme, oregano, sage, basil, cucumber, cantaloupe, and berries

Plants in a Pill: To Supplement or Not to Supplement?

Foods—broccoli, garlic, soy—can help keep cancer at bay. First, you hear about the potential disease-fighting powers of foods like these. Next thing you know, you see them in a pill bottle. Can popping the phytochemical components of foods in pill form actually help your health? "I generally discourage pills because most of the research data we have looks at whole foods not supplements," says phytochemical expert Cyndi Thomson, R.D., Ph.D., a clinical nutrition research specialist at the University of Arizona's Arizona Cancer Prevention Center in Tucson.

Supplements raise a bevy of yet unanswered questions, says Dr. Thomson. Is the component in the pill the active ingredient that fights disease? Does the pill component act alone or does it need the complex interaction of other substances found in food? (An orange alone contains more than 170 phytochemicals.)

Even if the pill component is the active ingredient, questions remain about how much is safe and effective, and whether it even survives processing. (One exception is garlic. Many studies showing garlic's cholesterol-lowering ability used garlic powder capsules instead of raw cloves.)

Until researchers sort out the answers, your best bet is to count on fruits, vegetables, and whole grains for your phytochemicals. If you take a phytochemical supplement, do not for a minute think of it as a substitute for the solid benefits of eating a plant-based diet.

Good Nutrition Q & A

You're concerned about preventing heart disease and cancer. You want to look good, feel good, and hold back the aging process. So you follow a diet low in fat and cholesterol.

Q What other diet changes can you make to decrease your risk of disease and stay healthy?

A **Think folic acid.** Mounting scientific evidence shows that getting enough of the B-vitamin folic acid decreases blood levels of the amino acid homocysteine. High blood levels of homocysteine appear to increase risk for heart disease.

Researchers don't know yet how much folic acid it takes to get this benefit, but the NAS recommends that adults get 400 micrograms each day for good health.

Leafy green vegetables, dry beans, wheat germ, and fortified grain products are good sources of folic acid. If you take a vitamin supplement, choose one with no more than 400 micrograms of folic acid. Getting too much folic acid can mask the symptoms of pernicious anemia.

Consider a vitamin E supplement. Research is strong that this antioxidant protects against heart disease. Problem is, protective effects are seen from intakes ranging from 100 International Units (IU) on up to 800 IU—well above the current recommended daily intake of 30 IU.

Ironically, vitamin E-rich foods are often those that health-conscious people are cautious of—vegetable oils, margarine, salad dressing, nuts, and seeds. Based on vitamin E's heart-protective effects and other potential health benefits, such as boosting the immune system in the elderly, the NAS is releasing new, higher recommended intakes for vitamin E in the fall of 1999, says Dr. Thomson. Taking a daily supplement of 200 IU is a safe and sound idea, she says. (Vitamin E should be taken in the form of mixed tocopherols.)

- **Eat more soy.** Eating 25 grams a day of soy protein as part of a diet low in saturated fat and cholesterol helps reduce risk of heart disease by lowering blood cholesterol levels. (Learn more about the health benefits of soy in Vegetarianism on page 267.)

Q What's the best diet to reduce high blood pressure?

A **Pump up fruits, vegetables, and low-fat dairy products.** This is the best dietary route to take, according to the results of a 1997 study called Dietary Approaches to Stop Hypertension (DASH), funded by the National Heart, Lung and Blood Institute (NHLBI).

During this eight week study, one group of participants (some with high blood pressure and some with normal blood pressure) ate eight to 10 servings of fruits and vegetables and three servings of low-fat dairy products each day as part of a diet low in fat and saturated fat. Though blood pressure fell in all participants following this diet, the results of those with high blood pressure were most impressive. Their systolic blood pressure (top number) dropped by 11.4 points and their diastolic blood pressure by 5.5 points. These drops began within two weeks and lasted for the remaining six weeks that subjects followed this diet.

To help prevent and treat high blood pressure, the NHLBI recommends eating DASH-style, along with reducing saturated fat and cholesterol, limiting dietary sodium to 2,400 milligrams a day, and including potassium-rich foods such as bananas, orange juice, and potatoes. The NHLBI also recommends these lifestyle strategies: shed extra pounds; drink alcohol only in moderation, if at all; and increase aerobic physical activities. (Go for a brisk walk every day.) And don't smoke.

set your sites high

The quality and credibility of nutrition information on the World Wide Web span from top notch to rock bottom. To untangle the good from the bad, go to the Tufts University Nutrition Navigator site at www.navigator.tufts.edu. This site rates and reviews Internet nutrition information to guide you to accurate and useful sites. It also provides links to the best of the bunch.

Q **Is there a breast cancer prevention diet?**

A **No diet can prevent breast cancer, but some eating habits may reduce your risk, says Dr. Thomson.** (Remember, Dr. Thomson conducts breast cancer research.) Here's Dr. Thomson's advice.

- **Load up on fruits and vegetables.** A study published in the *Journal of the American Dietetic Association* showed that women with increased risk of breast cancer who ate more fruits and vegetables had lower DNA damage levels than women who ate more beef and pork. (DNA damage is a measure of cancer risk.) Though the results are preliminary, Dr. Thomson says it's not too soon to up your fruit and vegetable intake.

"I recommend getting at least eight servings a day," says Dr. Thomson. That's more than 50 percent above the minimum recommendation of five servings a day. "The more different colors, the better, so you get a broader variety of nutrients and phytochemicals," she advises.

Make at least one serving a carotenoid-rich choice such as carrots, one a green leafy vegetable, and one a citrus fruit.

- **Make yours mono.** Research isn't clear yet whether the amount of fat in the diet influences breast cancer risk, says Dr. Thomson, but it does suggest that consuming mostly monounsaturated fats may offer some protection.

rate your weight

Use this formula to calculate your Body Mass Index (BMI):

Multiply your weight by 700, then divide by your height (in inches). Divide that number by your height again. For example, a 145-pound woman who stands 5' 6" tall has a BMI of 23:

145 pounds X 700 = 101,500, divided by 66 (5' 6")=1,538, divided by 66 = 23

Now compare your BMI to the chart below:

Body Mass Index (BMI)	
19 to 24.9	Healthful weight
25 to 29.9	Overweight
30 +	Obesity

Your physician can provide more information about your weight-related health risks.

Though researchers are still sorting out the fat issue, Dr. Thomson says that following a lower-fat diet that has about 20 percent of calories from fat may help. But make most of the fat you eat monounsaturated types such as olive, canola, and peanut oil. Another reason to go low-fat: High-fat diets increase risk for heart disease and for certain kinds of cancers.

- **Proceed with caution when it comes to soy.** Research results are mixed in terms of soy and breast cancer prevention, says Dr. Thomson. Researchers simply aren't sure whether consuming large amounts of soy helps or hurts women already diagnosed with the type of breast cancer that is estrogen-receptor positive. Her bottom line on soy: "Including some soy in your diet is fine, but a 'soy diet' is not."
- **Don't let the pounds creep up.** Dr. Thomson's research shows that gaining extra pounds during adulthood may increase breast cancer risk. Regular exercise can lower risk and help ward off those extra pounds, too.
- **Be a teetotaler.** Even one alcoholic drink a day may slightly increase breast cancer risk, according to the American Cancer Society. If you're at high risk for breast cancer, consider abstaining from alcohol completely.

Q How much does my weight figure in to my risk for disease?

A A lot, according to the NHLBI. Extra pounds increase your odds for suffering a litany of illnesses including heart disease, high blood pressure, stroke, diabetes, some cancers, osteoarthritis, gallbladder disease, and respiratory problems.

Bleak as this sounds, there is good news. Shedding even 10 to 20 of those excess pounds can begin to lower disease risk for even the most obese people. One factor for determining whether your weight puts you at risk for health problems is your Body Mass Index (BMI). You can calculate your BMI using the formula in "Rate Your Weight" (left). Your physician can provide a complete assessment by using your BMI and other factors such as your waist circumference and personal medical history.

- **Don't rely on fads or trick diets.** If you do need to lose weight, don't count on fad diets or "miraculous" fat-burning foods or pills. For lasting results, traditional methods work best: Trim some calories, engage in regular physical activity, and lose at a reasonable pace of about 1 pound per week.

Q Should I take fish oil capsules to prevent a heart attack?

A Fish oil capsules contain omega-3 fatty acids, a type of polyunsaturated fat found in fatty fish such as tuna, salmon, and mackerel. This kind of fat helps reduce blood clotting and may lower risk for heart attacks.

Getting omega-3s from pills is not recommended for the general public because research isn't clear about whether supplements are beneficial. Plus, they can cause several side effects such as digestive upsets, nosebleeds, easy bruising, and weight gain from extra calories.

The AHA recommends the capsules only for people with severely high triglycerides (a type of fat found in the blood) who are at risk of pancreatitis, and only under the care of a physician. For the rest of us, they say get your omega-3s from a few fish meals each week.

Q Do megadoses of vitamin C cure the common cold?

A Unfortunately, there still is no cure for the common cold, including taking extra vitamin C. Consuming enough vitamin C each day is important for fighting off infections, but research hasn't concluded that regularly taking high-dose vitamin C supplements boosts the immune system.

If you already have a cold, however, some extra vitamin C may have a mild antihistamine effect that helps shorten the cold's duration and makes symptoms milder. Boost your consumption with extra servings of citrus fruits and juices or a vitamin supplement containing 60 to 200 milligrams of C.

Q I'm prone to urinary tract infections (UTI). Can cranberry juice help?

A It looks that way, according to a 1994 Harvard study published in the *Journal of the American Medical Association*. Results showed that elderly women who drank 10 ounces of cranberry juice each day for six months were 58 percent less likely to have infection-causing bacteria in their urine than a group who drank a placebo (a look-alike drink with no therapeutic benefits). Cranberry juice seems to stave off infections by preventing bacteria from clinging to the urinary tract lining. Other infection-fighting steps to take: Drink plenty of water, go to the bathroom as soon as you feel the urge, and practice good hygiene habits.

Functional Foods: The Future Is Now

Functional foods are foods thought to provide health benefits above and beyond basic nutrition. Functional foods include foods in their natural state, such as fruits and vegetables, as well as specific components of foods that are added to other foods or packaged into dietary supplements. Think of calcium-fortified orange juice or calcium supplements.

As health-conscious consumers demand more options to safeguard their health, watch the number of functional foods explode. A few recent entries in the functional foods arena include:

- Broccoli sprouts sold as a concentrated source of sulforaphane—the phytochemical that gives broccoli its cancer-fighting punch
- Bread spreads containing plant stanol esters that lower total blood cholesterol and "bad" LDL cholesterol
- A product line of bread, cereal, pasta, frozen entrees, snacks, and desserts that contains psyllium, a soluble fiber that helps reduce risk of heart disease

Functional foods usually come with a premium price tag. Before you plunk down your hard-earned cash, keep in mind that they're not a substitute for a low-fat diet rich in grains, vegetables, and fruits.

Choose wisely. Calcium-fortified orange juice is a boon for healthy bones because it provides many other nutrients. But, do snack chips containing the purported stress-relieving herb kava kava really contain enough to make a difference? Probably not—nor is this the most efficient way to take kava kava.

Finding a Qualified Nutrition Expert

In the United States, there aren't national laws governing who can call themselves a "nutritionist" or "diet counselor." But at least 40 states do license or certify qualified nutritionists and dietitians to practice. In a few states, though, anyone can hang out a shingle and call themselves a nutritionist.

One way to make sure you're getting accurate nutrition information and sound advice on eating for good health, is to consult a registered dietitian, or R.D. (An R.D. may also be licensed or certified in the state).

R.D.s are highly trained food and nutrition experts. Earning the R.D. credential requires a bachelor's degree in nutrition or a related field from an accredited school, a supervised dietetic internship, and passing a rigorous national registration exam. To maintain their registered status, R.D.s must complete 75 hours of continuing education every five years.

When you meet with an R.D., she or he will customize an eating plan that's right for you by evaluating your current diet and exercise habits, your daily schedule, and your medical history.

To find an R.D. near you, call the American Dietetic Association (ADA) at 800/366-1655 or visit the ADA website at www.eatright.org.

nutrition news: take those headlines with a grain of salt

If you've glanced at a newspaper lately or watched the evening news, you know there's no shortage of reporting on nutrition news. Research on the relationship between what we eat and our health is occurring at a rapid pace, and the media rapidly reports these findings to satisfy the public's desire for new information. What's confusing—and frustrating—is that many reports sound as if they are the last word on an issue and warrant a change in eating habits.

Well, it just isn't so. Reliable nutrition recommendations are based on dozens and sometimes hundreds of research studies conducted over many years until a clear pattern emerges. During this process, each study provides a piece of the puzzle and results sometimes contradict each other. That's why you shouldn't overhaul your eating habits based on a study or two, or consider any single food the be-all and end-all for good health.

As research continues to unravel the fascinating connections between food and health, your best bet is to follow the solid nutrition advice from respected health authorities such as the American Dietetic Association, the American Heart Association, and the American Cancer Society. But do keep an eye on exciting developments as they unfold.

Another really good bet is to find an M.D. with special training in nutrition. Any of the university-based complementary and alternative medicine centers can steer you to an M.D. with solid training in nutrition.

Safety and Warnings

Have you ever been lured by a best-selling book, product, or potion that promised picture-perfect health—or even a cure for what ails you? Well, keep in mind the old saying, "If it sounds too good to be true, it probably is."

The next time you're tempted, check into websites for the National Council Against Health Fraud at www.ncahf.org and Quackwatch at www.quackwatch.com. These sites are packed with straight-shooting information about questionable claims, products, and treatments—from the silly to the downright dangerous.

You also can do your own test of questionable claims by measuring them against these "10 Red Flags of Junk Science" from the Food and Nutrition Science Alliance:

resources

Books

The American Dietetic Association's Complete Food & Nutrition Guide by Roberta Larson Duyff, R.D. (Chronimed, 1996)

Better Homes and Gardens Healthy Family Cookbook (Better Homes and Gardens, 1995)

Websites

Arbor Nutrition Guide: www.arborcom.com

The American Dietetic Association: www.eatright.org

USDA Food and Nutrition Information Center www.nalusda.gov/fnic

Magazines and newletters

Cooking Light magazine

Mayo Clinic Health Letter
800/333-9037

Tufts University Diet and Nutrition Letter
800/274-7581

University of California at Berkeley Wellness Letter
800/829-9080

- Recommendations that promise a quick fix
- Dire warnings of danger from a single product or regimen
- Claims that sound too good to be true
- Simplistic conclusions drawn from a complex study
- Recommendations based on a single study
- Dramatic statements that are refuted by reputable scientific organizations
- Lists of "good" and "bad" foods
- Recommendations made to help sell a product
- Recommendations based on studies published without peer review
- Recommendations from studies that ignore differences among individuals or groups

A couple of other notes on safety are in order:

- **Consider going organic.** Pesticides residues in food are an ongoing problem, according to Sam Benjamin, M.D., director of the Center for Complementary and Alternatuve Medicine at the State University of New York in Stony Brook.
- **Be careful with supplements.** Supplements are often inappropriately labeled, says Dr. Benjamin. It's a good idea to go with a company that has strict quality controlls. He suggests either Enzymatic Therapy or Mariposa Botanicals. (Dr. Benjamin has a financial connection to Mariposa.)

chapter 9

herbs

GREEN MEDICINE

I've personally seen medicinal herbs sucessfully treat conditions that high-tech pharmaceuticals couldn't touch.—*James A. Duke, Ph.D.*

When even talk show icon Larry King claims to be on the herbal bandwagon, you know it's getting crowded. More than a third of Americans now regularly use a medicinal herb of some type, spending more than $3 billion a year in the process, and sales are expected to increase by 20 percent a year into the foreseeable future.

Herbal medicine, in short, is enjoying its greatest popularity since ancient times when it wasn't considered alternative at all. Only in the past 80 years or so, in fact, have herbal remedies been upstaged by the more potent synthetic drugs that have become the mainstay of conventional medicine.

For thousands of years before that—since our caveperson days—herbs were conventional medicine, and they continue to be for an estimated 80 percent of the world's population even today.

"Far back into prehistory and in every part of the world, healers have used medicinal plants to treat a great variety of afflictions," says Steven Bratman, M.D., author of *The Alternative Medicine Sourcebook*. "What we call conventional medicine is a newborn baby by comparison."

The ancient Egyptians, for example, were making medicinal use of garlic, juniper, hemp, and poppy seeds nearly 2,000 years before the birth of Christ. And the Chinese were using herbal remedies even before that. Even the highly rational Greeks and Romans practiced herbal medicine, as did the more mystic healers of that period in the Mideast.

But do herbs work? That's the question we as health consumers need to ask ourselves today as herbal products now compete for shelf space alongside the aspirin and cough syrup as viable medicinal cures. Are we investing in remedies that are natural and therefore in some ways "better" than manufactured drugs when we buy an herbal product, or are we succumbing to wishful thinking?

Health for the Whole Body—and Safely, Too

To answer that question, we need first to identify exactly what it is herbal medicine can and cannot do. Unlike most synthetically manufactured drugs, which are designed to have a singular therapeutic effect on a singular medical problem, herbal medicine works in a more general way by strengthening the body's innate abilities "to deal with disease on its own holistic terms," says Daniel B. Mowrey, Ph.D, in his book *The Scientific Validation of Herbal Medicine.* Herbs do this by "energizing, stimulating, or otherwise recruiting the aid not just of one, but rather many systems within the body."

The healing power of herbs is generally not due to a single molecular compound—as is the case with most manufactured drugs—but rather to an herb's unique combination of compounds, the sum of which is thought to be considerably more effective than any of its singular ingredients alone. Herbal experts maintain that this "multiple action" of herbs makes them not only work better but also more safely.

Most herbs have numerous minerals, vitamins, and phytochemicals that work together to make the herb more effective, explains James A. Duke, Ph.D., former U.S. Department of Agriculture (USDA) botanist and author of *The Green Pharmacy.* This multibased action also serves to protect against many of the unwanted side-effects that often accompany more potent pharmaceuticals, he says.

While this multiactive, "nature knows best" characteristic of herbs may be beneficial to users, it has given fits to researchers looking to understand and validate the medicinal activity of herbs from a strictly scientific standpoint. "Often there are simply too many active or partially active ingredients to look at in order to be able to pinpoint which is really having the greatest effect," Dr. Duke explains.

Drugs No, Supplements Yes

But if herbs harbor such medicinal wonders, why don't herb companies simply bite the bureaucratic bullet and obtain for their products the government approval needed for them to be marketed more profitably as drugs? In a word, money.

The amount of research required by the U.S. Food and Drug Administration (FDA) to prove the efficacy of any product claiming medicinal value can take years and cost in the range of $350 million, Dr. Duke explains. That's far too much for an herb company to spend, given that their products (being naturally occurring plants) still could not be patented even if they were found effective.

Under pressure from the public, however, and to ease the burden on herb

green source of powerful medicines

The complex chemistry of herbs has been the bane of profit-driven pharmaceutical companies because what's available from Mother Nature cannot be protected by a patent. Only when a drug company can identify, isolate, then synthesize or somehow process a medicinally active plant compound in a way that is unique can the company obtain a patent granting exclusive rights to its sales.

Tinkering with a plant to make it unique and patentable was done first with the pain-killing narcotic morphine synthesized from poppy seeds by German scientists back in 1803. The same thing happened again with acetylsalicylic acid—the active ingredient in aspirin derived from the bark of the white willow tree by the Bayer Company 1899.

Dozens of other highly effective plant-based medicines have followed—digitalis, the heart medication derived from the herb known as foxglove, for example, and more recently the decongestant Sudafed modeled after a particular component of the common plant ephedra.

So fruitful can plant compounds be as molecular models for manufactured drugs, in fact, that even now pharmaceutical companies are scouring the rain forests to discover new drugs before the plants that contain them become extinct.

companies somewhat, the FDA did in 1994 approve legislation that allows herbal products to be categorized as "dietary supplements." This designation, while it does not permit herb companies to claim that their products are a cure for any specific medical condition, does allow them to claim a generalized effect, such as boosting energy or promoting restful sleep.

Unfortunately, this FDA legislation also excuses herb companies from having to provide scientific proof of such claims. And it absolves them of having to adhere to any standards of safety and quality control. The result of this hands-off policy has been an industry that is loosely controlled, to say the least. An investigation published in the *Archives of Internal Medicine* a few years ago, for example, found that the potency of one group of herbal products derived from the same basic plant varied by as much as 10,000 times!

This is why extra care needs to be taken when buying and using herbal products, Dr. Duke says. The difference between two seemingly similar products claiming the same basic effects can be as dramatic as night and day.

Herbs vs. Disease: What Scientists Say

Should such variability keep you from giving herbal remedies a try? No, but it does mean you'll need to make sure you buy herbal products from the most reputable sources.

As poorly regulated as the herbal industry may be, it does offer products that have, in fact, performed impressively in well-done scientific studies both in the United States and in Europe, where herbs can be advertised as remedies for a specific medical condition. The German government's expert panel for evaluating herbs (called Commission E), for example, has been especially active in the study of herbs as medicines, and many of their findings have been quite promising, reports Dr. Duke.

Personal experience, however, is what motivates Dr. Duke to give herbal medicine his most avid thumbs up. "I've been a botanist specializing in medicinal plants for most of my 30-year career, and I've personally seen medicinal herbs successfully treat conditions that high-tech pharmaceuticals couldn't touch," he says. Even in studies in which herbal therapies have fallen short of more potent drugs, "herbal medicine as a rule is safer than conventional medicine," maintains Dr. Duke. That's because "herbal remedies are more dilute and side effects tend to be less severe," he says.

Dr. Bratman voices a similar sentiment, though he's less enthusiastic about how effective some herbs are. "Compared to the dramatic powers of drugs, the effects of herbs are usually fairly subtle," he notes. "Occasionally an herbal treatment proves to be more effective for a particular individual than any currently available medication, but most of the time the effects of herbs are relatively modest." That doesn't mean they aren't good medicine. Because herbs generally produce so few unwanted side effects, "they are distinctly preferable to drug treatment when they do work," according to Dr. Bratman.

Making Herbs Even Safer

All is not totally roses with herbal therapy. "Herbal medicine is not risk free," says Dr. Duke. "To benefit from using herbs, you need to have confidence in the herbs you take and in any herbal practitioner you may consult. This is no different from conventional medicine, however, where you need to have confidence both in your practitioner and whatever medications he or she may prescribe."

Herbal medicine currently is practiced most reliably by herbologists (with widely varying degrees of training and expertise), naturopaths, nutritionists, chiropractors, and even some physicians. Once you've sought the advice of an expert you can trust, there still are some precautions you should take to be sure your herbal experience is safe and effective. (See "Resources" on page 124 for a list of organizations that can help you find a reputable herbal practitioner.)

Here are a few suggestions from Dr. Duke.

- **Beware of interactions with other medications.** Herbs *do* have medicinal effects, which means they can interact with other medications you may be taking. To avoid complications, therefore, be sure to keep your doctor informed of any herb you may be taking.

- **Watch out for side effects and allergic reactions.** Even an herb that is safe for most people may not be free of adverse side effects for you, so pay close attention when taking any herb. Cut back on your dosage or discontinue use entirely if problems such as headaches, dizziness, nausea, or any other abnormalities arise.
- **Don't try to be your own doctor.** With the rising popularity of herbs, many people have come to think they not only can treat, but also diagnose their own medical conditions. Be careful. Always notify your doctor of any condition for which you feel an herb may be appropriate. You need to be sure that you don't have a disease or condition requiring conventional medical treatment.
- **Keep no herbal secrets.** Studies show that the majority of people who take herbs (70 percent, in fact) do so without informing their doctors.

Don't be one of them, as any medical treatment you receive is likely to be affected in some way by an herbal regimen. Even if your doctor isn't knowledgable about herbs (most aren't), he or she still needs to know about the herbs you are taking.

Shopping for Herbs

Taking an herbal product, unfortunately, can seem easy compared to buying one. Currently more than 20,000 products are available, and because the herbal industry remains virtually unregulated, the quality and potency of herbal remedies can vary tremendously. We've already cited the study from the *Archives of Internal Medicine* that found the potency of various products prepared from the same basic herb to vary by as much as 10,000 times. Other studies have found some herbal products to contain virtually none of their advertised ingredients.

How can you protect yourself from such uncertainty? By observing the following precautions, says Varro E. Tyler, Ph.D., professor of pharmacognosy (the science of plants as medicines) at Purdue University in Lafayette, Indiana, and author of *The Honest Herbal*.

- **Know what you're taking.** This is especially true when picking herbs in the wild or buying dried herbs in bulk, but it applies to commercially packaged extracts, tinctures, and capsules as well. Some of these products may not contain what they claim, or they may contain ingredients other than what's listed on the label.

The solution is to buy herbal products from the largest, most reputable companies you can, because they have their reputations the most at stake, Dr. Tyler says. Generally, these companies tend to be those whose products are available at major retail outlets, such as pharmacies, supermarkets, and health food stores.

If you want to be doubly sure of a company's good reputation, you can refer to a book entitled *Rational Phytotherapy: A Physician's Guide to Herbal Medicine* by Schulz, Hansel, and Tyler. This volume lists herbal brands the reliability of which has been confirmed by solid scientific research. (At $49, this book is expensive. You might want to check it out through your library. This is a good book for doctors who are interested in herbal medicine to have on hand.)

- **Opt for standardized extracts when possible.** Because the quality and potency of bulk herbs can vary tremendously depending on where they've been grown, how they've been dried, and how long they've been stored, buying herbal products with standardized active ingredients is the safer and more reliable way to go, Dr. Tyler says.

When an herbal product is labeled "standardized" it simply means that the herb's most active ingredient or combination of ingredients has been measured and will be listed prominently on the product's label.

Standardized herbs usually are available as capsules, tinctures, or liquid extracts. Although they may be more expensive and lack some of the naturalistic charm of whole herbs, their dependability makes it worth it, most herbal experts agree.

- **Avoid "combination" products.** Herbal products touting multiple ingredients often contain inadequate amounts of those being boasted, so buy single-product herbs to play it safe. Any herbal product that claims a "secret formula" also should be avoided, Dr. Tyler says.

The exception to this rule is herbal combinations that are created by herbal practitioners just for you. Both traditional Indian ayurvedic medicine (see page 23) and traditional Chinese medicine (see page 69 rely heavily on customized herbal formulas.

herbs that work:

A Report on the 12 Most Common

Your 80-year-old aunt may tell you she hasn't lost a hand of bridge since taking ginkgo, but personal testimonials about herbs should be viewed with caution, Drs. Duke and Tyler agree. Far more trustworthy are the findings of well-done scientific studies, such as those conducted by respected scientific institutions in this country and Germany's Commission E. That said, here are the highlights of more than 80 scientific articles published over the past few years by the *Journal of the American Medical Association* and nine of the AMA's other *Archive* journals concerning the efficacy of 12 of the most common medicinal herbs being used in the United States today. (For an evaluation of other popular herbs, see "Different Herbs for Different Ills on page 119.)

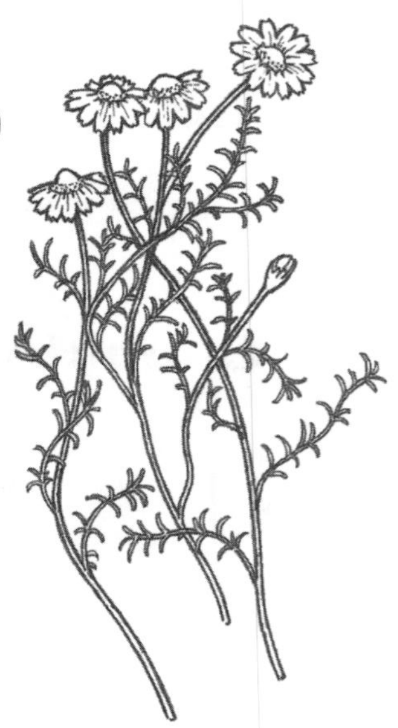

Chamomile
(Matricaria recutita)

Most common uses: to relieve anxiety, reduce inflammation of mucous membranes and skin, aid wound-healing, relieve menstrual cramps, ease indigestion and gas

Uses supported by scientific research: anxiety relief, inflammation reduction, relief of indigestion, and relief of cramps
How taken: as a tea, an inhalant, a bath additive, or applied topically as an ointment or lotion
Possible side effects: allergic reactions in people sensitive to ragweed
Potential drug interactions: should not be used with other sedatives such as tranquilizers or alcohol

Chamomile is a daisylike flower that for thousands of years has been used worldwide for so many afflictions that the German name for it *(alles zutraut)* means "capable of anything." Current scientific research would limit that claim a bit, and yet, studies with laboratory animals have confirmed at least several of the herb's alleged talents.

Research with mice has shown that chamomile's most active ingredient (apigenin) can help protect skin cells from inflammation produced experimentally by irritants. The compound also has been found to protect against stomach ulcers produced by medications, stress, and alcohol. A mild sedative, apigenin also appears to relieve anxiety while having a relaxing effect on the involuntary muscles of the intestines, thus helping to relieve cramps.

Chamomile is considered safe by the FDA even for children and pregnant and nursing women. It has no known side effects other than possible allergic reactions in people sensitive to ragweed. Because of the herb's sedating qualities, however, it should not be used in conjunction with other sedatives or alcohol.

In summary, chamomile's "beneficial effects seen in animals and its good safety record in widespread human use make it an acceptable home remedy for soothing mild skin irritation, intestinal cramps, or agitated nerves," the authors of the *Archives of Family Medicine* report conclude.

Echinacea
(Echinacea purpurea)

Most common uses: as an antiseptic, digestive aid, fever reducer, wound healer, and immune stimulant for the treatment and prevention of colds and flu
Uses supported by scientific research: immune stimulant capable of combating infections of the upper respiratory tract, including colds and flu, an aid to wound healing, and a treatment for infections of the urinary tract
How taken: as a tea, a tincture, or in capsules
Possible side effects: liver damage and suppression of immunity if taken daily for longer than eight weeks
Potential drug interactions: not to be taken with drugs known to be taxing to the liver (anabolic steroids, amiodarone, methotrexate, and ketoconazole)

First used by the Native Americans of the Plains to treat snake bites and the stings of poisonous insects, echinacea now is the top-selling herb in the country. As with chamomile, most studies (26 in all) done in this country with humans thus far have been inconclusive or lacking in proper

Herbs to Avoid

during pregnancy

The word here is ALL OF THEM.

As a general rule, women who are pregnant or who are trying to become pregnant should not be using herbs at all, according to Sam Benjamin, M.D., director of the Center for Complementary and Alternative Medicine at the State University of New York at Stony Brook. Herbs are real medicine and can have powerful effects, he says. Although they can be safe and effective in general, there is really no research that can tell us what effects they might have on a developing fetus. There are also a number of herbs that can cause miscarriage. The best bet is to stay away from herbs altogether, Dr. Benjamin advises. Wait until after you're done nursing to begin taking herbs.

scientific design. At least two human studies have produced impressive results, however.

One study found that echinacea was able to shorten flu symptoms in a group of 100 people by an average of 30 percent compared to a group given a placebo. Another study found that colds were reduced by 15 percent in a group of 647 college students given an extract of the herb.

Echinacea's most impressive performances have come in studies with animals, however, and in the area of immune response especially. Based on these studies, scientists have learned that components of the herb increase the number of circulating white blood cells (the body's first line of defense against invading organisms) while also enhancing the performance of other vital immune responses. These include antibacterial and antiviral activity as well as stimulation of cancer-fighting compounds (such as interferon and interleukins) known to combat malignant growth.

Applied topically, echinacea also has been shown in animal studies to fight infection, protect against radiation-induced skin damage, and help speed the healing of wounds by stimulating the production of cells (fibroblasts) known to be critical to the healing process.

As for the herb's safety, it's not been confirmed by appropriately designed studies, but no serious side effects have been reported in more than 2.5 million prescriptions a year in Germany and more than a century of use in the United States. (German doctors routinely prescribe echinacea.)

Research does show, however, that the herb may cause liver damage if used in conjunction with certain medications (anabolic steroids, amiodarone, methotrexate and ketoconazole) and that the herb also may cause a *decrease* in immune response if used daily for longer than eight weeks.

Feverfew
(Tanacetum parthenium)

Most common uses: treatment of migraine headaches and arthritis
Uses supported by scientific research: treatment of migraine headaches
How taken: as a tea, in a tincture, or in capsules
Possible side effects: mouth ulcers, gastrointestinal irritation, rare allergic reactions and rebound headaches if discontinued abruptly; also may cause adverse reactions during pregnancy
Potential drug interactions: not to be used in conjunction with other blood-thinning medications (Its ability to prevent migraines also may be negated if used in conjunction with other nonsteroidal anti-inflammatory medications such as aspirin or ibuprofen.)

Feverfew is a common roadside perennial of the daisy family that has been used for centuries for the treatment of arthritis and migraine headaches. So far only its use for migraines has been supported by well-controlled scientific research.

In one such study, 270 people with migraines found that the herb reduced both the severity and frequency of their headaches by an average of 70 percent. In another study frequent feverfew users experienced significant recurrences when they were given a placebo instead. So convincing has such research been, in fact, that encapsulated feverfew leaves have been officially approved for migraine prevention by health authorities in Canada.

Researchers suspect that the herb's active compound is parthenolide, thought to work by helping prevent undue constriction of blood vessels while keeping blood free-flowing. This compound may cause side effects, however—mouth ulcers and/or gastrointestinal irritation in 5 to 15 percent of regular users. Feverfew should not be used during pregnancy or by people taking other blood-thinning medications.

One important note. Herbal experts recommend taking feverfew on a regular basis to prevent migraines. The herb does *not* stop a migraine in progress. With this herb, it's especially important to look for a standardized product. "For patients who want to try feverfew, herbalists recommend a gradual dose increase up to 125 milligrams a day orally of encapsulated leaves standardized to contain 0.2 percent parthenolide," note the authors of the *Archives* report.

Garlic
(Allium sativum)

Most common uses: as an antiseptic; digestive aid; expectorant; and agent to lower blood cholesterol levels and/or high blood pressure,

treat blood-clotting disorders, and reduce risks of cancer
Uses supported by scientific research: as an agent to fight bacterial and viral activity as well as to lower cholesterol and blood pressure and reduce the tendency of the blood to clot; may also inhibit viral activity associated with cancer
How taken: raw, cooked, or as capsules
Possible side effects: allergic reactions in rare cases, bad breath
Potential drug interactions: may react adversely with large dosages of aspirin or other blood-thinning medications

So many health claims have been made for garlic lately that it's hard to know whether the herb belongs in your pantry or medicine chest. To make a long story short, it belongs in both.

Garlic's culinary talents aside, researchers have shown that it can lower blood cholesterol ("bad" LDL cholesterol, especially) by between 6 and 11.5 percent, and it can lower blood pressure by between 5 and 7 percent.

The herb also has demonstrated an ability to reduce blood clotting (and presumably risk of heart attacks) and has been associated with reduced risk of cancer in epidemiological research (studies of large populations of people).

Though definitive studies are lacking, scientific research suggests the herb also exhibits considerable antibacterial and antiviral activity, suggesting it may be of use in bolstering immunity to infectious diseases as well as cancer. "Pending conclusive evidence from additional, well-designed studies, it is reasonable for patients to take garlic, given that it is safe and relatively inexpensive," the *Archive* authors conclude in their journal report. It's considered safe by the FDA, even for pregnant and nursing women (although it will flavor the milk). Its only known side effect is rare—allergic reactions or irritation from contact.

People who decide to use garlic for medicinal purposes should be aware of a few caveats, however. Because garlic's main ingredient, allicin, is degraded by crushing, heat, and acid, the herb is best taken raw or in the form of coated tablets. The recommended amount is 300 milligrams (standardized to at least 1.3 percent allicin) taken two to three times daily. This equates to approximately one clove of garlic daily if taken fresh.

Do be aware that the potency of commercial preparations can vary widely. In one analysis of supposedly standardized garlic preparations, for example, 93 percent were found to be so lacking in allicin as to be no more valuable than a placebo.

Ginger
(Zingiber officinale)

Most common uses: to relieve indigestion, motion sickness, and flatulence
Uses supported by scientific research: relief of indigestion and motion sickness
How taken: as a tea, in tincture form, or as capsules
Possible side effects: none known
Potential drug interactions: none known

Ginger's alleged ability to settle the stomach goes back a long way. The ancient Greeks wrapped gingerroot in bread as an after-dinner digestive aid—the rationale for which stands up well to scientific scrutiny even today.

In addition to encouraging results from numerous studies with laboratory animals, one well-designed study with surgery patients found ginger to be as effective as a prescription drug in preventing nausea. Another study found the herb to be even *more* effective than the leading prescription drug for treating motion sickness.

"It is reasonable for patients to try ginger to treat nausea, not only because data supports its efficacy, but also because it is inexpensive, readily available, and safe," conclude the authors of the *Archives of Family Medicine* report. "Like garlic, ginger is not known to cause any serious side effects, despite world-wide culinary as well as medicinal use."

The usual adult dose for treating nausea or motion sickness is 250 milligrams to 1 gram of powdered gingerroot taken several times per day. (And yes, it really does help to sip ginger ale.)

Ginkgo
(Ginkgo biloba)

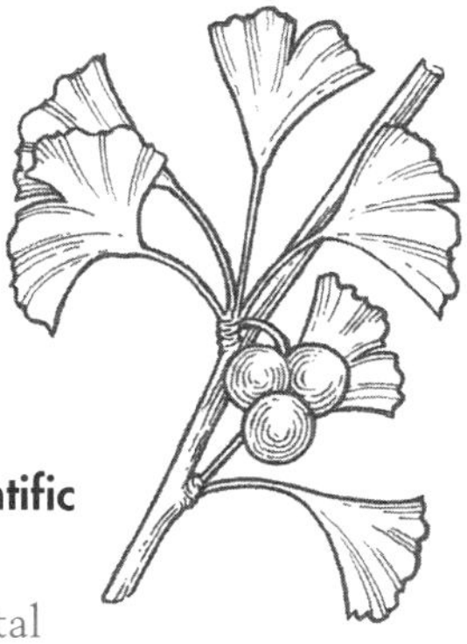

Most common uses: to improve memory, boost mental clarity, increase circulation, treat dizziness
Uses supported by scientific research: improves memory, improves mental functioning in elderly, increases circulation, relieves vertigo, helps protect cells against free radicals (naturally occurring molecules that damage the body)
How taken: as capsules
Possible side effects: stomach distress, restlessness, headaches
Potential drug interactions: may interact adversely with blood-thinning medications

Ginkgo has been used by the Chinese to treat brain disorders for thousands of years, but only in the past 20 years or so has the herb, deservedly, grabbed attention worldwide. So impressive has research into the efficacy of this herb been, in fact, that federal health officials in Germany have declared ginkgo safe and effective for treating circulatory disturbances (including memory impairment) throughout the body and brain.

Studies in this country have corroborated these German findings. In one year-long investigation, ginkgo was found to stabilize and in some cases even improve mental and social functioning in people suffering from Alzheimer's disease as well as other forms of dementia. More than a dozen European studies have shown ginkgo to be effective in reducing the symptoms of claudication (impaired blood flow), including one in which the herb helped people increase their pain-free walking distance by 50 percent.

The biological mechanisms responsible for ginkgo's effects are not fully understood but are thought to relate to its abilities to dilate blood vessels, keep blood free-flowing, block the release of inflammatory agents, and curb the activity of tissue-damaging free radicals.

The herb has no known side effects, other than mild stomach distress, restlessness, or headaches in rare cases. The dose shown to be effective is 40 milligrams taken three times a day (or 80 milligrams, taken twice daily) of an extract standardized to 24 percent flavanoid glycoside and 6 percent terpenoids. (Don't let these long chemical names throw you; this information will be clearly printed on the label.)

Ginseng

(Panax ginseng)

Most common uses: as a stimulant, aphrodisiac, antidepressant, stress reliever, protector against cancer, and cure for symptoms of menopause

Uses supported by scientific research: stimulant (mentally as well as physically) and possible inhibitor of cancer. Also may be helpful in the treatment of Type 2 adult-onset diabetes and infertility in men

How taken: as a tea from the powdered root or in capsules

Possible side effects: rapid heart rate, increases in blood pressure, insomnia, diarrhea, menopausal bleeding

Potential drug interactions: not to be used with estrogens, corticosteroids, or phenelzine sulfate

The claims made for ginseng are becoming as lofty as its price, which currently can exceed $20 per ounce.

In keeping with its reputation as an "adaptogen"—the herbal term for a substance that helps the body adapt to stresses of all kinds—ginseng has been reported to benefit virtually every system of the body while providing protection against heart disease, cancer, sexual lethargy, emotional stress, and even the aging process.

Such all-encompassing claims are difficult to verify from a scientific standpoint, of course, yet research has turned up some positive findings.

In one three-month study of 625 people taking ginseng, for example, researchers noted a significant increase in scores evaluating "quality of life." In another study with people of college age who took 100 milligrams of ginseng for 12 weeks, there was a significant increase in the speed with which they could perform difficult mathematic calculations.

Yet another study found an association (though not necessarily a causal one) between ginseng use and lower cancer rate; another showed the herb increased both the number and motility of sperm in 46 men whose sperm counts were low.

Most recently, ginseng was found to lower fasting glucose (blood sugar) levels in a group of people with Type 2 adult-onset diabetes while improving their sense of well-being.

What's the final word on ginseng? The scientific jury is still out, so in the meantime caution is advised.

"While laboratory and animal studies suggest that ginseng has beneficial effects on immune and hormonal functions, evidence

different herbs for different ills

Which herbs do the best job? Aside from those on pages 112 to 123, many others have come under scientific scrutiny. Here's a list compiled from the experiences and recommendations of the best herbal experts in the field. (Remember, always check with your doctor before treating any medical condition on your own.)

Medical Condition	Best Herbs to Try
Adult-onset diabetes	Fenugreek
Arthritis	Ginger, stinging nettle
Asthma	Turmeric
Backache	Peppermint, willow
Bladder infections	Cranberry, uva ursi
Bronchitis	Echinacea, turmeric
Burns and sunburn	Aloe
Bursitis and tendinitis	Willow
Colds and flu	Echinacea, garlic, ginger
Constipation	Flaxseed, psyllium
Cuts and scrapes	Aloe, comfrey
Depression	St. John's wort
Fever	Willow
Fungal infections	Garlic, licorice, tea tree
Headaches (migraine)	Feverfew
Heartburn	Chamomile, peppermint
Hemorrhoids	Butcher's broom, witch hazel
Herpes and cold sores	Echinacea, lemon balm
High blood pressure	Garlic
High cholesterol	Garlic, ginger
Indigestion	Chamomile, peppermint
Insomnia	Feverfew, lemon balm, valerian
Laryngitis	Cardamom, horehound
Liver problems	Dandelion, milk thistle
Menopause	Black cohosh, red clover
Menstrual cramps	Black haw, cinnamon
Premenstrual syndrome	Chasteberry, angelica, evening primrose
Prostate enlargement (benign)	Pumpkin seed, saw palmetto
Psoriasis	Red pepper
Toothache	Clove, willow
Ulcers (stomach)	Chamomile, ginger, licorice root, oregano
Vaginitis	Garlic, goldenseal, tea tree
Wrinkles (facial)	Cucumber, horse chestnut
Yeast infection	Echinacea, garlic, goldenseal

of its effects on humans is limited and contradictory," note the authors of the *Archives of Family Medicine* report. "Patients who take ginseng risk paying a high price without proven benefit."

The authors also caution users that commercial ginseng preparations can vary tremendously in quality. In one analysis of 54 ginseng products, 85 percent were determined to be "worthless," containing little or no true American or Korean ginseng at all. (Siberian ginseng is not a viable substitute. It bears little resemblance to the American or Korean varieties.)

If you do take ginseng, be sure you're getting a medicinally active product. Only preparations stating their content of "ginsenocide" should be used. As for the safety of ginseng, the FDA has put the herb on its GRAS (Generally Recognized as Safe) list. Yet rare cases of of insomnia, diarrhea, skin eruptions, and menopausal bleeding have occurred. Because it can be a stimulant, the *Archives* authors warn that it probably should not be used with other stimulants, as rapid heart rate or increases in blood pressure may occur.

Goldenseal

(Hydrastis canadensis)

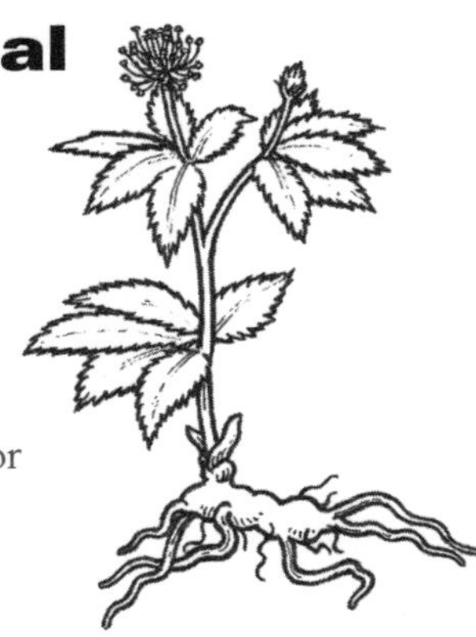

Most common uses: as a topical antiseptic, digestive aid, and treatment for yeast infections and diarrhea

Uses supported by scientific research: treatment of diarrhea (effective but not advised) and as an antiseptic for skin irritations and superficial wounds

How taken: internally as a tincture, a tea, or capsules; externally the tea is applied to the skin or used in ointments

Possible side effects: irritation of mucous membranes, gastrointestinal distress, uterine contractions, jaundice in newborn babies

Potential drug interactions: may interfere with the medicinal activity of heparin

Goldenseal was first used by the Cherokees as an antiseptic. It remains popular today for that same purpose.

Diarrhea, however, is the problem for which modern research has found the herb to be most effective. In one study, a single 400 milligram dose of what researchers suspect is the herb's most active compound (berberine) was found to be effective in treating diarrhea due to intestinal bacteria.

In the case of diarrhea, berberine blocks the adhesion of bacteria to the cells that comprise the intestinal walls. Due to the possible toxicity of goldenseal's other ingredients, however—especially one called hydrastine—the *Archives* authors do *not* advise using goldenseal for treating diarrhea attacks. Large amounts of hydrastine have been found to cause gastrointestinal distress, high blood pressure, contractions of the uterus, jaundice in young children, and in rare cases, even respiratory failure. The authors stress that goldenseal should never be used in any form, even topically, by pregnant or nursing women, young children, or people with cardiovascular disease, blood-clotting problems, or epilepsy.

Does the herb then have any use at all? Dr. Duke says that in tincture form goldenseal can be of value as an antiseptic applied topically to treat skin irritations, superficial wounds, yeast infections, earaches, ringworm, and athlete's foot.

Milk Thistle

(Silybum marianum)

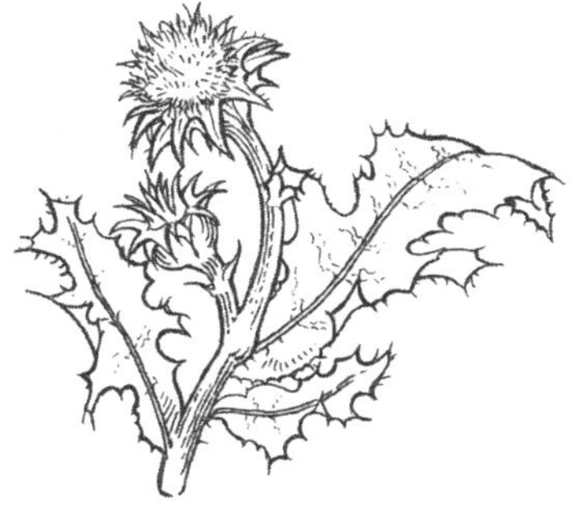

Most common uses: to treat liver problems, detoxifying the body
Uses supported by scientific research: protects the liver from toxins
How taken: as a tincture or capsules
Possible side effects: none known
Potential drug interactions: may effect blood sugar levels in diabetics taking insulin

Milk thistle has been used to treat liver problems for more than 2,000 years, and the most recent and well-designed scientific research offers encouraging evidence as to why. In one study, the mortality rate among liver patients receiving 140 milligrams three times daily of milk thistle's most active compound (silymarin) decreased by 30 percent. In another, people with liver disease experienced improved liver function after just one week of being given silymarin daily. So potent is silymarin that European physicians routinely treat mushroom poisoning by injecting it intravenously.

In studies with laboratory animals, silymarin has been shown to protect the liver from viruses, radiation, and a variety of toxins, such as alcohol and the popular painkiller acetaminophen (which is toxic to the liver in high doses). The compound is thought to exert its protection by binding to receptor sites on liver cells, thus beating toxins to the punch.

By scavenging tissue-damaging free radicals and inhibiting inflammation, silymarin also helps liver cells regenerate. Best of all, the substance has no known side effects other than lowering blood sugar levels in diabetics (people with diabetes need to monitor themselves closely if on a milk thistle regimen). Recommended silymarin dose is one 140-milligram capsule (standardized to 70 percent silymarin) taken two to three times daily.

St. John's Wort

(Hypericum perforatum)

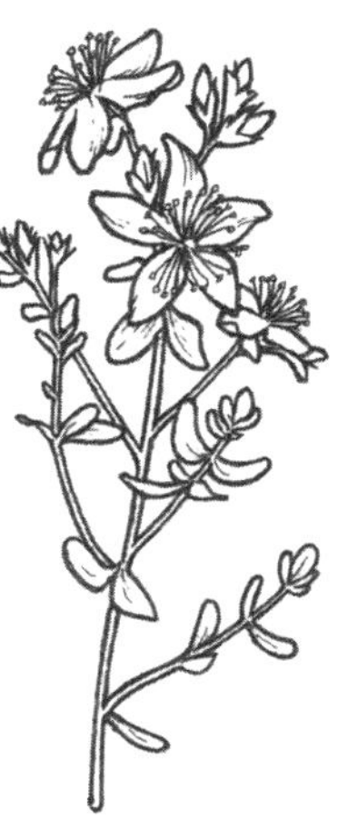

Most common uses: as an antidepressant, antiseptic, and remedy for diarrhea, indigestion, and nausea
Uses supported by scientific research: antidepressant and antiseptic
How taken: as a tincture or in capsules
Possible side effects: hypersensitivity to sunlight, especially in people with fair skin
Potential drug interactions: should not be used with other antidepressants

Touted as the Prozac for naturalists, this news-making herb increased in sales 20-fold between the years 1995 and 1997. It's currently Germany's antidepressant of choice, being prescribed over Prozac 4 to 1.

Used in ancient times to help people ward off evil spirits, the herb has stood up well to the latest round of investigation that comes with such fame.

Dozens of well-done studies have shown that St. John's wort works as well as prescription antidepressants and with significantly fewer side effects.

In progress is a $4.3-million, three-year study to determine such factors as long-term side effects, types of depression best treated by the herb, and optimal dosages. In the meantime, the light on this herb seems to be pretty much green—and not just for treating depression.

St. John's wort also has been shown to be an effective antiseptic in the treatment of wounds and burns. And its abilities to combat viruses and even cancer also are being researched.

The herb ranks high in safety, with its only known side effect being hypersensitivity to sunlight, especially in fair-skinned people. If you're taking the herb daily, be aware of this potential effect and make sure you protect your skin if you're in the sun for extended periods of time. (You could end up with a sunburn you won't forget in a hurry.)

The herb is not recommended during pregnancy, however, or in conjunction with other psychoactive medications.

People choosing to try St. John's wort should begin with the dosage levels used in most of the studies of its effectiveness. Most experts agree on 300 milligrams, three times a day, of an extract standardized to 0.3 percent hypericin.

Saw Palmetto

(Serenoa repens)

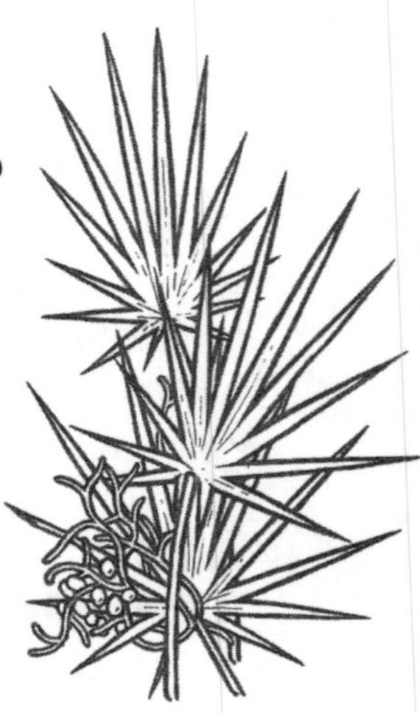

Most common uses: to treat benign prostate enlargement and increase breast size in women and sperm counts in men
Uses supported by scientific research: treatment of benign prostate enlargement
How taken: as a tincture or capsules
Possible side effects: gastrointestinal irritation and headaches in rare cases
Potential drug interactions: none known

The medicinal potential of this herb was first noticed by the Seminole Indians of Florida. Some of the men who snacked routinely on the herb's seeds began noticing improved urinary flow, and the herb's reputation as a friend of the male urogenital system was born.

Extracts from the fruit of this small, scrubby palm have since gone on to impress users and researchers alike. It improves urinary flow in men by helping to downsize the prostate gland if and when this small organ located in the groin begins to enlarge for reasons other than cancer. Prostate enlargement is a problem for as many as 50 percent of all men by the age of 50. The herb works by preventing the hormone testosterone from being converted into a compound known to stimulate prostate growth.

And work it does. In all but a few of the well-done studies of saw palmetto's effectiveness in treating benign (noncancerous) prostate enlargement, results have been impressive. Not only has the herb generally worked as well as the leading prescription drug Proscar, but it has significantly fewer side effects. Proscar's possible side effects include impotence and lack of sexual desire.

As for saw palmetto, only mild headaches or gastrointestinal irritation have been reported as possible side effects, and even these are rare. One more plus: Saw palmetto is considerably cheaper than the prescription drug.

The recommended dose of saw palmetto for treating benign prostate enlargement is 160 milligrams of an extract (standardized to contain 85 to 95 percent fatty acids and sterols) taken twice daily until the condition improves, which is usually one to three months.

Valerian
(Valeriana officinalis)

Most common uses: as a mild sedative, antidepressant, and treatment for insomnia, high blood pressure, and excess gas
Uses supported by scientific research: mild sedative and treatment for insomnia and intestinal cramps
How taken: as a tea, a tincture, or capsules
Possible side effects: restlessness and heart palpitations with prolonged use
Potential drug interactions: not to be used with other sedatives

It's been rumored among historians that it was not the Pied Piper's flute music that lured the rats out of Hamelin, but his pockets full of the tranquilizing herb valerian. The odiferous plant, which herbalists don't mind admitting smells all too much like dirty socks, is highly intoxicating to rats and cats alike.

Valerian's attraction to humans over the centuries, however, has been its abilities to relieve anxiety and help induce restful sleep—both of which have been convincingly confirmed by well-controlled scientific research. In studies of the herb's ability to aid sleep, participants reported neither the dependency nor the residual "grogginess" characteristic of many medications used for this purpose.

Laboratory experiments have shown that valerian works by binding to the same receptor sites on the brain as tranquilizers like Valium, but with milder and thus fewer negative effects. The herb's only drawback, oddly, seems to be restlessness and heart palpitations in rare cases and particularly with long-term use.

The herb is not advised for use during pregnancy. Nor should it be used in conjunction with other sedatives or before activities requiring one to be alert, such as driving. Recommended dosage of the herb is 400 to 450 milligrams taken an hour or so before bed.

resources

So what's the best way to give herbal medicine a try?

It's not—NOT—by diagnosing your own condition or running out to the nearest drugstore for a bottle of whatever has worked for your grandmother or neighbor. You should take the time to consult an experienced professional in the field. Herbal medicine is practiced by herbologists, naturopaths, chiropractors, nutritionists, some M.D.s and—least reliably—by employees of herb shops and health food stores.

There is no single standard for the certification of herbal practitioners, unfortunately, but several reputable herbal organizations do exist that can help you find an herbalist you can trust. These are listed below, along with some excellent books to help educate you in this up-and-coming but centuries-old field.

Organizations

The American Herbalist Guild
P.O. Box 1683
Soquel, CA 95073

The Herb Research Foundation
1007 Pearl St., # 200
Boulder CO 80302
303/443-0949

Sage (Rosemary Gladstar's Educational Foundation)
P.O. Box 420
East Barre, VT 05649
802/479-9825

Books

The Healing Power of Herbs by Michael Murray, N.D. (Prima Publications,1995)

The Green Pharmacy by James A. Duke, Ph.D. (Rodale Press, 1997)

Herbal Healing for Women by Rosemary Gladstar (Fireside Books, 1993)

The Scientific Validation of Herbal Medicine by Daniel B. Mowrey, Ph.D. (Keats Publishing, Inc. 1986)

The Complete Medicinal Herbal by Penelope Ody (DK Publishing, 1993)

Healing Plants by Ana Nez Heatherley (Lyons Press, 1998)

The Complete Illustrated Holistic Herbal by David Hoffmann (Element Books, 1996)

chapter 10

homeopathy

TRIGGERING THE BODY TO HEAL

For 200 years, homeopaths have watched people get better with our remedies.
—*Richard Jenkins, M.D., San Francisco homeopath and internist*

When Bill Gray, M.D., first entered medical school at Stanford University, he dreamed of saving people's lives. "I wanted to be the hero in the white coat," he says now. But as he progressed through his training, he became disenchanted with the limitations of Western medicine in healing chronic disease. Dr. Gray eventually traveled to Greece to study with one of the world's leading homeopaths, George Vithoulkas. Now one of the top homeopaths in the United States, Dr. Gray coordinates a booming practice in the San Francisco Bay area.

Homeopathy Goes Mainstream

"Homeopathy was once considered quackery, real fringe medicine, but now I find it's being increasingly accepted even by conventional physicians," Dr. Gray says. "They're now sending me patients with illnesses as serious as Lyme disease. They know I can cure people."

Homeopathy shows signs of entering the medical mainstream, mainly due to the public's increasing interest in alternative health. Many major drug chains, such as Walgreen's and Rite-Aid, carry homeopathic medicines. In fact, sales of homeopathic drugs, which are now found in the aisles of major grocery, drug, and health food stores, totaled more than $300 million in 1998. What's going on here?

Less Is More

Homeopathy is a system of medicine developed by German physician Samuel Hahnemann during the early 19th century. While researching Peruvian bark, an extract that contains the drug quinine—the treatment for malaria—Hahnemann tried taking bark extracts himself and, as a result, developed the debilitating symptoms of malaria. After many similar experiments, he developed the theory of homeopathy, proposing that natural substances that bring on symptoms in healthy people could actually heal the same symptoms in someone who is ill.

The reason for the healing effect, Dr. Hahnemann said, is that symptoms are an expression of the body's effort to heal itself. By stimulating these same symptoms, you could activate the body's healing response—its complex defense systems.

Homeopathy and allopathic (conventional Western) medicine coexisted for more than 100 years but were always bitter rivals. During the early 20th century, both groups began vying with even more intensity for political power. In 1910, the Carnegie Foundation released the Flexner report, an evaluation of medical schools authored by allopathic doctors in the American Medical Association (AMA), which gave most homeopathic medical schools poor ratings.

In the ensuing years, homeopaths were also prevented from belonging to the AMA or publishing in conventional medical journals. That, combined with the discovery of antibiotics by allopathic medicine, sounded a death knell for homeopathy's growing popularity. But homeopathy re-emerged in the 1970s, along with the growing interest in natural health care.

Homeopathy remains one of the most controversial areas of alternative medicine today. And while it's been increasingly accepted by the public—according to a 1998 study in the *New England Journal of*

homeopathy helps heal

Most homeopaths treat a wide range of conditions ranging from migraines to asthma and carpal tunnel syndrome.

A study published in a 1997 issue of the British medical journal *Lancet* found that homeopathy was most effective for these conditions:

- Agitation or anxiety
- Allergies
- Asthma
- Chronic pain
- Cough
- Cramps
- Labor pain in women
- Migraine headaches
- Rheumatoid arthritis
- Sprains and strains

Homeopaths interviewed for this book also reported significant success with treating these conditions:

- Attention deficit disorder
- Chronic fatigue
- Chronic problems from long-lasting head injury
- Colds
- Depression
- Digestive problems
- Drug or alcohol addiction
- Lyme disease
- Sore throat

Medicine, Americans made almost 2 million visits to homeopaths in 1997—most traditional physicians have been more than critical, maintaining that homeopathy is ineffective and doesn't make scientific sense.

"The idea that homeopathy works is simply a delusion on the part of the clinician practicing it and the patient," says Wallace Sampson, M.D., a professor at Stanford University and a member of the American Council Against Health Fraud. "Every study I've seen that's purported to prove that homeopathy works is either erroneous or falsified."

Yet one of homeopathy's most vocal supporters, Dana Ullman, M.P.H., a Berkeley, California, writer and homeopathic drug formulator, says that this alternative medicine actually works by scientifically verifiable rules. "There is still a lot of 'homeo-phobia' out there. To be a critic of homeopathy just means you don't understand it."

Basic Principles

Homeopathy is based on three major principles that underlie and explain its healing potential:

- **The law of similars.** This theory states that natural substances that bring on certain symptoms in the healthy can heal the same symptoms in ill people. Exposing ill people to these same substances in extremely tiny doses, often substances to which the patient has a supersensitive reaction, triggers the immune system, helping the body to heal itself, homeopaths believe. Some allopathic medicines, such as allergy shots, work in a similar fashion to rev up the body's immune system.
- **Individualization.** Most homeopaths believe that a single remedy will be enough to heal all of a patient's symptoms. For instance, an individual suffering from migraines and depression can be healed of both these symptoms by one substance. Homeopathic drugs are classified according to the "symptom picture" they alleviate. Every patient is prescribed drugs based on their individual symptoms.

So, several people with the same disease—such as premenstrual syndrome (PMS)—but having different symptom pictures, might each be prescribed a different remedy.

- **The law of infinitesimals.** One of the most crucial tenets of homeopathy states that a person's symptoms can be cured by small doses of natural substances that are diluted in water and shaken many times. The diluting and shaking action actually makes these natural substances more potent, homeopaths say.

Treatment with Tiny Doses

The first step manufacturers take to create homeopathic drugs is to dissolve a natural substance in 10 or 100 parts of distilled water and shake the resulting solution. One part of the resulting solution is then diluted and shaken again, and the process is repeated until the right dilution results. The more the remedy is dissolved and shaken, the more powerful it becomes, homeopaths say. All homeopathic medicines today are made by drug manufacturers certified by the U.S. Food and Drug Administration (FDA).

Labels on homeopathic medicines tell you how diluted the remedy is. "X" denotes that the first dilution was 1 in 10 and "C" means a 1 in 100 dilution. A 10X dilution would be a remedy with one part natural substance and 10 parts water in the first dilution then diluted and shaken nine more times. A 10C solution begins life as one part extract and 100 parts water, then is diluted and shaken nine more times.

Even homeopaths acknowledge that most of the drugs they use are so dilute that they contain no remnant of the original substance. But the original substance's imprint or "essence" remains, they say, and such solutions are made powerful through the movement and clustering of water molecules during the diluting and shaking process.

Recently, some homeopathic adherents and researchers have also theorized that homeopathic medicines may act through an electromagnetic charge in the solution. This charge results when the natural ingredient is dissolved in solution and shaken, and water molecules begin to move and reorient themselves.

Shui-Yin Lo, Ph.D., physicist at the American Technologies Group in Monrovia, California, published scientific papers in 1996 revealing that when substances are dissolved and vigorously shaken in water, unique molecular structures or clusters that maintain an electrical field are formed. These clusters remain stable even at very high temperatures and seem to have the ability to increase immune response, important in the cure of infections and cancer.

Dr. Lo, who is not a homeopath, says that these solutions *are* created by diluting and shaking natural substances, but they are far different from homeopathic remedies.

"Our solutions are only diluted one to 13 times, while homeopaths may dilute their medicines up to 300 or 1,000 times," he says.

Dr. Lo does not believe that his research in any way proves the theories that underlie homeopathy. Nevertheless, proponents of homeopathy point to his research findings as potential evidence of the ability of water to somehow pick up an imprint from a material it is mixed with.

Science and Homeopathy

Despite such controversy, Dr. Gray and other homeopaths say their medicines *do* work. Dr. Gray maintains that 70 percent of his patients feel that they are cured within the first year of treatment. And a survey taken in the Los Angeles area found that 60 percent of people who visited homeopaths experienced significant improvement of their chief complaint within four months, according to a paper in the journal *Alternative Therapies.*

Still, results of studies on homeopathy published in major Western journals have been mixed. It was only in 1994 that the first meticulously done (double-blind, placebo-controlled) study on homeopathic medicine was published in an American medical journal. Before then, many studies on homeopathic medicines had been poorly executed, mostly because they were under-funded or performed by homeopaths with a bias toward the medicine. Homeopathy is also difficult and expensive to test in scientific studies, its supporters say, because its remedies are individualized for each patient.

That first meticulously done (double-blind placebo-controlled) study, published in *Pediatrics* in 1994 and directed by homeopath Jennifer Jacobs, M.D., of Edmonds, Washington, revealed that homeopathic treatment for life-threatening diarrhea in Nicaraguan children had a significant advantage over placebo. (A placebo is a look-alike preparation with no therapeutic benefit.)

Diarrhea in Third World children frequently has no effective treatment except rehydration fluids, though antibiotics are often used inappropriately, Dr. Jacobs said in her study. But her research on 81 children revealed that children treated with fluids and homeopathy had a 15 percent, or about one day, decrease in the duration of diarrhea compared to those treated with only fluids. The usual duration of such diarrhea episodes is about five to six days. The treatment was not only cost-effective, but might potentially contribute to reduced symptoms and death from the disease, Dr. Jacobs said.

Homeopathy and Addiction

Though homeopathy is not well known for its ability to aid people with drug and alcohol addictions, an as yet unpublished study by homeopath Susan Garcia-Swain, M.D. of Seattle, Washington, has turned up some striking results. During the 18-month study, more than 700 people with addictions received a homeopathic remedy, a placebo, or no remedy at all, in addition to standard medication and therapy at the Starting Point detoxification and recovery center in Sacramento, California.

The results? At the end of 18 months the relapse rate for the homeopathic group was only 32 percent. By contrast, the relapse rate for the other groups was much higher—ranging from 68 to 72 percent.

"This was a study that was made simple enough so that non-homeopaths could repeat it; it is entirely reproducible," says Dr. Garcia-Swain. "Physicians are now calling me from all over the world—even non-homeopaths—asking me to help apply the study to their patients. That's very encouraging."

Two independent addiction centers are now planning to repeat the study, she says, and Dr. Garcia-Swain is working on getting it published.

There have been other well-executed studies that have shown homeopathy to be effective, but few of these have been repeated successfully by different independent research groups. Only when a successful study had been repeated does the scientific community consider a treatment effective.

In 1997 a landmark review published in the respected medical journal *Lancet*, researchers analyzed 89 of the most well-done studies on homeopathy, but its conclusions were mixed. The researchers found that homeopathy was almost two to three times more effective than placebo remedies. At the same time, the authors said they could not find enough scientific support to say that homeopathy is effective for any single condition. That is, they could not find treatments that had been tested in stringent studies done by at least three independent scientific groups. The researchers rated only 26 of the studies as "high quality."

"The public worldwide continues to use homeopathy at increasing rates, despite the lack of definitive evidence to support its worth," says Wayne Jonas, M.D., one of the *Lancet* study's authors and former director of the National Institutes of Health Office of Alternative Medicine. "So homeopathy is an area that should be systematically investigated in order to determine its potential role in the American health-care system."

How to Find the Best Practitioner

Many people feel that they can't wait for absolute proof that homeopathy works. They need help for a medical problem—and now.

"Studies show us that people who go to homeopaths are frustrated by traditional Western medicine. They've already seen two to three doctors for conventional treatment, usually for a chronic disease," says Ted Chapman, M.D., a homeopath, researcher, and family practice physician in Boston, Massachusetts.

But how do you find a good homeopath? One good way to start is by asking your own physician. Some doctors are open to homeopathic treatment, and even if yours is not, he or she should be aware that you are looking into this form of alternative therapy.

Another good approach is to ask your friends if any of them have tried homeopathy. Question them about how long the treatment took and whether or not it was a success. The National Center for Homeopathy also publishes a directory of licensed homeopaths in paper form and on their web site.

The organization's phone number is 703/548-7790 and the web site is www.homeopathic.org.

The directory includes a list of homeopathic study groups, groups of lay people who get together regularly to discuss the science of homeopathy. They're often good sources for finding the best homeopaths in town. Other good sources for referrals include alternative medical clinics and homeopathic pharmacies.

In most states, homeopaths need to be licensed medical professionals to practice. So any traditionally trained medical doctor could open shop as a homeopath. And so could a chiropractor, acupuncturist, or nurse licensed by the state. Only three states—Arizona, Nevada, and Connecticut—license homeopathy separately. Many lay homeopaths also practice throughout the United States illegally. (Most state authorities don't seek out or vigorously prosecute such clinicians.)

Even though lay homeopaths are not licensed, they may still be well trained.

homeopathic checklist

To check whether your homeopath is a good one:

- **Get some specifics.** Ask if the clinician specializes in homeopathy as a primary therapy. Ask your clinician where he or she received training and how long he or she has been in practice. Your homeopathic practitioner should have at least two years of training in homeopathy.
- **Note how you are interviewed.** Notice whether your homeopath asks for lots of details about your physical symptoms and psychological state. Proper individualized homeopathic diagnosis requires a lot of information.
- **Make sure you're viewed as unique.** Your homeopathic practitioner should prescribe medicines for *your* constitution, the whole array of your "symptom picture," not just an isolated acute or chronic illness.
- **Ask about sources.** Find out whether the homeopath uses a computer or a book called a "repertory" to find the correct medicine.

They may have apprenticed to a homeopath or gone through a homeopathic medical training program. But since there is no state or national board that licenses lay homeopaths, you should consider that you may have less legal recourse if something goes wrong.

There are national board certification tests—through the Council of Homeopathic Certification and the National Board of Homeopathic Examiners—that provide proof that a homeopath is qualified. Naturopathic physicians can obtain doctoral certification in homeopathy through the Homeopathic Academy of Naturopathic Physicians. Physicians and osteopathic physicians may also obtain doctoral certification through the American Board of Homeotherapeutics. But these national certification tests and doctoral programs do not guarantee a homeopath the license to practice in any state.

Using the Therapy

Your first visit to a homeopath may last anywhere from one to several hours. The reason? Most homeopaths take a detailed history, involving a much more extensive discussion than even a yearly checkup with your family doctor. "We talk about every limitation that the patient experiences in his or her life—whether that's physical or emotional," say Dr. Gray. In fact, much of the time during the visit will be taken up with talking about your psychological state.

The homeopath's questions will delve into your personal and family history—asking not only about inherited physical disease, but also events that have affected you psychologically, even changed your life. The homeopath often tries to get a sense of your personality type, too. Emotions and personality, most homeopaths believe, play a large part in the development of many chronic illnesses.

Later visits will often be shorter and last about an hour.

It's important that you clearly express your symptoms—physical, mental, and emotional—to your homeopath.

"Self-observation is very important. Being able to pay attention to your body and express that to your homeopath; it's a vital skill," says Dr. Gray. It may help to jot down some of your observations about your physical and mental state before your first visit.

Medically licensed homeopaths will also perform a physical exam during the first visit. Most often, a homeopath will prescribe a remedy, too. Most homeopaths keep a large variety of such medicines on hand.

Homeopathic medicines are usually sugar-coated granules or powders that you take by mouth. Your homeopath may also give you a prescription to be filled at a pharmacy that dispenses homeopathic remedies, if it's one he or she doesn't carry. Mail order is available for people without a homeopathic pharmacy nearby.

What to Expect

Visits to a homeopath usually cost $50 to $400 for the first time and $30 to $200 for follow-ups. Your medical insurance may reimburse visits, if your homeopath is an M.D. or other licensed professional. The cost for homeopathic medicines, though, is hardly ever reimbursed. But these medicines do tend to be inexpensive. They're over-the-counter drugs and generally cost between $5 and $15 in health food stores or drugstores.

If your remedy works, you shouldn't need more than a few follow-up visits each year—at the most, just once a month.

You should expect with an acute illness, say, a sore throat or flu, to see a significant improvement from a remedy in, at the most, a few hours, homeopaths say. Chronic illnesses can take up to several years to heal, but you should experience steady and significant improvements within the first few months and at least a 50 percent reduction of symptoms in the first year, sometimes more. Dr. Gray says he heals most people within the first year.

"We certainly can't cure everybody," adds Richard Jenkins, M.D., a homeopath and internist at the Complementary Medicine Clinic at California Pacific Medical Center in San Francisco. "But most of our patients respond well and can go on to live their lives with much fewer symptoms. As a result, they need medical treatment less often."

The time it takes to see improvement may be longer for difficult diagnoses. Dr. Gray says he has seen some difficult chronic conditions improve greatly only after six or more years of treatment.

Other factors that can slow down the effectiveness of remedies include conventional drugs, which are often taken for chronic conditions. Your homeopath should not insist that you give up medications prescribed by your conventional doctor, however. If your homeopath is a good one, he or she should try to wean you from traditional drugs slowly—and only when it's safe to do so.

Conventional drugs slow down the healing process of homeopathy because they mask symptoms instead of attacking the underlying cause of the illness, homeopaths believe.

"Most of my patients are eventually able to go off all their drugs," Dr. Gray says. "I wouldn't consider them cured if they didn't."

Safety and Warnings

Besides taking Western medicines, there are other things that can counteract homeopathic remedies. These include coffee, camphor (such as in ointment rubs for muscle aches), and tea tree oil, which is sold in health food stores for skin conditions and wound healing. Being exposed to mothballs and using an electric blanket can also counteract a homeopathic remedy. So can a visit to your dentist if he or she uses a drill on your teeth, though the reason is unknown.

"We don't recommend that people stop seeing dentists. But you have to make a judgment as to whether drilling is absolutely necessary. And if it is, you may need another dose of your remedy afterward," Dr. Gray says.

You should also know that some remedies can make symptoms worse—most often just for a few days—before you start getting better. That's called a "healing crisis." If a healing crisis is more than just mildly bothersome, you should phone your homeopath for advice.

It's important to follow your homeopath's advice—or in the case of over-the-counter remedies, the instructions on the bottle—about how long to take a remedy. You can actually make your symptoms worse by taking some remedies for too long, Dr. Jenkins says.

If your symptoms don't improve or if they come back after a short time, then you may have the wrong remedy.

"That's when you need to go back to your homeopath, so he can get more details about the case. It doesn't happen very often, but sometimes the remedy may be close to what you need—just not on the money," Dr. Jenkins says.

As for Dr. Jenkins, he's sure that his patients are benefiting from homeopathy. In fact Dr. Jenkins first came to believe in homeopathy when he himself was cured of debilitating cluster headaches by a homeopath.

"Homeopathy is a science based on the time-tested experience of clinicians," he says. "For 200 years, homeopaths have watched many people get better with our remedies."

Over-the-Counter Homeopathic Relief

Most of the homeopathic medicines you see sold over the counter in the local drugstore are not true classical homeopathic remedies. Over-the-counter remedies are, in fact, often combinations of the most frequently used homeopathic substances for certain individual illnesses, say cold or flu. In contrast, most homeopaths prescribe and dispense remedies containing just one substance that is meant to heal someone with a wide range of symptoms and conditions. Do the over-the-counter mixtures work? Even clinicians within the homeopathic community disagree.

"These medicines are not representative of what homeopathy does," says Dr. Gray. "In classical homeopathy the remedy is always individualized for each patient. There's no science to the way these combination medicines are put together. They may not be harmful, but most are not effective."

Yet many people have found relief from their ailments by using combination medicines, such as those for teething pain and allergies, says Ullman, who's a formulator of homeopathic over-the-counter medicines as well as a writer and researcher. "Combination medicines are a user-friendly way to try homeopathic remedies," he adds. "It is more effective to individualize remedies. But not everyone who needs a remedy has access to a practicing homeopath or knows how to find or use an individualized remedy."

Single remedies are also available in health food stores and homeopathic pharmacies, but it's best to purchase them only on the advice of a homeopath.

resources

Books

Many self-help books on the market provide advice for using homeopathic medicines at home. But the most reliable self-help books give detailed prescriptions for different symptom pictures. They should also provide specific directions for how much of a remedy to take and for how long.

Healing with Homeopathy by leading homeopaths Wayne Jonas, M.D., former director of the NIH Office of Alternative Medicine, and Jennifer Jacobs, M.D. (Warner, 1996)

The Consumer's Guide to Homeopathy by Dana Ullman, M.P.H. (J.P. Tarcher, 1996)

Web site:

Dana Ullman's web site: www.homeopathic.com

chapter 11

hydrotherapy

LIQUID RELIEF

> This is an area that is so safe and so potentially useful that ... you should not hesitate to try any form of hydrotherapy that's suggested for whatever ails you. —*Isadore Rosenfeld, M.D.*

Who hasn't iced an injury, inhaled steam to clear clogged sinuses, or soaked in a hot tub just to relax? These are all forms of hydrotherapy, sometimes known as water therapy. The main techniques of hydrotherapy include compresses, ice rubs, poultices, saunas, showers, soaks, and whirlpool baths. Even drinking a glass of water may qualify under certain circumstances.

Hydrotherapy is simply using water in any form—liquid, ice, or steam—for healing purposes. It can be taken internally or applied externally in a sauna, shower, or tub, through a jet spray, hose, or compress, to heal.

What It Is, What It Does

The main principle behind hydrotherapy is that applications of moist heat and cold promote circulation of blood and other body fluids and soothe or stimulate the nervous system. Ice can act as a tonic and an anesthetic as well as reduce swelling. Heat can relax muscles and nerves and promote blood flow. Most physicians usually stop there. But naturopathic physicians stress that water can also assist the body's natural defenses by detoxifying the body of accumulated poisons.

It is possible, naturopaths maintain, to detoxify the body by drinking water, irrigating the colon (or other orifices, such as an infected ear or nose), or using steam so that perspiration carries away toxins through the skin. Where the conventional medical approach uses drugs to fight disease, the naturopath supports the body's natural defenses to banish germs and toxins.

Hydrotherapy offers psychological benefits, too. While a psychiatrist might prescribe a drug and talking or behavior therapy to allay anxiety, a naturopath might prescribe a regimen of meditation, exercise, dietary changes, herbal remedies, and supplements as well as hydrotherapy.

According to Jamison Starbuck, N.D., a naturopathic family practitioner and health writer based in Missoula, Montana, naturopaths use hydrotherapy as part of a holistic treatment program, not as a cure in itself. (N.D. stands for Doctor of Naturopathy.)

"We also look at what other parts of this person we need to improve besides the site of injury or disease," says Dr. Starbuck. "We also use hydrotherapy to promote the 'vital force' (what Chinese medicine calls *qi*) or the immune system and energy level—that which keeps a person alive and moves them toward healing."

Isadore Rosenfeld, M.D., professor of clinical medicine at New York Hospital/Cornell Medical Center and attending physician at New York Hospital and Memorial Sloan-Kettering Cancer Center, offers a different view. "The fundamental difference between the orthodox practitioner and the complementary physician is that the latter makes grander claims for hydrotherapy," he says.

But Dr. Rosenfeld, author of *Dr. Rosenfeld's Guide to Alternative Medicine: What Works, What Doesn't, and What's Right for You,* concludes, "this is an area that is so safe and so potentially useful that—regardless of the theoretical disputes between the two camps—you should not hesitate to try any form of hydrotherapy that's suggested for whatever ails you."

Does Hydrotherapy Hold Water?

Because hydrotherapy has been so widely used throughout history, there has been little urgency to study it scientifically. Most applications help heal a whole host of ailments with little chance of harm. But several current studies have addressed the safety and effectiveness of water therapy across a broad variety of health conditions.

Nurses and other therapists who work with the physically and mentally disabled lend support to the psychological benefits of water exercises. A 1992 study of the role of hydrotherapy in people with learning disabilities concluded that hydrotherapy offers an opportunity for exercise, socializing, and stress relief. The researcher added that patients with physical disabilities enjoy moving more freely in water than they can on land.

A 1996 study published in *Arthritis Care Research* looked at 139 people with chronic rheumatoid arthritis. They were randomly assigned to one of four experimental treatments: hydrotherapy (in this case, water exercises), seated immersion in water (not technically considered hydrotherapy in this case because a specific area of the body wasn't targeted), land exercise, or progressive relaxation. All attended 30-minute sessions twice a week for a month. The study participants were all tested physically and psychologically before and after the study and followed up three months later.

The researchers found that all the people in the study experienced some benefit, but hydrotherapy produced the

hydrotherapy helps heal

What conditions do naturopaths treat with water? "That's like asking an M.D. what they use drugs for," says Douglas C. Lewis, N.D., instructor of physical medicine at Bastyr University in Seattle. "We treat anything drugs can be used for with hydrotherapy." When a physician or physical therapist mentions hydrotherapy, they are generally referring to water exercise or first aid for injuries. The main conditions most successfully treated by naturopaths and conventional medical doctors are:

- **Arthritis:** Moist heat relieves pain by increasing blood flow. It can relax painful joints and weak muscles so they can be exercised and strengthened.
- **Cardiovascular conditions:** Water exercises strengthen the heart and lungs and promote muscle strength in the chest wall, diaphragm, and extremities.
- **Infections:** These range from bowel, gastrointestinal, and genitourinary to respiratory and skin disease.
- **Sports injuries/first aid/rehabilitation:** Treatments include everything from compresses and ice packs to water exercises. Conditions that water can treat include sprains, strains, bruises, cramps, and spasms, as well as circulatory problems arising from paralysis.
- **Wound care:** Whirlpool treatments and compresses speed healing of burns, wounds, and ulcers in both rehabilitative medicine and naturopathy.

Naturopaths also use water therapy for immune support in preventive medicine and to treat:

- **Anxiety and panic disorders**
- **Chronic fatigue syndrome**
- **HIV/AIDS**

Colonic irrigations and sweat baths may be used to treat:

- **Food poisoning**
- **Drug overuse, including smoking or drinking alcohol**
- **Multiple chemical sensitivities**
- **Exposure to environmental toxins**

These applications may not be endorsed by many allopathic doctors and have not been well documented in mainstream medical literature in this country. There is scientific support for these uses, however, from European clinical studies, as well as laboratory studies and clinical practice by naturopaths.

greatest improvements, physically and emotionally. Not only did the people getting hydrotherapy show significantly greater improvement in joint tenderness, but females in the group showed improvement in the ability to move their knees through a greater range of motion. (Further study may explain why the men failed to improve on this measure.)

In another study, Australian researchers found no difference between treating chronic low back pain with hydrotherapy versus land exercises, but both groups improved significantly, so the study supports hydrotherapy's effectiveness. A British study of patients with osteoarthritis of the hip found similar results.

Hydrotherapy is also an important part of wound care in many medical settings. One study conducted by Harvard Medical School researchers found that pressure ulcers in rehab patients improved significantly faster when daily 20-minute whirlpool treatments were added to a conservative treatment of relieving pressure and applying moist saline compresses.

One Japanese study found that people with chronic pulmonary emphysema were helped by underwater breathing exercises. Not only did the carbon dioxide-oxygen exchange in their blood improve, but their hearts grew stronger too.

In Sweden researchers tried alternating cold and hot showers on the legs of people with intermittent claudication (a fancy term for exercise-induced leg cramps from poor circulation). They found that hydrotherapy significantly improved the people's ability to walk. Improvements in ankle blood pressure measurements were sustained up to a year later. The researchers recommended adding hydrotherapy to conservative treatment of this condition.

Also, Viennese researchers have found preliminary evidence that hydrotherapy may provide relief for people who have varicose veins.

How to Find the Best Practitioner

If you want to take advantage of the healing potential of hydrotherapy, your physician can refer you to a physical therapist or physiatrist. Many YMCAs and community recreation programs offer hydrotherapy (water exercise) for arthritis patients, pre- and postnatal care, senior fitness, back pain treatment, and more. Bruce E. Becker, M.D., a physiatrist and associate professor at Wayne State University in Detroit, says that he helped his community pool in Eugene, Oregon, sponsor more than 70 different classes at various fitness levels. (A physiatrist is a physician who specializes in helping people recover from injury.)

You also can use hydrotherapy for treatment by working with a naturopathic physician. Naturopaths are licensed only in certain states. (For more details on naturopathy and the physicians who practice this form of medicine, see page 185.)

Tapping into Home Hydrotherapy

Hydrotherapy is as accessible as the nearest faucet, and there are hundreds of ways to use it.

Naturopaths almost never recommend heat treatment without cold, and heat should be applied first, ending with cold. Here are a few basic techniques:

- **Try using hot baths.** These can ease joint pain and respiratory ailments or induce sleep. Herbal baths can relax as well as soothe and heal the skin. Soak for 20 minutes, adding water as needed to maintain the temperature. Dr. Starbuck advises a cold rinse or a rub with a cold washcloth afterward.
- **Use a hot sitz bath (hip bath).** This form of hydrotherapy is useful for treating pelvic pain and infection. Sit in a tub (or basin) in navel-high water with your feet up over the edge of the tub. The idea here is that only the hip and pelvic area is submerged.

  Soaking for five minutes or so in warm water (or for longer periods at higher temperatures) relieves anal and vaginal irritation, hemorrhoids, and anal fissures as well as easing pain of prostatitis, colitis, diverticulitis, menstrual cramps, and lower abdominal pain due to inflammatory bowel disease. Whenever you sit in a hot bath long enough to sweat, cool your face with a washcloth dipped in cold water.
- **Try a cold sitz bath.** Short (no more than two minutes) cold sitz baths (brrrr!) can improve pelvic muscle tone in cases of stress incontinence.

  Avoid cold sitz baths if you have a vaginal discharge or circulatory disorders.
- **Try a little contrast.** Naturopaths recommend contrast sitz baths, using separate basins of hot and cold water, to improve circulation in the pelvic region, speed healing of vaginal and urinary tract infections, reduce pelvic pain, and even treat ovarian cysts. Try a three- to four-minute-soak in hot water, followed by a 30- to 60-second cold soak (or dip a towel in a basin of ice water and use it like a diaper). Repeat three to five times, ending with cold.
- **Get relief for feet.** Foot baths can relieve swelling in the feet and legs. They also can divert blood from other areas, providing relief for head and chest congestion and menstrual cramps. Soak your feet in comfortably hot water for 10 to 30 minutes, adding water as needed to maintain the temperature. Rinse your feet with cold water afterward. Hot foot baths are not recommended for people with arteriosclerosis, Buerger's disease, or diabetes.
- **Use heat and cold for feet.** Contrast (alternating hot and cold) foot baths may relieve ankle swelling, headaches (used along with a cold compress on the head), foot infections, and toothaches among other conditions. Steep your feet and ankles in hot water for three minutes, then plunge your feet into cold water for 20 to 30 seconds. Repeat three times, ending with cold water, then dry your feet.
- **Try steam.** Inhale steam to ease breathing by loosening mucus in the chest. You can use a vaporizer or simply hold your face no closer than a foot away from a pot of steamy water and cover your head and shoulders with a towel to trap the steam. Continue for up to an hour, reheating the water as needed. Dr. Starbuck warns that for some people who are sensitive to heat, a foot may be close enough to burn your skin, so err on the side of caution.
- **Get relief with compresses.** Small hot compresses can relieve pain from muscle

the history of hydrotherapy

The first documented use of water therapy was by Hippocrates, the father of medicine, in the fourth century B.C. And water has formed part of almost every civilization's healing traditions, from the baths of ancient Greece and Rome, Native American sweats, Turkish baths, and Finnish saunas to modern European spas.

In the 19th century, cold-water cures were popularized in Europe by a poor, uneducated farmer named Vincent Preissnitz. Preissnitz cured himself and others using only water. He opened the famous Grafenberg spa, to which people flocked from around the world. The German priest Sebastian Kneipp brought Preissnitz's practices to America around the turn of the 20th century. Others using this therapy at the time included John Harvey Kellogg (of cereal fame) and Dr. Robert Hay Graham (of graham cracker fame).

Dr. Kellogg opened the Battle Creek Sanitarium in Michigan in 1876, eventually absorbing a nearby hydrotherapy center opened by Seventh Day Adventist followers of Dr. Graham. Benedict Lust, founder of the first naturopathic school in America, incorporated Kneipp's water cures in his training. This camp advocated hydrotherapy as a staple of healing along with fasting, vegetarian diet, herbal medicine, and other holistic natural treatments.

Until the advent of antibiotics during World War II, doctors in this country commonly used hydrotherapy to treat anything from local infection or diseases like pneumonia and typhoid to mental illness. But with the increasing power and sophistication of medical technology and organizations, hydrotherapy has largely become the domain of physical therapists, rehabilitation specialists, and alternative health-care practitioners, especially naturopaths.

Today conventional doctors prescribe hydrotherapy mainly as an adjunct to physiotherapy or first aid to heal injuries and relieve pain, while holistic practitioners still use water therapy to treat anything from ear infections to chronic fatigue syndrome. And many modern spas still offer water therapies as an integral part of their holistic health regimes.

spasms and certain types of arthritis. They create soothing warmth in the affected area and speed healing by attracting nutrient- and oxygen-rich blood to the affected site.

Cool compresses can ease the pain of varicose veins after a long day on your feet. If you suffer from diarrhea, a cold compress on the abdomen or lower back for 10 to 15 minutes every hour may slow the runs to a crawl, according to Dr. Rosenfeld. A cool compress on the face or forehead prevents your body from overheating in a sauna or hot bath.

- **Switch back and forth.** Alternating hot and cold compresses stimulates circulation to help heal joint and muscle injuries. They also can relieve migraines. Try three to four minutes of heat followed by 30 to 60 seconds of cold. Repeat three to five times, ending with cold.
- **Use ice appropriately.** Ice packs (ice wrapped in a towel, a frozen gel pack, or even a bag of frozen peas) can minimize swelling from bruises and sprains by narrowing blood vessels to reduce blood flow, swelling, and inflammation. Limit cold applications to 20 minutes at a time to prevent damage to the skin.

An ice pack acts as a mild local anesthetic and can relieve headaches, toothaches, nosebleeds, sprains, bruises, or muscle spasms. Both M.D.s and N.D.s recommend "RICE" as the best first-aid treatment for muscle strains and sprains: Rest, Ice, Compression, Elevation.

Don't use heat on such an injury until after the first 24 to 48 hours. After that, contrast baths or compresses are more effective for bringing nourishment to the injury and driving out toxins, Dr. Lewis explains.

- **Use body heat.** Naturopaths sometimes recommend double compresses—cold compresses covered with a layer of dry cloth. These are usually left in place several hours or overnight until the body's heat warms them in a reflex reaction to the coldness.

Naturopaths use double compresses to treat sore throats, ear infections, chest colds, joint pain, and digestive problems. Here's a remedy they recommend: To treat a cold, wear cotton socks soaked in cold water and wrung out, completely covered with dry wool socks to seal out air. Wear the socks an hour or two or overnight until your body heat warms and dries the inner sock.

Treatments That Won't Soak You

Treatments by natural means generally cost less than conventional drugs and other medical procedures. (In Germany, the government requires physicians and pharmacists to study naturopathic methods and botanical medicine to help control costs.)

The exceptions to this generally low-cost form of treatment might be spa visits or treatments such as saunas and whirlpool baths that require special practitioners or equipment. Dr. Rosenfeld notes that the expense of a hot tub or a trip to a spa might be tax-deductible or reimbursable if your doctor is willing to prescribe the treatment and your insurance carrier is willing to foot the bill. But insurance reimbursement for hydrotherapy for conditions like AIDS or chronic fatigue syndrome is unlikely.

Safety and Warnings

Most water therapies are helpful and not harmful. But there are a few precautions to be aware of.

- **Seek professional advice.** You should discuss hydrotherapy with your doctor before taking the plunge. Anyone with a heart condition or circulation problems could have a bad reaction to really hot water. In fact, there are a few treatments that should be done only in a clinical setting with qualified professional supervision. Long cold baths relieve fever and combat fatigue. Neutral baths (immersion in water slightly cooler than body temperature) are used to treat insomnia, emotional agitation, and menopausal hot flashes. They also reduce excessive fluid retention in people with mild heart conditions and cirrhosis of the liver. While both are used in clinical settings, they are not recommended for home use.
- **Insist on cleanliness.** It is important that any equipment used in hydrotherapy be thoroughly sanitized before you use it. (This is especially important for colonic irrigations and enemas, which technically fall into the realm of hydrotherapy, although not specifically recommended in this book.)
- **Don't share germs.** People who have open wounds should not go into public pools that are used for hydrotherapy. "The water in the tanks and tubs they use should be drained and cleaned each time," says Dr. Becker. "I tell patients to avoid the pool if they have a fever or are acutely ill, have urinary tract infections, or are incontinent."
- **Insist on cleanliness. Watch for reactions.** Dr. Lewis advises newcomers to hydrotherapy to use moderation and educate themselves on the effects of heat and cold. Very young and very old people and those with circulatory problems, such as those that can occur from diabetes, should exercise caution in using extreme temperatures.

"When I prescribe contrast sitz baths to older women with pelvic infections, I tell them to have someone in the room with them," he says. "There's a danger that the lowered blood pressure from sitting in a hot tub then standing to apply the cold towel like a diaper will cause dizziness, and they can slip in the tub."

resources

Books

There are a number of books that offer clear, cogent guidance on hydrotherapy:

Home Remedies: Hydrotherapy, Massage, Charcoal, and Other Simple Treatments by Agatha Thrash, M.D., and Calvin Thrash, M.D. (Thrash Publications, 1981)

The Complete Book of Water Therapy by Dian Dincin Buchman, Ph.D. (E.P. Dutton, 1979)

Alternative Medicine: The Definitive Guide compiled by The Burton Goldberg Group (Future Medicine Publishing, 1997)

chapter 12

light therapy

BRIGHT RAYS OF HEALING

And God said, let there be light: and there was light.... And God saw that it was good.—Genesis 1:1–10

Ever since ancient times, light has been used to heal a whole spectrum of ills. Herodotus, a fifth century, B.C., Greek historian, was responsible for the first documented instances of solar therapy. And light was used to treat depression and lethargy thousands of years ago in ancient Egypt.

Today, light therapy—controlled exposure to bright light—continues to play a role in conventional medical practice as well as its alternative cousins. Its most typical applications operate by absorption through the skin: Doctors expose newborns to blue light to cure jaundice. And dermatologists frequently prescribe sunlight or ultraviolet light to heal psoriasis and certain kinds of dermatitis.

Lasers offer a form of light therapy on the cutting edge of medicine, so to speak. Their highly concentrated light beams are now used to perform surgical procedures and dentistry without damaging surrounding tissues and so are less invasive than the most finely honed scalpel.

But the core of phototherapy, as light therapy is also called, capitalizes on light's effects on the central nervous system, especially the body's clock. This form of light therapy, which focuses mainly on circadian (daily) and seasonal biorhythms, is under active investigation by researchers around the world. Mainly used to treat seasonal affective disorder (SAD), it may one day become part of standard treatment for nonseasonal depression, insomnia, jet lag, problems adjusting to working different shifts, premenstrual syndrome (PMS), menstrual irregularity, and other conditions.

Most of this newer form of light therapy involves short periods of exposure to an intense form of artificial light that simulates daylight. Its effectiveness results more from the light absorbed through the eyes than through the skin. The artificial lights used to regulate body rhythms need to be intense, because typical indoor lighting is far too weak to affect the hormones involved.

For treatment purposes, exposure may be only to part of the light spectrum, depending on its purpose. Most light therapy is administered by means of fluorescent light fixtures specially mounted in a light box. But newer devices have also been developed for improved portability and convenience. One is a visor that sheds light on the face and eyes. Another is a lamp timed to switch on before dawn and brighten gradually, like the rising sun.

Treating SAD

Until the invention of electric lighting, human beings tended to spend most of the day outdoors. Only in the last century or so have we spent significant time under artificial light, which is far dimmer than sunlight. So even when we work all day in light that's bright enough to see by, we may be operating in biological darkness as far as our nervous system is concerned. Some researchers believe that this historic change in light exposure may have resulted in throwing some of our biological functions off kilter because these functions evolved in response to natural light cycles.

Treating seasonal affective disorder (SAD) is currently the leading application of light therapy. This form of treatment really straddles the boundary between alternative and mainstream medicines. SAD, also known as winter depression, occurs during the fall and winter months and lifts in the spring and summer. Its key symptoms are lethargy and fatigue, which lead to oversleeping and intense carbohydrate cravings, which promote overeating and weight gain. This picture differs from the typical forms of depression, characterized by insomnia, loss of appetite, and weight loss.

An estimated 6 percent of Americans—that's 10 million people—are thought to have SAD. Another 14 percent may have a milder form of winter blues. Women who have SAD, especially those in their reproductive years, outnumber men who have it by about 4 to 1.

No one knows exactly why some people are vulnerable to SAD or how light therapy works. But researchers believe that vulnerability to SAD may be at least partly genetic. They speculate that light may relieve seasonal depression by resetting our body's clock, which times many of our key biological functions.

Why Light Matters

Theories abound on how and why light therapy corrects SAD and other circadian disorders. Norman E. Rosenthal, M.D., senior researcher at the National Institute of Mental Health (NIMH) and clinical professor of psychiatry at Georgetown University, lists more than half a dozen in his book *Winter Blues*, but none has been definitively established.

According to Dr. Rosenthal, we know that light travels from the retina along the optic nerve to a group of cells in the part of the brain known as the hypothalamus. This group of cells is thought to act as our body's clock. The hypothalamus regulates sleeping, eating, temperature, sex drive, and mood—the very functions disturbed in people who are depressed. The hypothalamus also helps regulate the release of hormones, including melatonin—the hormone secreted by the pineal gland, a tiny pinecone-shaped gland at the center of the brain—as well as the brain's chemical messengers, such as serotonin and dopamine.

When we're not exposed to enough bright light each day, our circadian rhythms can lose their beat. This reaction is fairly common in northern latitudes between late fall and early spring, when the days are short and nights are long.

But our body's clock can also lose time by inappropriate use of melatonin supplements, traveling across several time zones, or by working odd hours. Such desynchronization may bring on symptoms of depression, PMS, problems working different shifts, jet lag, and sleeping and eating disorders.

Any disorder affected by our body's clock, including those caused by changing seasons, may be correctable by light therapy. And even nonseasonal disorders with symptoms that overlap the seasonal disorders, such as nonseasonal depression and PMS, may be helped.

No One Knows Why SAD Happens

You don't really need to know all the complicated theories behind SAD in order to benefit from light therapy. So you can skip this next section if you find the science daunting. It is interesting, however, to occasionally step back and look at the volume of intellectual work and theory that underlies doctors' understanding of new treatment options. Exactly what is SAD and why would it respond to something like light therapy?

Originally, researchers speculated that SAD was caused by an abnormality related to melatonin. Light suppresses secretion of this hormone. One theory, based on findings that light governs lower animals' circadian rhythms, states that turning off melatonin would cure SAD. The evidence for this theory remains clouded by contradictory findings, however.

A second hypothesis says that light corrects the timing of our circadian rhythms, shifting them ahead or behind their usual pattern. Morning light exposure makes us feel like waking up earlier and falling asleep earlier. Evening light exposure turns us into night owls, making us want to stay awake longer and wake up later. But until recently, studies have found mixed results on this score.

A third theory focuses on the eye's sensitivity to light. Some researchers have found subtle abnormalities in the electrical patterns generated by the eyes of people with SAD. They speculate that people who have this disorder may be less sensitive than normal to light perception. But scientists at NIMH have found no substantive differences between the eyes of people with SAD and those of people without seasonal disorders.

Yet another hypothesis states that people with SAD may have physiologically abnormal stress responses. People with this disorder don't feel depressed if left alone to rest. It's when they're stressed that they feel depressed. In one study at NIMH, Dr. Rosenthal and his colleagues found that people with SAD, when under stress, responded by releasing abnormally low

light therapy helps heal

- Psoriasis
- Seasonal affective disorder (SAD)

Promising experimental applications:

Bulimia
People with SAD often gain weight in winter, and light therapy curbs the appetite for sweets and starches. There is some evidence that light therapy may be useful in treating bulimia, an eating disorder that involves bingeing and purging. Bulimia occurs mainly in winter.

Insomnia
Certain sleep disturbances improve with light exposure. Morning light is useful for night owls who can't wake up early. Evening light works best for those who fall asleep early and wake up too early.

Jet lag
Light therapy is best used for relieving jet lag after short trips that involve crossing one to five time zones.

Lupus
Preliminary studies at Louisiana State University Medical School have found promising relief of symptoms for those exposed to certain light rays (UVA-1 rays). This treatment is currently under U.S. Food and Drug Administration review for clinical application.

Mental illness
Psychiatric conditions such as obsessive-compulsive, panic, and eating disorders tend to worsen during winter, so light therapy is being used experimentally to treat them.

Nonseasonal depression
Research shows that light is as valuable for treating nonseasonal depression as for seasonal depression, but it has not been as widely used in the United States as abroad. Light therapy may be useful in enhancing the effects of antidepressant drugs while reducing their dosages and side effects.

Premenstrual syndrome (PMS) and infertility due to menstrual irregularity
Preliminary studies show that light has some influence on menstrual regularity and in improving symptoms of PMS. A few studies even show promise in using light to regulate fertility, but such treatment is still experimental.

Preventing heart disease, breast and colon cancers, and bone thinning
Exposing the skin to ultraviolet rays helps the body synthesize vitamin D, promoting absorption of calcium. Research backs the disease-preventive effects of such light exposure.

levels of hormones from the adrenal glands when they were injected with a hormone that normally stimulates its release. Light therapy restored this response to a more normal level. But this is only a partial explanation of how light therapy may work, according to Dr. Rosenthal.

One theory that Dr. Rosenthal favors focuses on serotonin—a chemical that transmits signals in the parts of the brain responsible for governing circadian rhythms and secreting certain stress hormones. Abnormalities in the brain's use of serotonin may explain the hormonal response to stress and circadian abnormalities in people who have SAD.

There is plenty of evidence to support this particular theory. Serotonin levels in the hypothalamus reach their low point during winter. Dietary carbohydrates increase production of serotonin, and people with SAD feel energized by eating sweets and starches. And drugs that keep the body's serotonin levels high, such as Prozac, reverse SAD symptoms.

Dr. Rosenthal suggests that light therapy may reduce the dosage and side effects of drug therapy for both seasonal and nonseasonal varieties of depression. The combination is better than either treatment alone. Comparisons of Prozac to light therapy in treating people with SAD found them equally effective.

One study, reported in *Science*, further complicates this already complex picture. Researchers at Cornell University found that light exposure to the skin behind the knee may reset the body's clock. As study participants lounged on a reclining chair, light from a quartz lamp was transmitted to the back of each of their knees for three hours. The rise and fall of their body temperatures and melatonin levels in their saliva were measured hourly. These measures clearly responded to the stimulus.

Remember, the study participants were not able to see the light. How can it be that their body chemistry responded to it? The researchers speculated that light might alter blood gases that act as nervous system signals, much the way blue light shined on the skin changes bilirubin, the toxic substance that causes jaundice.

Dr. Rosenthal cautions that these findings have not yet been replicated in another study. But he also cites NIMH studies that suggest that UV rays in sunlight acting on the skin promote the body's production of helpful substances—beta-endorphin and vitamin D. Either or both of these substances may make our mood sunnier.

Still other research suggests that light hitting the blood vessels in the eye may activate a substance in the blood (hemoglobin) that might combine with certain other chemicals the blood carries to the hypothalamus, where they can affect our body's clock.

Obviously, this is a complicated picture. Further study is needed to sort out the biological roots of SAD and the specific effects of light on them. But even though light therapy has been clearly established as effective, and SAD has been accepted by the American Psychiatric Association's diagnostic manual since 1987, some insurance companies still treat light therapy for SAD as experimental and fail to reimburse patients for its costs.

More Light on Phototherapy

Scientific studies show that at least three-quarters of people who have SAD improve when they are treated with light. But until quite recently, researchers have been unable to rule out the placebo effect as the reason why light therapy works.

A placebo is a treatment with no inherent therapeutic value. Sometimes, however, placebos do have some healing effect because of the belief and expectations of the people receiving them.

This positive response to a placebo is known as "the placebo effect." Why would researchers have a hard time ruling out the placebo effect when they're studying light therapy?

For one thing, much of the research has been conducted on small numbers of people, so individual differences between them could skew the results. Some studies failed to include a similar group not receiving the therapy (a control group), which would offer a baseline against which to measure the experimental results. And many studies have tested the same subjects under two different conditions (say, bright versus dim light exposure), so the order in which they were exposed to the light could have clouded the results.

Also, most experiments using light therapy have compared bright light to dim light. Since the people in the experiment naturally expect the bright light to work better, it's hard to rule out those expectations as a factor in the results. Another problem plaguing these studies is that light in the environment is hard to control. As one researcher put it, "It's like studying Prozac with Prozac occasionally in the drinking water."

But three studies reported in 1998 affirm the value of light therapy and help refine science's ideas of how it works. Two of the new studies used a negative ion generator as a placebo device.

People in the study were told that negative ions are thought to improve mood. The third experiment used people with no symptoms of SAD as controls. Taken together, the three studies included 341 people—the largest yet to compare morning versus evening light exposure.

All three studies found that morning light was superior to evening sessions, and either one was more effective than the placebo treatment.

In the largest study, 54 percent of the people in the study who were treated with morning light for two weeks experienced significant relief, compared with 33 percent of those who used evening light.

The two other studies found similar results, although in one study it took three weeks of treatment before benefits were evident.

The Best Ways to Brighten Your Days

If you suspect that you have SAD, it's a good idea to get an evaluation for depression, suggests Dr. Rosenthal. A qualified physician or therapist should take a careful medical history and do a physical examination to confirm your diagnosis. Your

how to find the best practitioner

If you're uncertain about whether your depression falls into the category of seasonal affective disorder or clinical depression, you might want to check with a psychiatrist who specializes in light therapy.

To find one, contact your nearest university's department of psychiatry for a referral to a qualified practitioner, suggests Norman E. Rosenthal, M.D., author of *Winter Blues*. Light box manufacturers (listed on page 154) may be able to supply you with a list of practitioners in your area. You can also consult Light Therapy Products on the Web—www.lightherapyproducts.com—or call at 800/486-6723.

evaluation will serve as a baseline so your doctor can monitor your progress and decide how well your treatment is working.

It will also help rule out other possible diagnoses with similar symptoms, such as a sluggish thyroid, low blood sugar, chronic fatigue syndrome, or fibromyalgia. If the light therapy fails to work, the therapist can recommend or prescribe alternative or supplementary treatments.

Many researchers recommend taking an eye exam before starting light therapy to determine whether you have any retinal problems.

While this is not mandatory and many people have been treated without an eye exam, it is a simple and relatively inexpensive precaution.

What can you expect when you start light therapy? Dr. Rosenthal says that your first sensations may be physical: a sense of lightening of the body, calmness, or increased energy. Some people even experience butterflies in the stomach or pins and needles in the hands. Many people report that they feel more alert and energized and have an easier time waking up in the morning.

More than 75 percent of people with SAD benefit from light therapy, but that doesn't mean that all your winter difficulties will disappear. Ideally, your SAD symptoms should disappear one by one. You should feel more energetic, experience fewer cravings for sweets and starches, and be able to think more clearly. In short, you should feel less like a hibernating bear and more like a human again.

what to do about side effects

Side effects from light therapy are few. Those that do develop can almost always be handled by shortening the time you spend under the light, rescheduling your treatment time to an earlier or later slot, or sitting a bit farther from the light source.

- **If you get headaches or eyestrain:** Restart treatment with shorter exposures and build up gradually over a week or two. Sit slightly farther from the light source until symptoms subside.
- **If you feel irritable or hyperactive:** Decrease your exposure in terms of either brightness or time. This may happen to people who often feel hyped up in summer.
- **If you feel tired or can't sleep:** Shift your treatment to an earlier time. Fatigue may occur after several days of therapy, especially if your sleep time has changed to accommodate treatment. This problem is usually temporary.
- **If your eyes, nose, and sinuses feel dry:** The heat generated by the light box can dry out the surrounding air, parching your eyes and nasal passages. This can be especially hazardous for contact lens wearers, since dryness can abrade your corneas. Use artificial tears (available at your local pharmacy) and place a humidifier near the light box. Try drinking hot beverages.
- **If your skin burns:** Apply sunblock before your treatments.

The Nuts and Volts Of Treatment

If your symptoms are mild and a qualified professional is not readily available, Dr. Rosenthal endorses a two-week trial period for self-help. "If you see absolutely no effects after two weeks of giving light therapy a good shot, get to a doctor," he advises. It is possible that you are not dealing with depression or SAD.

Those who benefit most from light therapy are people whose mood brightens with greater light exposure under natural circumstances, such as traveling toward the equator and working or living in bright rooms. The symptoms that respond best to light therapy are oversleeping and late-day sweets cravings, according to Dr. Rosenthal. Those who lose sleep, eat less, and lose weight during winter depressions do least well with light therapy, though it's still worth trying, because these predictions are not exact.

Some people experience improved mood and energy after a single session, though this is unusual. For most, it takes two to four days to experience a sustained sense of well-being. Research shows it may take several weeks for some people to register the full effects.

If your doctor or therapist has not prescribed a specific regimen for you, your best bet is to experiment. You can try a single light exposure session in the morning, use an extra dose during the afternoon or evening to prevent a slump in energy then or break up the sessions into morning and evening. For treatment to remain effective, you must keep it up as long as light is scarce in your environment. Many people find that if they skip more than one day, their symptoms creep back.

Even high-intensity light boxes give out no more light than you would receive from the sky just after sunrise. Many studies and treatment regimens are based on exposure to 10,000 lux (a measure of light intensity), equal to 20 times ordinary indoor lighting but far dimmer than outdoor sunlight. That's the amount of light that would reach your eyes outdoors under clear skies just after sunrise but far less than that on a sunny day at the beach. Some boxes and visors have a three-way switch that allows the user to turn it on by degrees at the beginning and end of a session.

"The amount of exposure you'll need varies by individual, latitude, equipment, and time of year," says Dr. Rosenthal. A typical person with SAD using the 10,000-lux fixture in the northern United States might start treatment in mid-September with 15 minutes in the morning. In October and November that person would increase exposure to 30 minutes, divided into two 15-minute sessions, one in the morning and one in the afternoon.

Those who begin treatment in midwinter do best starting with about 45 to 60 minutes of light a day, divided between morning and evening. After about a week, you can judge whether this seems like too little or too much. The minimum effective dose may be as low as 20 minutes a day.

The light box should be placed at eye level on a flat surface, such as a desk or table. If you use a slanted fixture, your eyes will be exposed to enough light if you look down at the desktop rather than into the light. Many people use the time for reading, crafts, chores, or watching TV. The most important consideration: Create a schedule that works for you, otherwise you won't stay with it, and you won't benefit. Dr. Rosenthal gives more detailed recommendations for light therapy in his book *Winter Blues*.

Light Therapy Basics

One light therapy basic to be aware of is that not everyone needs equipment to benefit. Remember, the sun is the best possible source of light. If you can't move farther south during the winter, here are some practical measures to try, including some tips on equipment.

- **Take morning walks.** Mild cases of SAD may improve with daily walks outdoors, even on partly cloudy days. Gazing up at the sky may deliver several thousand lux of light to the eyes. (Never stare directly at the sun, even during winter.)
- **Brighten your surroundings.** Trim bushes around your windows and keep the curtains

open. If you work in an office, try to sit near a window. Maximize daylight by getting up early.

- **Take a winter vacation in a sunny resort.** If you can, getting away for even a week to 10 days will give you an extra boost of light during the gloomy time of year.
- **Exercise outdoors.** Walking or skiing are two great ways to get lots of sun. If you exercise indoors, try to work out near a window.
- **Rent a light box.** Some light-box companies have rental programs for home-use equipment. These programs rebate part of the cost of the box if you find the therapy doesn't help. Or the weekly rental fee may offset the purchase price if you decide to buy. You should have some sense of whether you will benefit within the first few weeks, if you use the lights diligently.
- **Choose light sources carefully.** Overly concentrated light, such as from halogen lamps, can cause headache, eyestrain, or other side effects. Don't rely on tanning lamps or plant lights for your light ration. They emit UV rays that can cause serious eye damage.
- **Check your equipment and yourself.** If no benefits become apparent within the first four days, ask yourself the following:

- Are you using the right kind of fixture?
- Is it placed at eye level?
- Are you seated at the proper distance from it?
- Are your daily sessions long enough?

Try shifting treatments to a different time of day. If it's still not helping, consult a professional.

If the treatments become less effective:

- Is it due to changes in your life circumstances?
- Is there less environmental light?
- Is your treatment inconsistent?
- Do you have more stress?

You may need to increase light or add a supplemental treatment.

Dr. Rosenthal urges that you seek professional care if:

- You experience marked depression.
- You develop problems at work.
- You need a lot more sleep in winter.
- You lose control over food and weight in winter.

Safety and Warnings

Think of light as a drug with few side effects. Light therapy for seasonal disorders has only been around since the early 80s, so it's hard to assess long-term side effects. Actually, so far there have been no reports of adverse long-term side effects.

A survey of more than 50 people from early NIMH studies found that none reported any eye problems. In a Canadian study eye exams were performed on 71 patients treated annually with light therapy for five years and no evidence of retinal damage was found in anyone. Still, here are some reasonable measures you should consider in beginning light therapy:

- **Reduce UV rays.** Be sure any fixture you purchase contains UV-reducing features. Researchers have found no evidence that full-spectrum light is any better than ordinary white fluorescent light. In fact, UV rays are neither necessary nor beneficial in treating SAD. Their potentially harmful

light therapy for the skin

There are times when light therapy is so mainstream that it can't even be thought of as "alternative." Sometimes it's just plain old good medicine.

"Phototherapy is standard medical treatment for psoriasis, especially when it's severe," says Steven R. Feldman, M.D., Ph.D., associate professor of dermatology at Wake Forest University in Winston-Salem, North Carolina. It is also used for a wide variety of inflammatory conditions and a few rare conditions like skin lymphoma and certain kinds of acne.

"UVB phototherapy has been around for 50 years, maybe even millennia. We know it works, though not why," adds Dr. Feldman, who is also director of the Westwood-Squibb Center for Dermatology Research.

- **Preparation is important.** Phototherapy is typically administered by a dermatologist, says Dr. Feldman. The patient undresses and slathers mineral oil on the itchy, scaly skin that characterizes this condition. The patient then stands in a 6-foot-tall light box surrounded by 32 fluorescent tubes that emit a form of ultraviolet rays known as UVB. The first session may last 10 to 15 seconds.
- **Progress is slow.** Over a period of weeks, the patient works up to a couple of minutes. People with psoriasis may have three to five sessions a week for 15 to 25 treatments. Light treatments can put psoriasis into remission for about six months or so.
- **Medications might be used.** There are a number of variations on light therapy for skin disorders. One is PUVA, which combines a drug called psoralen with exposure to another form of ultraviolet light, called UVA. The psoralen makes the skin (and all body tissues, including the eyes) more sensitive to light, enhancing the light's effects.
- **Home treatment is possible.** People on UVB treatment can rent or buy a home unit, a single 6-foot-tall light panel. A unit costs about $1,500.
- **Precautions are important.** Phototherapy is not recommended for people with HIV. Those who have diseases that might get worse with exposure to light—such as lupus—or those who are sensitive to light because they take certain medications are not good candidates for this form of light therapy.

Light therapy for skin disorders is considered safe, if done with proper medical supervision, despite a small risk of skin cancer with prolonged light exposure. In fact, a study by Dr. Feldman and colleagues at the Bowman Gray School of Medicine at Wake Forest University in Winston-Salem, North Carolina, found that even visits to a tanning salon could be helpful for people who can't easily get to a doctor's office.

resources

Equipment

The best-tested alternative for light therapy is a 10,000-lux light box. Light boxes come in various designs adaptable to home or office use. You can exercise on a stationary bike or a ski machine in front of an upright box attached to the wall or mounted on a stand. It also takes up less table space. Some boxes can be used tilted or upright. The light visor uses lower-intensity light and is less well tested, but many people swear by them for their portability and convenience. A dawn simulator acts as a bedside lamp that gradually brightens like a summer sunrise to help you wake up energized and on time.

Alaska Northern Lights makes light boxes that sell for about $250.
800/880-6953
www.akms.com/nlights

American Environmental Products in Fort Collins, Colorado, sells light boxes, costing $300 to $500.
970/493-6914
www.sunalite.com

Bio-Brite, Inc., in Bethesda, Maryland, makes a state-of-the-art light visor.
301/961-8557

The SunBox Company in Gaithersburg, Maryland, creates an information packet on SAD that can be obtained by calling 888-SAD-AWAY (723-2929). Their light boxes start at $250. A light visor retails for about $370. A dawn simulator retails for $150 and up. A sunrise-simulating alarm clock goes for about $100.
800/LITE YOU (548-3968)
Email: sunbox@aol.com
www.sunbox.com

Books

Winter Blues: Seasonal Affective Disorder; What It Is and How to Overcome It by Norman E. Rosenthal, M.D. (The Guilford Press, 1998)

effects to skin and eyes are, in fact, a disadvantage.

- **Consider your overall health.** Bright light may activate certain conditions, such as AIDS and lupus. People who have these conditions are poor candidates for this form of light therapy.
- **Protect your eyes.** People with diseases of the retina, such as macular degeneration or retinitis pigmentosa, and those on certain medications that sensitize the retina to light share a high risk of eye damage. If you fall into this category, consult an ophthalmologist for regular monitoring.

chapter 13

magnet therapy

POLARIZED TREATMENT

Just because we don't understand how something works doesn't mean that it can't work. —*James D. Livingston, Ph.D., professor of engineering at the Massachusetts Institute of Technology*

Senior golf whiz Jim Colbert, a self-proclaimed "cripple" in 1994, went on to be voted Player of the Year in 1996 with the aid of magnets strapped to his ailing back. And now an estimated 70 percent of senior golf pros have joined him in using magnets to help improve their games.

The Miami Dolphins football team has gone so far as to put magnetized seat pads on the team bench during games in hopes that players might revive more quickly and thoroughly between plays.

Obviously, magnets are not just for holding finger paintings to refrigerators anymore. Magnets are now being used to treat arthritis, foot pain, back problems, and headaches, not to mention all the other ailments that aging athletes mention in their enthusiastic endorsements for these products.

The recent attraction to electromagnetic energy for health and healing is nothing new. The Romans felt there was a healing power in the electrical charge produced by eels, which they applied to people suffering from arthritis and gout. Egypt's legendary beauty Cleopatra reportedly wore a magnetized lodestone on her forehead in hopes of preserving her good looks and youth.

Centuries of experimentation followed by such luminaries as Germany's infamous hypnotist Franz Mesmer, our own Ben Franklin, and Louis Pasteur of France. Their investigations, as we've found today, produced positive as well as negative results. For a period in the late 1800s, before drugs came along to steal their thunder, magnets had become quite a rage, finding their way into hats, belts, girdles, and (when ground up) even liniments and salves.

Today, the alleged healing power of magnets continues to attract enthusiastic users. An estimated 2 million Americans now use magnets for medical purposes, and sales of magnetic products (everything from headbands to foot pads and even mugs for magnetizing what we drink) is now a global industry pulling in an estimated $2 billion dollars every year.

Opinions Are Polarized

All of which raises the inevitable question: How well—if at all—do magnets actually work?

It's a difficult question to answer, most doctors and scientists agree, because some studies have shown results that are impressive, but others have shown no results at all. Part of the problem with magnetic therapy, its critics say, is that the kind of magnets used for therapy are capable of exerting a measurable force only millimeters away from their surface. Move a magnet more than a centimeter (about 3/8 of an inch) away from an area being treated, and there's no measurable magnetic field at all. Products such as mattress pads or car seats in which magnets have been embedded, therefore, might be thought of as little more than comfortable placebos, critics say. (A placebo is a therapy or treatment that has no therapeutic value beyond that which comes from the patient's belief in its healing abilities.)

Complicating the picture further is the uncertainty surrounding how magnets may work. Some experts feel magnets may reduce pain and speed healing by increasing blood flow, which draws more oxygen and other healing nutrients to a painful or injured area.

Other investigators feel nerves may be affected in ways that simply make them less capable of transmitting pain impulses to the brain, while yet another theory proposes that magnets may beneficially reduce the acidity of bodily fluids.

One doctor from Japan has gone so far as to maintain that magnets simply help combat a condition he's labeled "Magnetic Field Deficiency Syndrome"—a problem that plagues everyone, he says, given that the earth's magnetic field is said to have decreased by as much as 30 percent over the past 1,000 years.

So What's a Potential User To Do?

"Many doctors seem to be convinced that magnets can relieve pain, so if more conventional approaches haven't solved the problem, magnets might be worth a try," says James D. Livingston, Ph.D., author of *Driving Force: The Natural Magic of Magnets* and a professor of engineering at the Massachusetts Institute of Technology in Cambridge. Based on his training as well as 30 years of research for General Electric, Dr. Livingston has his well-educated doubts about the medical benefits of stationary magnets, but he encourages the public, just as he's trying to do, to keep an open mind.

"Personally, I feel the force emitted by the types of magnets being sold simply can't produce the kinds of changes being claimed," he says. "And yet, results produced by magnetic therapy, or by any medical treatment for that matter, should not depend on our ability to understand the biological mechanisms. What counts most are the therapy's effects, whether due to its own inherent value or simply a placebo effect we bring to the therapy on our own."

Paul J. Rosch, M.D., a clinical professor of medicine and psychiatry at the New York Medical College and the president of the American Institute of Stress takes a similar view. "Physicians and patients alike need to keep both eyes wide open when it comes to evaluating these treatments," he says. "Some promotional efforts take advantage of a general lack of knowledge about what magnets can and can't do, and regulatory authorities do not have the manpower to enforce rules that prohibit companies from claiming medical benefits. The future of permanent magnets looks very bright, and it would be unfortunate if it were tarnished by irresponsible claims."

Research Both Positive And Negative

When Dr. Rosch says "bright," he's expressing not just his personal opinion but rather one based on some pretty encouraging evidence derived from scientific research. Back in 1991, as an example, Robert R. Holcomb, M.D., Ph.D., of the Vanderbilt Medical Center in Nashville, Tennessee, found that magnets significantly reduced levels of discomfort in people suffering from pain in their lower back and in their knees.

More recently, magnets performed impressively in a 1997 study directed by Carlos Vallbona, M.D., of the Baylor College of Medicine in Houston. The study examined the effects of magnets on 50 people who had a condition known as postpolio syndrome, which is characterized by painful muscle spasms and stiff joints. Magnets of either 300 or 500 gauss (a measurement of a magnet's strength) were applied to painful areas or certain key trigger points thought to mediate pain. Within just 45 minutes, more than three-quarters of those tested reported reductions in pain averaging more than 50 percent. By comparison, only 19 percent of a control group treated with placebo magnets reported pain reduction averaging only about 15 percent.

More good news for magnets came in 1998 when cosmetic surgeon Daniel Man, M.D., of Boca Raton, Florida, reported at a meeting of his peers that magnetic devices had helped patients recover faster and with less discomfort from face-lifts and other cosmetic procedures. This came on the heels of another positive study reported in 1998 by Michael Weintraub, M.D. Dr. Weintraub found that people with diabetes who wore magnetic foot pads for four months experienced significant relief from a condition known as diabetic neuropathy, which is characterized by pain or numbness in the feet.

Two other studies done in 1998 also produced decidedly positive results. One found that a magnetic device was effective in helping men suffering from excessive snoring or sleep apnea, and the other demonstrated positive effects on wound healing. In the latter study, done at the Toledo Hospital in Ohio, a magnet brought about complete healing in just one month of a wound on the abdomen of a 51-year-old woman who previously had not healed in an entire year.

But then there's the flip side. As proof that magnetic therapy certainly is not fool-proof, a 1997 study reported in the *Journal of the American Medical Association* by researchers from the New York College of Podiatric Medicine found that magnetic foot pads used to treat people with painful heel spurs had been of no use at all. Another study done in 1982 of magnetic jewelry advertised to ease neck and shoulder pain showed it to be as useless as it was unattractive, Dr. Livingston reports.

Why such conflicting results? "Whether the effect is placebo or not," says Dr. Livingston, "for some people and some conditions magnets may simply work better than others."

Just Ahead of Its Time?

Dr. Livingston's words touch on an important point that applies not just to magnetic therapy, but to many alternative therapies still in the process of being understood from a strictly scientific standpoint.

"Just because we don't understand how something works doesn't mean that it *can't* work," says Dr. Livingston. "Not until recently was it understood how aspirin works, and look at all the good that it has done."

Two other experts in agreement with Dr. Livingston's thinking are Dr. Rosch and Ron Lawrence, M.D., Ph.D., the president of the North American Academy of Magnetic Therapy. They feel that magnetic therapy is simply in a stage of acceptance similar to where acupuncture was 30 years ago.

"Magnetic therapy suffers from the same lack of early standardization, scientific credibility and regulation," they maintain in their book *Magnet Therapy: The Pain Cure Alternative.* These doctors insist it works, however, and go on to give an impressive array of evidence to that effect. In addition to muscular aches and pains and the discomforts of arthritis, they report that magnets have been useful in treating back and spinal disc problems, asthma and allergies, hard-to-heal wounds, fibromyalgia, carpal tunnel syndrome, diabetic neuropathy, fatigue, depression, insomnia, and anxiety due to stress.

As encouraging as some of the new research on magnets has been, however, Dr. Livingston cautions people not to be overly optimistic, especially if their enthusiasm is based on anecdotal evidence such as the claims made by celebrities and athletes past their primes. Not only are these people usually being paid for their opinions, he points out, but the magnetic devices they tout may owe their effects to factors other than a magnetic one.

The magnetic back braces used by many senior golfers, for example, may reduce pain simply by giving support or by producing localized warmth to an injured or painful area. Then, too, the device by virtue of its very presence may simply act as a reminder to the aging athlete that he or she should not be making certain pain-producing movements in the first place, Dr. Livingston says. Regardless of the current, somewhat foggy status of magnetic therapy, however, trust that the picture should be coming into better focus shortly.

Dr. Holcomb currently has 12 studies in progress. And Dr. Man is conducting additional studies regarding the possible role of magnets in speeding recovery from cosmetic surgery.

Using Magnet Therapy

As if the research on magnets weren't confusing enough, there are the additional questions about the type of magnet to be used. There are unipolar and multipolar magnets. Then there's the question of products sold in magazines versus products sold at health food stores or, worse yet, by network sales people door to door. Short of getting a Ph.D. in electrical engineering—and an internship with the Better Business Bureau—what's a consumer to do?

Let's answer the type question first. Unipolar products have their magnets arranged so that all their south-seeking poles face toward the body while their north-seeking poles face away.

In a multipolar (also sometimes called bipolar) product, however, magnets are arranged so that their north and south poles face the body in an alternating pattern. Is one type superior to another, as manufacturers of *both* types claim?

Dr. Livingston says that while the effects of both types have yet to be definitively shown, the multipolar products would be less likely to be effective because of their reduced depth of penetration.

"The field from even unipolar magnets decreases very rapidly with increasing distance from the magnet, but the field from multipolar magnets decreases even faster," he says. "If a multipolar magnet were to have any measurable effect on the body, it would be limited to a depth of only a few millimeters, or less than about an eighth of an inch."

It's wise, therefore, to apply any magnetic product so that it remains as close to the surface of the skin as possible.

Brand? All things considered, it probably doesn't make much difference, Dr. Vallbona says, based on what he's learned from his experiments.

During his research, he has employed as many as four different brands with no significantly different effects. Because no two people are identical in their body chemistries, however, many experts recommend that if one brand doesn't work, you might consider trying another.

As for the question of strength, stronger is not necessarily better, experts also agree. Any product with a rating of at least 400 gauss, if it's worn consistently, should do the trick, if it's going to work at all. And don't expect immediate results, especially if your condition is a chronic one. Although some ailments may respond almost immediately, others can take several weeks.

Safety and Warnings

So could magnet therapy be for you? Baylor College of Medicine's Dr. Vallbona offers some advice: "Go to your doctor first and identify the problem behind your pain. Then discuss magnet therapy and ask whether he or she thinks it's worth a try."

It's worth noting that while the U.S. Food and Drug Administration (FDA) has issued no warnings to makers of magnetic devices sold for health purposes, the agency has not approved any of these products as effective either. The FDA has, however, had cause to take legal action against certain manufacturers for making unproven claims.

That brings up one important warning: "I would hate to see these products being used when other more conventional treatment would be needed," says Dr. Livingston.

Buying Magnets

Here are some things to keep in mind if you decide to give magnet therapy a try:

- **Expect to pay a high price.** Small magnets for local application usually sell for about $25; mattress pads can cost as much as several hundred dollars.
- **Leave yourself an out.** If the product is of the more expensive variety, make sure it comes with a 30-day, money-back guarantee.
- **Get all the facts.** Ask for scientific evidence of the product's effectiveness if you're dealing with a salesperson. And be skeptical if it isn't forthcoming.
- **Don't be taken in by the "expertise" of a salesperson visiting your home.** Take your time in making a decision and don't let yourself be pressured.
- **Give it time.** Use the device as often as possible, but do discontinue if any adverse reactions, such as an increase in pain, occurs.
- **Don't expect instant results.** Often a week or so is required, especially if the condition being treated is chronic.

resources

Books

Magnet Therapy: The Pain Cure Alternative by Ron Lawrence, M.D., Ph.D., and Paul J. Rosch, M.D. (Prima Health, 1998)

To request information beyond what's in this book you can contact either author by e-mail:
Dr. Rosch: stress124@pol.net
Dr. Lawrence: neurodoc@pol.net

Driving Force: The Natural Magic of Magnets by James D. Livingston, Ph.D. (Harvard, 1996)

Magnet Therapy: Balancing Your Body's Energy Flow for Self-Healing by Holger Hannemann (Sterling Publications, 1990)

Organizations

North American Academy of Magnetic Therapy 800/457-1853

chapter 14

mind/body medicine

MENTAL MAGIC

After Louis Pasteur demonstrated that specific bacteria could cause specific diseases, doctors increasingly disregarded the importance of beliefs and mind/body interactions.—*Herbert Benson, M.D.*

Anyone who's ever cried at the movies, stirred at the sound of a loved one's voice, or salivated at the mere mention of "chocolate chip" needs no introduction to the relationship between mind and body.

We all know that the thoughts we think and the emotions we feel can make our bodies do lots of unexpected things. But it might seem like a pretty big leap to go from cookies and three-hankie movies to the idea that the mind can prevent a heart attack or rid the body of cancer. Or that praying to or simply believing in a higher power—whether it's God or the Buddha or Mother Nature—can make you live longer.

Indeed, one of the most hotly debated classes of alternative medicine is the group of therapies lumped under the heading of mind/body medicine: methods such as imagery, meditation, and spirituality that involve no pills or potions, no massage or needles or physical contact of any sort. Perhaps the most natural of all the natural therapies, mind/body medicine looks to the patient—or more specifically, the patient's mind or spirit—to do all the healing.

The Major Impact Of Mind

"Mind/body medicine is based on the idea that a person's mind—their emotions and experiences, their psychology, their habits of thinking—

affect their body, for good or for bad," says Harold G. Koenig, M.D., author of *The Healing Power of Faith* and associate professor of psychiatry and behavioral sciences and director of the Center for the Study of Religion/Spirituality and Health at Duke University Medical Center in Durham, North Carolina.

mind/body medicine helps heal

Conditions that respond to mind/body therapies run the gamut of stress-induced problems. They include:

- Anxiety
- Depression
- Heart disease
- High blood pressure
- Immune disorders
- Menstrual irregularities (including PMS)

These therapies can change negative thinking patterns, which create stress and can lead to unhealthy habits and bad decisions—drinking too much, acting out of anger—and impair immune function. And they can help someone facing a serious crisis—the loss of a loved one, chronic pain, even a terminal illness. But they're also helpful for garden-variety, day-to-day stress, says Dr. Koenig. "Normal life involves lots and lots of stress, disappointments, and interactions with others that create resentment and hurt and wear your body down," he says. "Mind/body therapies relieve stress to keep you healthy and increase your quality of life."

"Mind/body approaches are really just formalized ways of using the mind to explore different aspects of who we are," explains Marty Sullivan, M.D., a cardiologist at Duke University, who has studied mind/body treatments on cardiac patients.

Dr. Sullivan, who also is codirector of Duke's Integrative Medicine Program, admits that, while mind/body medicine is being validated in study after study, experts don't understand exactly how it works. We don't know what the mechanism is, and there are a lot of theories out there—that mind/body therapies have a direct impact on immunity, that they're involved in the involuntary control of bodily functions, even that they're associated with all of the things that are not very well explained by the Newtonian universe. The answer, he says, is that we don't know. Yet.

Studies have linked various mind/body therapies to an array of health benefits. But among the most compelling research of all is a metanalysis of studies involving more than 23,000 people that found, no matter the disease or condition, a person's own opinion regarding his or her health is a better predictor of their long-term prognosis than virtually any objective factors, including physical exams and laboratory test results.

Mind/body treatments vary widely, but all share the common trait of fostering positive effects in the physical body—greater resistance to disease, speedier healing, improved mental health—by encouraging the mind to be calm. They're big news in medicine now for several reasons, including the realization among health care providers that the vast majority of the conditions that bring people to their doctors every year aren't caused by microbes or car accidents. They're caused by stress.

Science and the Mind/Body Connection

What's going on here? Why are scientists only now considering the relationship between the physical and the emotional? Haven't we always known that the brain can influence the body?

Actually, the theory of a mind/body connection is as old as medicine itself. Indeed, virtually every major culture and medical system in the world has recognized the interrelationship between the two.

Most cultures, including our own, see another element at work within us, the spirit, that can't be explained by either psychology or physiology. These things—mind, body, spirit—work in synch to create health or disease.

In Western medicine, until the mid-18th century, the doctor and spiritual advisor were often the same person—until the advent of drugs and surgical interventions put the focus of healing squarely onto the body. With the rise of penicillin and anesthesia (and modern theories of mental health), medicine dissected its patients: Physicians took custody of the body. Psychiatrists and therapists took the mind. And the spirit was left to organized religion. The three components might still reside in the same person, but their care was assigned to three decidedly different custodians.

In the past few decades, the medical community has rediscovered the mind/body link. Doctors and researchers are actively exploring the impact that psychological, even spiritual, stress can have on all of the aspects of an individual's well-being—including susceptibility to disease, mental health, and longevity.

Herbert Benson, M.D., a cardiologist and pioneer in the field of mind/body medicine, contends that the vast majority of common health complaints—as many as 90 percent—are caused by stress and other mind/body interactions. This is a big step back (or forward, depending on your point of view) to a more traditional approach to health—caring for the whole patient, says Dr. Benson.

"After Louis Pasteur demonstrated that specific bacteria could cause specific diseases, doctors increasingly disregarded the importance of beliefs and mind/body interactions," explains Dr. Benson, who now serves as director of the Mind/Body Medical Institute at Boston's Beth Israel Deaconess Medical Center and a professor at Harvard Medical School. "Modern remedies were so dramatically effective that they became the sole treatments used, and that completely changed the attitudes toward the nature of healing."

These specific treatments made enormous improvements in society, Dr. Benson says, yet they effectively eliminated the use of nonspecific methods, such as prayer (and its components of visualization and affirmation).

Dr. Benson is among several well-respected doctors who have focused their attention on mind/body healing. And if acceptance among the medical community is any indication of a therapy's promise, then mind/body therapies most certainly represent a school of medicine with a big future.

In the past few years, mind/body therapies have entered the curriculum at more than half of the nation's medical schools—including the prestigious programs at Harvard and George Washington University in Washington, D.C. Furthermore, studies and articles showing the effectiveness of mind/body therapies have appeared in major medical journals, including the *Journal of the American Medical Association*.

Pressure from the Public

As the medical community is embracing mind/body theories, consumers are following suit. In fact, it might be argued that consumers are way ahead of the conservative establishment. The Mind/Body Medical Institute estimates that a full 86 percent of Americans believe that mind/body therapies can help people who are ill to recover. A full 41 percent of the population say that they have been cured or have gotten better because of their own mind/body practices.

Spirituality, one of the better-researched areas of mind/body medicine, shows even higher approval ratings: More than 90 percent of Americans say they believe in God, and more than half report that religion is "very important" in their lives. Dale A. Matthews, M.D., an associate professor at the Georgetown School of Medicine in Washington, D.C., reports that physicians and mental health practitioners are, on average, about half as likely as their patients to say that religion is critical to their lives.

In essence, mind/body treatments work to stimulate the brain in order to create physical changes. Evidence is mounting that these methods can treat or prevent many major diseases. They also can make people feel healthier and happier, live longer, and spend less time in the hospital.

Mind/body medicine incorporates many healing modalities, including cognitive therapy, visualization and imagery, meditation, and religious or spiritual practices. Quite often, these therapies are used together. (For example, meditation typically uses visualization. And many religious practices incorporate visualization and meditation, plus positive thinking and affirmations.)

All of these practices are designed to encourage the mind to focus on positive things, which triggers a host of physiological changes that, in turn, foster better health. By getting the mind to be quiet, mind/body therapies get the body quiet, too. And that allows it to manage psychological and physical stress, fend off infection, and heal itself much more efficiently.

The Best of the Therapies

Mind/body medicine is based on the simple belief that the mind has powerful effects on the body—both positive and negative. When the mind is focused on negative things, or when the spirit is clouded with despair, it creates stress in the body that can be just as destructive as any disease or accident.

Stress—the kind that comes from prolonged worry or a sense of powerlessness in the face of life's challenges—has been tied to the deadliest diseases we know, including cancer and coronary heart disease. But when mind and spirit are calm, they can help your body resist disease, heal itself after injury, and cope with trauma without falling apart. Thus, all of the diseases and problems associated with stress can be addressed with mind/body therapies.

Here is a brief discussion of the most popular mind/body therapies.

Cognitive Therapy

Most often considered a conventional, not alternative, treatment, cognitive therapy is one component of psychotherapy in which an individual is taught to change habitual thought patterns in order to change behavior. It has long been accepted as a legitimate method of healing the mind.

When used in the context of mind/body medicine, cognitive therapy also can produce profound changes in the body. For example, psychotherapy treatments that included cognitive therapy have been shown to help reduce the length of hospital stays in elderly people with hip fractures. People who were treated with cognitive therapy also had fewer rehospitalizations and spent less time in physical therapy.

Cognitive therapy and other aspects of psychotherapy are getting increasing attention as the discipline of mind/body medicine evolves—and physicians are recognizing the prevalence of psychological disorders and the interrelationship between mental and physical health. The empathy and support—along with the cognitive therapy—that people get through psychological counseling has been proved effective at relieving depression. One study, which screened leukemia patients for depression, found that everyone who was diagnosed with depression died in the following year. The patients who were not depressed all survived.

Imagery and Visualization

Imagery is the technique of using one or more of your senses to mimic in the brain the effects that seeing (or smelling or touching) the real thing would have. Visualization is a type of imagery that uses only visual elements—you picture something in your mind's eye. The two techniques work in much the same way, providing the mind with input that it will translate into a message of healing and deliver to the rest of the body.

Although the process of converting an imagined scene or scent into altered brain chemistry and better well-being involves a complicated neurological process, imagery itself is actually a fairly simple exercise. "Ask yourself how many windows you have in your living room," says Stephen M. Kosslyn,

Ph.D., a professor of psychology at Harvard University and an associate in the neurology department at Massachusetts General Hospital in Boston.

You probably won't pull that number directly out of your memory bank, as you would if you'd been asked your phone number. "To answer that question, you'll probably visualize the walls in your living room, then mentally scan over them to count the windows," explains Dr. Kosslyn. "That's creating a mental image."

These mental images are handled in the brain in much the same way that actual images are, Dr. Kosslyn explains. Thus, just as seeing a positive image can make you feel calm, "seeing" a conjured-up image can activate the same parts of the brain to create the same effect. Imagery and visualization are often key components in meditation and are used in various forms of psychotherapy.

Both imagery and visualization can create profound changes in various body systems. Studies show that they can affect circulation, heart rate, body temperature, and blood glucose (sugar) levels. Visualization has been studied in people with cancer—with dramatic results. The people instructed to picture themselves healthy, visualizing the cancer cells going away, experience improvement in their conditions. Imagery also can help people with cancer bolster immunity, combat the nausea and other side effects of chemotherapy, and control their pain.

Meditation

Meditation is an ancient practice that allows the practitioner to calm his or her mind, generally by repeating a meaningful phrase or "mantra." It's a self-directed practice that requires you to focus on a single thought—a word, phrase, image, your breathing, whatever—and eliminate all other thoughts. It's designed to quiet mental chatter and distractions, to allow the mind to become still.

Meditation is an ancient practice that originated in the spiritual traditions of China, India, and Japan. It also factors heavily in Western religions (the "Hail Mary" recited by Catholics). One school of Indian meditation, Transcendental Meditation (TM), has been studied extensively and tied to improvements in health ranging from reduced chronic pain to lowered cholesterol and blood pressure.

Other types of meditation, such as South Asian *vipissana* (or "mindfulness meditation") also have been shown to relieve pain.

A new school of meditation, called the relaxation response, was developed by Dr. Benson at Harvard University after he had begun studying meditation and its effects on the body. Dr. Benson's research has found that meditation can alter oxygen consumption and blood chemistry, blood clotting, and brain functioning. He has found that the relaxation response can improve diseases ranging from high blood pressure and cardiac irregularities to insomnia and premenstrual syndrome (PMS). It's also been used to relieve the symptoms of cancer and AIDS.

therapy for healthy people

Although mind/body therapies can certainly be applied to a host of modern Western woes, they also have a basis that's more Eastern and old-fashioned.

Mind/body medicine is on many levels a long-term approach to health, while our culture is decidedly "outcome-oriented," says Marty Sullivan, M.D., a cardiologist, associate professor of medicine, and codirector of the Integrative Medicine program at Duke University in Durham, North Carolina. "When people get sick, they think, 'OK, I have this disease. What can I do to change it?' So they look into the mind/body stuff and suddenly a lightbulb goes on. And the whole way they look at life changes: What's important? What has meaning and value?"

Perhaps the most fundamental question of mind/body medicine is this: What does life mean to you? "No matter what happens, there's one thing that's never taken away from you," says Dr. Sullivan. "That's your inner world, your inner work. All the wisdom traditions would say that this inner work determines who we are as people. That's something that our culture, generally, has not emphasized."

Thus, whether you're facing an immediate crisis or are looking to bolster your overall health, you can look to mind/body therapies to help you build your inner defenses. "Everyone should have a mind/body approach to life—not just to disease management," says Dr. Sullivan. "It's like somebody asking, 'Do you do any financial planning?' If you only do it when you're broke, it's not gonna help much."

Spirituality and Religion

Spirituality and religion often go hand in hand, as religious practice usually incorporates a sense of spiritual involvement with a higher being and an earthly community. Yet spirituality and religion are not necessarily the same thing, says Christina Puchalski, M.D., assistant professor of internal medicine and geriatrics at George Washington University School of Medicine and director of education at the National Institute for Healthcare Research, both in the Washington, D.C., area.

"I think everyone is spiritual, whether they're religious or not," she says. "And I define spirituality as a search for a transcendent or deeper meaning in life. In some ways, religion is really just organized spirituality."

David B. Larson, M.D., adjunct professor of psychiatry and behavioral science at Duke University Medical Center in Durham, North Carolina, and president of the National Institute for Healthcare Research in Washington, D.C., also separates religion from spirituality. "Spirituality is what gives you meaning and purpose, a sense of something that's more important than yourself," he says. "Most of the time we don't need meaning and purpose, but when you're facing big life events or chronic illness or loss, you call on higher powers and forces."

Spirituality and religion contain many components, he says, which help foster motivation, compassion, and coping. Spirituality can be attached to organized religion, he says, but also to almost anything you find inspirational: music, art, community. "Religion is just one of the houses within which it can fit," he says.

The key to reaping health benefits from your faith is to put it to work, says Dr. Larson. Be active in your church. Make a commitment to practice your faith. "Being part of a religious community gives real social support, which also reduces stress," he says. "And that community gives you a world view, a mental coherence that lets you see things with a broader perspective." The acts of prayer and visualization are important, too, but the real key, he says, is the belief model itself.

Research is showing that a person's belief system, including their sense of hope about the future and about a larger meaning behind life's trials and tribulations, determines to a large extent how well they handle tough situations. "You cope better, physically and psychologically, if you can see things in a longer view, and people who are religious tend to have that longer view," explains Dr. Puchalski.

Religious belief is in many ways the easiest type of spirituality to measure, so for scientists and researchers, church attendance is often used as a benchmark of someone's spirituality. And as imprecise a measure of devotion as this may be, it has given us some compelling evidence for the healing powers of spirituality.

People who attend religious services at least once a week, for example, have stronger immune systems and much lower rates of high blood pressure, cardiovascular disease, and cancer. And when they do get sick, people with a strong faith cope better, get well faster, and have fewer complications. They also live longer—an average of seven years—than their nonreligious counterparts.

Statistically speaking, religious people are less likely to have risky health habits, like smoking and drinking alcohol. But even after researchers adjust their findings to reflect these differences, the numbers show that being active in your faith spells better health.

Another component of spirituality is the element of prayer. Studies have shown that people who are actively religious—and pray—are healthier. But what if someone else was using his or her own faith to help you?

Believe it or not, there is research to show that having other people pray for you can improve your health—and it can even help you cope with a lethal disease like AIDS.

Larry Dossey, M.D., author of *Prayer Is Good Medicine* and several other books on the power of spirituality, says that virtually any condition could be improved by prayer. "The research shows clearly that there is probably no disease off-limits," he says. "As a matter of fact, the most famous study in this century shows that prayer works in cardiovascular disease, which kills more Americans than any other disease."

What to Expect

Unlike many therapies, alternative or conventional, mind/body methods typically produce almost imperceptible immediate effects. You might feel more relaxed or centered, but you most likely won't see an instantaneous response. And you shouldn't expect to, says Dr. Dossey. "There are people who get God mixed up with vitamins. But you can't treat these transcendental, spiritual interventions like you would a pill. This is a different dimension and should be treated with respect."

With the exception of cognitive therapy, which often is included in conventional psychotherapy and so will be covered by some—but certainly not all—insurance plans, mind/body treatments are not covered by insurance. Nor are they regulated by the government, meaning anyone can hang out a shingle proclaiming a mind/body practice. Thus, you need to be particularly careful in selecting any individual who is going to provide your training in any of these areas.

Beyond that, here is a bit of advice on what to expect from the various treatments:

- **Cognitive therapy.** This practice follows the classic psychotherapy model. You'll meet with a therapist, discuss your goals, and chart your course. Cognitive therapy can be practiced by licensed psychologists, psychiatrists, and counselors.
- **Imagery and visualization.** You might learn visualization from an expert, or you could just pick up a book on the subject. The experience might feel awkward at first, as you try to master the skills of determining your intention, centering and quieting your thoughts, and cleansing your mind.
- **Meditation.** If you see a practitioner, you might get a quick introduction in the practice of meditation. Dr. Puchalski, for example, offers lessons in the relaxation response to any of her patients who ask.

"In the first session, I teach them to breathe very slowly and deeply, using the diaphragm, then pick a word that has some deep connotation to them," she explains. "Then they'll close their eyes, relax, and breathe, saying the word. The trick is to train your mind to focus on the word and passively disregard any other thoughts that pop up. You're training your mind to keep your attention on your word."

- **Spirituality and religion.** When it comes to spirituality and prayer, there's no universal experience, says Dr. Dossey, but there is one common denominator in effective spiritual practices: love. "I have spent 15 years looking at prayer and science, and I think the best predictor of success is the empathy and compassion that people bring to their practice," he says. "The operative term is love. In all of the studies that have been done on prayer, for example, you see that if you take away the love, it just doesn't work."

Practicing prayer is actually easier than it sounds, Dr. Dossey promises, even if you're new to the whole idea. "Begin in ways that feel natural, like giving silent thanks before meals or saying a quick prayer of gratitude in the morning. From there you can go on to pray for things: a quick recovery, better health. The idea is that prayers of gratitude are more natural for almost everybody than asking for something."

Safety and Warnings

Although mind/body therapies are among the safest medical procedures you could find, there are a few precautions you should take before you try them.

- **Pick the right practitioner.** "You're looking for someone who can guide you to do things that are going to help you, not to impose their ways on you," says Dr. Larson. He warns against "gurus," a sentiment echoed by other experts.

"Reputable mind/body practitioners don't require that people buy into a specific set of beliefs," he says. "They allow them to explore their own avenues of healing in a way that respects them."

"If it smells like, looks like, and talks like evangelism, it's probably evangelism," adds Dr. Dossey. If the evangelism happens to belong to your own chosen faith, that's fine. But if you sense that someone is using your illness to pull you into a religious practice, you should question that.

"I would steer clear of someone who wanted to help me with my illness but wanted me to join their church or charge money for their prayers," says Dr. Dossey. "That ought to make bells and whistles go off."

If you belong to an established religion, the best guide can be your minister, priest, or rabbi.

- **Keep it positive.** Like any other lifestyle change, mind/body therapies will work the best if they're performed with relish. That means if it feels good to you, do it. "Things that are opening and freeing, things that make you feel better and inspire you to try new things—those are things that you want to stick with," says Dr. Larson.

Be true to yourself. If you're feeling uncomfortable or threatened in any way, you should look elsewhere, says Dr. Larson. "Watch out for any therapies that don't respect your value system or where you feel that your autonomy isn't respected." Even though you're going to an expert or practitioner for their guidance, you should feel that the process involves a free exchange of ideas.

chapter 15

music & art therapy

THE RIGHT NOTES

> Musical vibrations may help restore regulatory function to a body out of tune during times of stress and illness. —*Jane F. Brewer, R.N., senior lecturer at the University of Plymouth in England*

It's no secret that music can strike a powerful chord with our emotions, evoking everything from tears to goosebumps as it plays our heartstrings.

But recently it's been music's ability to affect our bodies that has researchers whistling Dixie. Researchers have found that premature babies gain weight faster when sung lullabies by Brahms. People with rheumatoid arthritis feel less pain after listening to music by Mozart. People with Parkinson's disease walk more steadily and feel better after singing, humming, or just beating on a drum.

It's not just humans that respond to music. Animals also have been found to respond positively to music. (Cows that have Mozart played for them produce more milk.) And even plants seem to get a rise from a good tune, though they can be a little fussy.

Flowers and vegetables in one study flourished when played classical music, showed no response to country and western, and withered to rock and roll. Why such profound effects from something that would seem to go in one ear and out the other? (Or in one tendril and out the other?)

Because music doesn't just go in one ear and out the other. It makes a powerful impact on our bodies and brains—an impact so powerful that music currently is being used to treat conditions as diverse as strokes, asthma, high blood pressure, learning disabilities, headaches, menopause, depression, Alzheimer's disease, cancer, and even AIDS.

Music may even help boost our intelligence, as shown in a study done in 1993 at the University of California at Irvine, which found that college students who listened to just 10 minutes of a Mozart piano sonata before taking an IQ test were able to improve their scores by an average of more than eight points.

Getting Your Cells Aligned

"Like a potter shaping clay, music shapes us both inside and out," says Don Campbell, composer and founder of the Institute of Music, Health, and Education. Although there is some controversy surrounding the conclusions that he draws from research on music therapy, Campbell's groundbreaking book *The Mozart Effect* has been opening the ears of many doctors to music's healing powers. He likens music's effects to the process of getting the wheels aligned on your car, explaining that not just cellular activities in the body but also thought processes in the brain become less random, and more efficient, as they begin to be swayed by music's intrinsic compliance with order.

Music works toward this "alignment" in several ways, he says, which is why its effects are thought to be so powerful. At its most basic level, music consists of sound waves (vibrational energy) that have an impact on our bodies just as the sound waves of any nonmusical noise would, Campbell says.

"Music in this sense is comprised of the same basic energy that can cause windows to rattle during a thunderstorm, or that a good vocalist can use to shatter a piece of fine glassware," explains Clive Robbins, D.M.M., cofounder of the Nordoff-Robbins Music Therapy Center in New York City. (D.M.M. is a German medical degree.)

But music takes this basic vibrational energy and refines it by adding both rhythm and harmony, thus creating a synchronization of sound waves that has more power to produce bodily changes. It's a little like one of those garden hose attachments that boosts the cleaning power of a stream of water by giving it both a pattern and a pulse. Music does the same thing to sound waves, organizing them in terms of both pace and pitch, Campbell says. The result is a highly organized onslaught of sound waves with greater power to impart its sense of order to whatever it may encounter. Studies have shown, for example, that music can be made to create highly intricate geometric patterns in mediums such as liquids and gases. So why should the fluids and other highly sensitive components of our bodies be any different?

They aren't, research suggests. "We absorb music's vibrational energies, and they subtly alter our breath, pulse, blood pressure, muscle tension, and other delicate functions within our bodies," Campbell says. This ability of music to "set us straight" may be especially true when we're feeling emotionally upset or physically ill and are in a sense "out of tune," says Jane F. Brewer, R.N., senior lecturer at the University of Plymouth in England.

"Musical vibrations may help restore regulatory function to a body out of tune during times of stress and illness," she says. Music "may also help maintain and enhance regulatory function when we're feeling well and are in tune."

Good for the Brain, Too

These same energies that have positive effects on the cellular activity of our bodies also appear to bring greater harmony to the workings of our brains. This is why music is thought to be so helpful for children with learning disabilities, people who have had a stroke, and senior citizens suffering from memory loss. It also may be why music has been found to have such a positive impact on creativity, concentration, feelings of well-being, and just the simple ability to relax, says Dr. Robbins.

Listening to music has been shown to help coordinate the activity of the two hemispheres of the brain such that the left, more analytical portion, begins to coordinate better with the right, more intuitive side, Dr. Robbins explains. The result, he says, may be a more balanced and competent thought process overall.

This effect of improving brain function has been suggested not just by the IQ study mentioned above, but also a survey done in 1996 by the College Entrance Examination Board. This survey found that students who played a musical instrument scored an average of 39 and 51 points higher than nonmusical students on their math and verbal SATs respectively. Another study done at the Chinese University of Hong Kong in Japan found that college students who had received musical training before the age of 6 did significantly better than nonmusically trained students on a test that asked them to recall as many words as possible from a list of 16 that researchers read to them out loud. "Music training in childhood may have long-term positive effects on verbal memory," notes researcher Agnes S. Chan.

Research shows that music study does, in fact, have an impact on the structure of the brain itself. MRIs show that the brains of people who play music for a living are in fact larger in an area known as the corpus callosum—the portion of the brain that links the right hemisphere with the left, thus coordinating analytical with intuitive thought.

Music for the Health of It

But music's cerebral effects aside, its benefits to the body are what have given scientists reason for optimism. Music has been used to combat illness in a variety of ways by cultures from all over the world for thousands of years, but not until the early part of the 20th century did scientists begin to explore its healing potential in earnest.

Aided by the invention of the phonograph around 1900, doctors began noticing that music could be used to help patients sleep and to reduce their anxieties prior to surgery. Encouraged by the results, doctors at Duke University Hospital in Durham, North Carolina, soon were making earphones available to all patients so they could tune in to their favorite tunes on the newly developed radio.

By the end of World War II, music was a mainstay at veteran's hospitals as a way of boosting patient morale, and by the end of the 1940s major colleges and universities began offering courses teaching how music might be used as a legitimate healing therapy. That trend continues today, with degree programs in music therapy now being offered by more than 70 major educational institutions nationwide.

"The field has exploded, and throughout medicine we have learned of music's amazing power to heal," says John S. McIntyre, M.D., former president of the American Psychiatric Association, commenting on music's emergence as a valuable new medical treatment.

Currently, an estimated 5,000 therapists certified by the American Music Therapy Association practice in hospitals, rehabilitation centers, schools, and nursing homes nationwide, and many services provided by musical therapists are now covered by Medicare, Medicaid, and other health insurance programs.

Who is benefiting from music's therapeutic charms?

"Patients of musical therapy include children and adults of all ages and levels of intelligence suffering from a wide range of problems including learning disabilities, physical handicaps, autism, sensory impairment, emotional disturbances, psychiatric problems, brain injuries, and terminal illnesses," says George D. Lundberg, M.D., the former editor in chief of the *Journal of the American Medical Association*.

Therapy sessions differ according to the patient and the problem being treated, but "music therapy is essentially the building of a relationship between a patient and a specially trained therapist using music as the basis of communication," Dr. Lundberg says. "Both the therapist and patient take an active part in the therapy sessions through playing, singing, or listening. The therapist does not teach singing or playing an instrument. Rather the instrument and voice are used to explore the world of sound and create a common musical language."

Different Songs for Different Wrongs

Music therapists generally work with music of two basic types, depending on the mood and medical condition of the person being treated, Dr. Robbins says. There's sedative music with flowing rhythms and soothing melodies used to help people overcome anxiety disorders, lower blood pressure, recover from surgeries, convalesce from major illnesses or heart attacks, or simply become more open and trusting during psychological counseling.

More stimulating music, on the other hand, characterized by jauntier rhythms and more dynamic melodies, is used to pep people up. This kind of music is helpful for people who have had a stroke or who have Parkinson's or Alzheimer's disease.

sonic nutrition

Mozart is still number one after all these years! Although music of nearly all styles has been found to have healing potential (yes, even rap and thunderous rock and roll have demonstrated therapeutic value for the right audiences), the music of one particular composer clearly has stood out from all the rest. The composer is Wolfgang Amadeus Mozart, the 18th-century prodigy who amazed the royalty of Western Europe with piano concerts at the age of 5 and wrote his first symphony by the time he was 8 years old.

His "music from God," as one envious contemporary is alleged to have described it, has been found to invigorate not just people, but even animals and plants. (Don Campbell, author of *The Mozart Effect*, makes the claim that yeast used in Japan to make the rice wine known as sake increases in density—a measure of quality—by a factor of 10 when Mozart is played in the yeast's presence.)

Why should Mozart's music shine so clearly above all others with respect to its physical as well as emotional effects?

Researchers speculate that Mozart's music has a sense of order and an emotional purity that make it universally stimulating for people of all ages, races, and ethnic heritage. Campbell reports, as an example, that when officials from the Department of Immigration and Naturalization softly play Mozart during English classes for new arrivals, immigrants learn faster regardless of what country they're from.

Mozart's music also has been shown to facilitate learning in children, as evidenced by studies in which students in public schools performed better when Mozart was played in the background during classes. City officials in Edmonton, Canada, have found that Mozart tunes piped through loudspeakers seem to lend a sense of order even to pedestrian traffic.

But perhaps the most amazing display of the seeming magic of Mozart has been demonstrated in tests of intuitive and spatial reasoning. Researchers from the University of California at Irvine found that Mozart's music helped students improve their scores on a test of spatial reasoning by 62 percent. By comparison, students who listened to other forms of music or simply sat in silence for equal periods of time upped their scores by only 11 and 14 percent respectively. In the words of world-famous music therapist and physician Alfred Tomatis, M.D., of France, Mozart's music "has a liberating and healing power that exceeds by far what we've been able to observe in his predecessors ... his contemporaries, or his successors."

"Mozart's music does what many systems of alternative healing try to do," notes Campbell. "It helps give people's internal energy flow a sense of balance. It's not too fast or too slow or too complex or too simple either. Somehow it's just right."

the top 10 medical conditions music treats best

In China music albums often bear the names of medical problems they help treat, according to Don Campbell, author of *The Mozart Effect.* Leading the hit parade over the past few years are such scintillating titles as *Obesity, Insomnia,* and *Constipation.*

While Americans might not buy musical albums with diseases for titles, American research does point to a number of diseases and conditions that respond particularly well to music's mellifluous powers.

1. Alzheimer's disease. Researchers from Tennessee Technological University in Cookeville have found that people with Alzheimer's disease displayed significantly fewer episodes of aggressive behavior during bathing activities when they were listening to music of their choice. Studies have shown that music also can help restore some of the mental functioning lost to this age-related disease.

2. Neonatal care. Music's soul-soothing capabilities seem to extend to the very young as well as the old. According to a 1998 report published in *Pediatric Nursing,* premature babies sung Brahms' *Lullaby* for 15 to 30 minutes at least once a week were less fussy, gained more weight, and were able to leave the hospital sooner than infants who convalesced without music.

3. Nausea for chemotherapy. The stomach, too, seems to take comfort from the sounds of music as evidenced by one study done at Ohio State University in Columbus. The study found that music helped reduce nausea and vomiting in people undergoing chemotherapy for cancer.

4. Attention deficit disorder (ADD). What better test for music's calming powers than this attention-robber? Music came through nicely in a trial reported in 1995 in the *International Journal of Arts Medicine* showing that listening to Mozart three times a week produced significant improvements in both ability to concentrate and physical restlessness. These effects were still significant six months after therapy was stopped.

5. Brain injury. Researchers at the Pennsylvania State University College of Medicine in University Park found that 10 weeks of music therapy produced improvements in emotional responsiveness, social behavior, and mood in 15 people suffering from brain dysfunction due to injury.

6. Pain. There's not a country-western singer alive who would question that music can help assuage a heartache, but studies show that music can be an effective antidote for physical pain, as well. This was shown convincingly in one study in which half of a group of women who listened to music during childbirth required less anesthesia.

7. Anxiety. Would music be able to reduce the anxiety associated with breathing with the help of a respirator? Researchers from the University of Iowa College of Nursing in Iowa City asked this question in one study. They found that people who listened to music for 30 minutes prior to receiving their respiratory treatments were more relaxed, based on decreases in both heart rates and respiratory rates alike.

8. Parkinson's disease. In one 1998 Italian study, 16 people with this neurological disorder (characterized by impaired muscle control and sometimes emotional disturbance) received music therapy. After just 13 sessions lasting two hours each, they scored better on tests, not just of muscular function, but also emotional stability, happiness, and quality of life in general. Drumming in particular helped patients coordinate their movements.

9. Headaches. We all know that music can cause headaches. Just think of a son's or daughter's beginning efforts on the violin or drums. But music also has been shown to be effective in controlling severe headaches in at least two major studies. One study combined music with relaxation techniques and guided imagery while the other, done in Poland, simply had people attend concerts of their choice for six months.

10. Recovery from heart attack. Optimal recovery from a heart attack depends on correcting as many of its causes as possible, and music seems capable of taking on a sizable share of those. In a study reported in the medical journal *Heart and Lung*, music therapy sessions that also incorporated relaxation techniques produced significant drops in blood pressure, resting heart rate, and perceived levels of stress.

These people benefit from the music's energy psychologically as well as physically, when it's used as an impetus for rehabilitative exercise.

"There's a basic rule, however, that whatever works best for an individual patient is what should be used," Dr. Robbins says. "A younger person, for example, might not respond as well to Bach as to someone like Madonna or the Spice Girls, so we try to work within the patient's basic musical tastes as much as possible."

A University of Miami study done in 1998 found that adolescent girls suffering from depression produced less of the stress-related hormone cortisol after listening to 23 minutes of rock and roll than when they were asked just to sit and relax in silence for that same period of time.

"People shouldn't feel they have to follow any set rules when it comes to using music for therapeutic purposes," Dr. Robbins says. "They should keep an open mind, however, and expose themselves to as many different styles of music as possible to see which has the most beneficial effects."

Often people respond positively to classical music, for example, even though they may be listening to it closely for the first time. But some energetic pop music by artists such as the Beatles or Michael Jackson also can have therapeutic effects on older people who may be hearing it for the first time, too, especially in situations such as rehabilitative exercise programs where stimulation is the goal. "The appropriateness of any piece of music really depends on the situation and the therapeutic purposes for which it's being applied, " Dr. Robbins says.

Then, too, certain types of music can be better than others, depending on the listener's mood, Dr. Robbins adds. Someone who's feeling melancholy, for example, is unlikely to want to receive a sudden jolt of unbridled happiness as delivered by a rousing rendition of "Oklahoma," but probably would prefer something more thoughtful and serene. Someone who's just won the lottery, on the other hand, probably is not going to be comfortable listening to a brooding classical fugue. "If the goal is to alter an unwanted mood such as sadness, often it's best to match the mood first, then progress to happier music gradually," Dr. Robbins says.

Stressed Out or In Pain? "Tone" It Down

If you'd like to put music's curative powers to a test, you can try dusting off a technique known as "toning," which dates all the way back to the 14th century. Toning is defined as the technique of "making a sound with an elongated vowel for an extended period." This chant-like procedure has been used medically to lower blood pressure and respiratory rate in cardiac patients and to reduce anxiety in people undergoing surgeries and MRIs. But it also can have practical applications for all of us, says Campbell. Toning can be an effective way to calm ourselves before stressful events or simply to help ease everyday pains such as minor burns, sprains, or hammer-whacked thumbs.

Start by closing your eyes and focusing on the source of your pain, Campbell advises. Then simply begin to make a continuous "ah" or "oo" (as in "soup") sound, imagining your pain leaving your body through your voice as you do. For especially acute pains, you may want to raise the pitch of your voice using "ee" or "ay" sounds (which also can be helpful in releasing pent-up anger, Campbell says).

Never strain your voice while toning. And feel free to take short rests every 60 seconds or so to replenish your breath. Your pain should be gone or at least significantly reduced within a few minutes, Campbell says.

Another technique similar to toning can be a quick, convenient way to relieve stress, such as the kind encountered during traffic jams, family squabbles, or problems at work, Campbell says. With this strategy, you simply sit as quietly as possible, close your eyes, and hum, not a tune but rather just a single note that's comfortably within your range of pitch. Bring the palms of your hands to your cheeks, notice the vibrations. You'll be able to feel the vibrations more strongly if you put your fingers in your ears. Try to imagine your body being given a gentle, internal massage, Campbell says. You should feel noticeably more relaxed within just a few minutes.

Listening Versus Playing

If listening to music can produce such pronounced health effects, might performing music amplify these effects even more? Both Campbell and Dr. Robbins think so. Campbell, in fact, often uses performance exercises in his classes and seminars to make the benefits of performing quite clear. He reports that a group of conservative computer executives participating in one of his seminars recently felt significantly more creative after banging paper plates together as mock cymbals in accompaniment to an Irish folk song.

Dr. Robbins reports similar results from his experiences as an instructor in his center in New York. "There's obviously a closer connection to music when it's played, so it would certainly seem logical that this connection would produce greater physiological as well as emotional effects," he says. "We do know that stroke victims and people with Parkinson's disease or certain learning disabilities frequently do better when they actually participate in singing, drumming, or playing, so that would certainly lend credence to the benefits of performing."

Some credence might also come from the survival of more than a few rock-and-roll stars of 1960s vintage who have held up surprisingly well despite alleged histories of less-than-perfect lifestyles.

When we tap into the musical parts of our brains, we're also tapping into the parts responsible for imagination, intuition, and fantasy—essentially youthful ways of thinking, Dr. Robbins says. Who's to say, he asks, what the effects on our bodies might be if we can use music to take a more creative, optimistic, and generally less-stressed approach to life?

It's important when considering music's health benefits, however, to consider how music is approached, Dr. Robbins says. As the pursuit of music becomes less enjoyable, unfortunately, it's probably also going to become less beneficial from a health standpoint. Parents funding music lessons for their children might want to keep this in mind. If the experience is clearly producing less music than frustration or stress, it might be a good idea to look for a different approach to instruction or perhaps simply to postpone lessons for a while, Dr. Robbins says. Unfortunately, children can be scarred by negative musical experiences as well as they can be healed by positive ones.

How to Find a Music Therapist

Should you decide to try music therapy, experts in the field advise the following precautions to assure you're getting the best treatment possible:

- **Check those credentials.** Make sure your therapist is board-certified or at least registered with the American Music Therapy Association.
- **Try for a close match.** Seek out a therapist who has had experience in treating your particular condition, if possible.

Get the specifics. Ask what therapy sessions will involve, the results you can expect, and the success rates your therapist generally has achieved in treating your particular concern.

- **Be demanding.** Don't settle for a therapist who simply plays some nondescript music in the background and calls it therapy. Your therapist should devise a program that is tailored specifically to your individual needs, whether it's in the form of listening to music, playing an instrument, singing, or simply beating on drum.
- **Exercise your vision.** Be prepared to participate in a form of therapy called "guided imagery." This technique—in which the imagination is called upon to envision relaxing or healing images designed to help the body heal itself—has been shown to be an effective adjunct to music therapy.
- **Consider insurance.** Make sure your therapist has both the knowledge and interest to help you obtain whatever insurance coverage may be available for your treatment.

Safety and Warnings

Finally, you may be thinking, a therapy that's 100 percent danger-free! Not quite, but the positive note is that music therapy's hazards are 100 percent preventable.

- **Don't get carried away.** The greatest danger comes simply from listening to or playing music too loud, Dr. Robbins says. Habitual exposure to sound levels in the range of 80 decibels (the approximate volume of most vacuum cleaners) can produce irreversible hearing loss. And much music as it's played today (either in concert, on car stereos, or through headphones) can exceed this threshold. Most rock concerts, for example, are performed at levels between 100 and 130 decibels, studies show.

resources
for music therapy

Organizations

American Music Therapy Association
8455 Colesville Rd., Suite 1000
Silver Springs, MD 20910
301/589-3300
www.musictherapy.org

The Mozart Effect Resource Center
3526 Washington Ave.
St. Louis, MO 63103
800/721-3177

Institute for Music and Neurologic Function
Beth Abraham Hospital
612 Allerton Ave.
Bronx, NY 10467
718/920-4567

Nordoff-Robbins Music Therapy Clinic
New York University
26 Washington Place
New York, NY 10003
212/998-5151

The Bonny Foundation
2020 Simmons St.
Salinas, KS 67401

Music to Try

Music for the Mozart Effect, Vols. I–IV
Spring Hill Music
P.O. Box 800
Boulder, CO 80306
800/427-7680

The Mozart Effect: Music for Children, Vols. I–IV
1400 Bayly St., No. 7
Pickering, Ontario, L1W 3R2
800/668-0242
In Canada: 800/757-8372

- **Watch those headphones.** There's also the very real danger that comes from listening to music through headphones while exercising outdoors. The music is a distraction that increases the chances of being assaulted and/or having an accident, studies show.
- **Be aware of responses.** It is important to match music with mood, however. "Music can aggravate as well as ameliorate," says Dr. Robbins. So be sensitive to how music is being perceived, whether you're playing it for someone else or for yourself. Nor are there any hard, fast rules about who should listen to what and why, he adds. "We all have very individual tastes in music," he says, "and it's the effect the music produces that's more important than any explanation of why." Other than those potential pitfalls, there may not be a safer healing therapy going, Dr. Robbins says.

art therapy
helps heal

- AIDS
- Alzheimer's disease
- Cancer
- Depression
- Diabetes
- Drug addiction
- Grief
- Learning disabilities
- Stress
- Strokes

Art Therapy: Drawing from Within

There was a time when Carla's childhood was too painful for her to remember, much less talk about, so she escaped into her own idea of reality and developed a multiple personality disorder as a result. But then Carla met art therapist Cathy Malchiodi, author of *The Art Therapy Sourcebook*, and slowly her true personality began to take shape.

Carla didn't talk much during their sessions, at least not in the beginning, but she did draw—pictures rife with violence and fear, thus expressing in images what for so long she had been unable to say in words. "Carla's art became a way for us to begin to understand the defense mechanisms she had adopted over the years to help her cope," Malchiodi says. "Today she's much improved with a much better understanding of who she is and what she wants to do with her life."

And so goes art therapy, a medical practice that now employs an estimated 4,000 licensed practitioners working with people of all ages to treat conditions ranging from drug addictions to cancer.

"Therapists frequently work as part of a team of other health-care professionals such as physicians, psychologists, and physical therapists, but many function as primary therapists in private practice as well," says Edward J. Stygar, Jr., executive director of the American Art Therapy Association.

Not for Artists Only

What might the goal of art therapy be? Not, Malchiodi says, to treat artists only, as is mistakenly thought by some people. "Nothing could be further from the truth," she says. "Art therapy can be for everybody because, as Freud observed, our ability to think and to express ourselves in visual terms is even more basic than our ability to express ourselves through language. In art therapy, therefore, people are encouraged to express what they may not be able to say in words through drawings, paintings, or other visual forms."

This isn't to say that patients don't discuss what they produce with the therapist, but discussion usually is based on the artwork rather than the patient directly, thus making sessions less intimidating. "Therapy sessions typically employ traditional art techniques such as drawing, painting, and sculpting, but with an emphasis on getting patients to express images that come from inside them rather than from the outside world, thus giving insight to their problems," Malchiodi says. "Input from the therapist is important, but there are very few other forms of therapy in which patients are so actively or creatively involved."

What sort of problems might such involvement be used to treat? In the language of the American Art Therapy Association's official position statement: "Art therapists use drawings and other art media and imagery to assess, treat, and rehabilitate patients with mental, emotional, physical, and/or developmental impairments."

Satisfying A Basic Need

If that seems to encompass an ambitiously wide range of disorders, it's important to keep in mind that art therapy, like many alternative health strategies, embraces the concept of a strong connection between body and mind. The concept supports the idea that whatever attends to our emotional well-being also is going to produce positive effects physically. Therein lies the basis for the extensive list of conditions art therapy is used to treat. In addition to myriad psychological disorders including depression, intense grief, learning disabilities, and cases of physical abuse such as Carla's, art therapy is proving itself to be valuable in assisting people with such physical ailments as heart attacks, cancer, strokes, Alzheimer's disease, tuberculosis, kidney disease, diabetes, and AIDS.

"Any time a medical condition produces anxiety or stress, art therapy can be a useful therapeutic tool," Malchiodi says.

She notes, too, that people often "come to life" during therapy sessions, becoming more animated and joyful and exhibiting more self-esteem.

"Making something unique with one's own hands is a powerful experience with undeniable therapeutic benefits," she says. "The creation of art, in fact, may be among our most basic needs. Despite the constant shelling and sniper fire in Sarajevo in the early 90s, as an example, people continued to express themselves through art. They maintained their orchestras and choirs, continued to hold concerts, and actually turned a destroyed theater into an exhibition space for art created of debris from the city's ruins."

Art Therapy for the Do-It-Yourselfer

While it's true that art therapy seeks to guide artistic expression with particular therapeutic goals in mind for particular people, the act of creating art in and of itself can be therapeutic for anyone willing to invest the time and emotion it takes to do it, says Bruce Moon, Ph.D., the director of the art therapy graduate program at Merrywood University in Scranton, Pennsylvania, and the author of five books on art as therapy.

"People get sick because they keep things in, not because they let things out,"

Dr. Moon says. "The creation of art can be very cathartic regardless of the talent or experience of who's creating it. I wouldn't want to see people turning to art instead of their doctors for conditions requiring medical attention, but at the same time I do feel that art can be a very healthy release for a wide variety of emotional states, whether it's loneliness, anger, or simple day-to-day stress."

You might want to pick up a pencil or a paint brush after a harrowing day with that in mind. "Just create what you feel like creating," Dr. Moon suggests, and don't worry about how "good" it is. "It's good if it expresses your innermost feelings."

resources
for art therapy

For more information on art therapy or how to find a licensed art therapist in your area, contact:

American Art Therapy Association
1202 Allanson Rd.
Mundelein, IL 60060-3808
847/949-6064
www.arttherapy.org

Journals

Art Therapy: The Journal of the American Art Therapy Association
1202 Allanson Rd.
Mundelein, IL 66660
847/949-6064
Fax: 847/566-4580
E-mail: arttherapy@ntr.net

Books

The Art Therapy Sourcebook by Cathy Malchiodi (Lowell House Publishers, 1998)

The Dynamics of Art as Therapy by Bruce Moon, Ph.D. (Charles C. Thomas, 1998)

Art and Soul: Reflections on Artistic Psychology by Bruce Moon, Ph.D. (Charles C. Thomas, 1997)

chapter 16

naturopathy

THE NATURAL PATH

The body is amazing. If you can give it what it needs, it can fight off almost anything before it becomes a problem.—*Lorilee Schoenbeck, N.D.*

Alternative medicine is about choices. It's about realizing that Western medicine—while indispensable in many cases—is not always the only way to get well. Most importantly, it's about taking charge of your own health, choosing what's right for you instead of just swallowing a pill and hoping for the best.

Yet blazing your own trail to well-being can be confusing. What's the best way to treat an illness or improve your overall health? Homeopathy? Hydrotherapy? Herbal remedies? Massage? All of the above? None of the above? Sometimes it helps to have a guide, a Sherpa to lead you up that tricky health-care hill.

That's where naturopathy comes in. A naturopathic physician is trained in any number of complementary-care therapies and also has a scientific background similar to that of medical doctors. In fact, in a growing number of states you can even use a naturopath as your primary-care physician.

Nature's Way

"We can be the best of both worlds," says Lorilee Schoenbeck, N.D., a naturopathic physician at the Champlain Center for Natural Medicine in Shelburne, Vermont. "We can choose the best from alternative and conventional medicine and help create a program that can make you truly healthy." (N.D. stands for naturopathic doctor. It's a medical degree involving four years of special training that will be described later in this chapter.)

Naturopathy isn't the perfect path to health and happiness, however. For one thing, there's not a large body of scientific evidence proving that naturopathy's integrated approach really works. It also can be hard to find a qualified practitioner. Though the field is growing, there are still only 1,000 or so naturopathic physicians in the entire country. Unfortunately, there are also a number of under-qualified people calling themselves naturopaths, so you'll have to be careful.

naturopathy helps heal

In the 11 states that license them, naturopathic physicians (N.D.s) can treat a vast array of health problems. That's because they're considered primary care physicians—just like medical doctors. N.D.s, however, cannot perform major surgery or cure advanced problems like end-stage kidney diseases or cancers. Here's a list of common conditions that an N.D. is likely to treat:

- Allergies
- Anemia
- Arthritis
- Asthma
- Chronic pain
- Common colds
- Depression
- Digestive problems
- Fatigue
- Flu
- Headaches
- Hemorrhoids
- Hypertension
- Insomnia
- Menopause problems
- Menstrual pain
- Obesity

"That's not the optimal situation," says Thomas Kruzel, N.D., a naturopathic physician in Portland, Oregon, and past president of the American Association of Naturopathic Physicians (AANP). "In states that don't do licensing, just about anyone can call themselves a naturopath. Yet, if you take the time to look into things, you can find the right fit for you—and find a whole new way of looking at your health."

Basic Tenets

Naturopathic medicine is as old as history itself. For as long as people have used herbs, water, and other natural medications, healing specialists have guided others in their proper application.

Most naturopaths today look to the ancient Greek physician Hippocrates as the father of naturopathy—the same man whose teachings led medical doctors to create the Hippocratic oath.

Hippocrates lived more than 2,000 years ago, yet his philosophy of healing has a distinctly modern ring to it. The basis of his teaching—and the basis of naturopathy—is summed up in one phrase, *vis medicatrix Naturae.* Translated, this means, "the healing power of nature."

Naturopathic physicians believe that the body is its own best healer, provided it gets the proper rest, nutrition, and natural assistance. Some naturopaths call this innate healing ability "vitality," a phrase you may hear frequently when talking with a caregiver. The idea behind naturopathy is to use treatments that remove whatever's causing problems—be it stress, poor diet, infection, or any other agent—so that vitality can allow the body to repair the damage itself and get on with the task of being healthy.

Naturopathic physicians believe in five other main tenets as well.

- **Treat the whole person.** The human body is made up of dozens of organs and systems, from blood and brains to bones and bowels. But it's a mistake to look at the parts individually, Dr. Schoenbeck says. "Everything is interconnected. You can't go about trying to treat one thing without taking into account all of the others," she says. For example, headaches may come from tense muscles in your neck—but what's causing the tense muscles? An out-of-whack skeletal system? Poor posture? High blood pressure? Stress?

"It takes time to get to the bottom of things sometimes," Dr. Kruzel says. "But we have to be thorough. It does no good to treat a problem halfway, because it's just going to come back if you do."

- **Find the cause, not the symptoms.** "This is where we differ greatly from medical doctors," Dr. Kruzel says. "If someone comes to me with a symptom, like a stomachache, I'm not just interested in making the symptom go away. I'm interested in what the underlying cause is, because fixing that is where true health comes from.

"After all, a symptom is nothing more than your body's way of telling you that something is wrong. If you just hush up the symptom, you've done nothing to really help the body get better."

Walter J. Crinnion, N.D., a naturopathic physician in the Seattle area, puts it another way: "If you want to get rid of a dandelion in your yard, you don't pull off its leaves. You have to pull it up by the roots."

- **Prevent illness before it happens.** The best way to treat disease is to keep it from ever taking hold. That's why naturopathic physicians are keenly interested in prevention. "I talk to people about diet, lifestyle, exercise, stress management, family history, and other things every time I see them in my office," Dr. Schoenbeck says. "The body is amazing. If you can give it what it needs, it can fight off almost anything before it becomes a problem."

The emphasis on prevention is another major departure from Western medicine, Dr. Kruzel says. "How many people go to an M.D. when nothing is wrong with them?" he asks. "There's no point, since an M.D. is not going to take the time to really discuss prevention." A dedicated naturopath, on the other hand, will talk with you at length about how to make yourself more disease resistant and resilient.

- **Teach.** Though it's often forgotten, "doctor" and "teacher" used to have the same meaning in ancient languages. If you're accustomed to being told *what* to do by a doctor, but never *why* it's a good idea, naturopaths may be a pleasant change of pace.

"We want people to understand what's going on," Dr. Schoenbeck says. "It's the only way to show patients how to take care of themselves." If you're overweight, for example, you're going to get more than a terse "don't eat so much" from the doctor. You'll get loads of advice on which foods to eat, how much to eat, when to eat, and what supplements might serve you best. You'll also be reminded that the person most responsible for your health and well-being is you—not your physician.

- **Do no harm.** The main goal of naturopathy is to help the body help itself. In many cases, that means giving the body a little nudge in the right direction then getting out of the way. "Our emphasis is always on natural, nontoxic treatments," Dr. Kruzel says. That can mean bodywork like massage, hydrotherapy, relaxation, nutrition, and other modalities—none of which use powerful, chemistry-changing drugs.

"I'm not saying that drugs and surgery are never an option. But they are not the first option in naturopathic medicine," Dr. Kruzel says. "Even the herbs we use have been tested over centuries and are safe and gentle."

Naturopathy Makes a Comeback

While natural remedies have been around since the dawn of man, the term "naturopathy" is relatively new. In fact, it was introduced to America in the 1890s by a European man named Benedict Lust. Lust was convinced of the power of natural medicine. Lust himself claimed to have been cured of tuberculosis by bathing in the Danube River.

Naturopathic medicine enjoyed early success in the United States. Lust founded the American School of Naturopathy in 1902 and also founded the AANP. By the 1920s, there were more than a score of naturopathic medical schools and thousands of practitioners nationwide. But the tide turned against naturopathy in the middle of the century, thanks in large part to the growth of what is now called "conventional medicine." Scientific breakthroughs like antibiotics—plus the growing political and social clout of medical doctors, led to a dramatic decline in the number of naturopathic physicians.

Today, there are about 1,000 naturopathic physicians in the United States and three colleges with accredited naturopathic medicine programs. But that number is increasing again—thanks in no small part to the public's disenchantment with conventional medicine. "Despite all its fantastic discoveries, it still doesn't have all the answers," Dr. Schoenbeck says. "People now see that it has limits, and they are much more willing to look at natural approaches to wellness."

The State of Research

But what about the effectiveness of naturopathic medicine? Do its natural remedies and lifestyle changes really help cure and prevent disease? To a large extent, the jury is still out. Scientists have already begun looking at the methods naturopaths use—hydrotherapy, bodywork, herbal medicine, homeopathy, and others—to see how effective they are in curing and preventing diseases. Some of this work has been promising and is discussed in other chapters in this book.

But to date, there hasn't been much research into the naturopathic approach as a whole. So, there's really not an answer to the most basic question: Does a naturopathic approach that uses a combination of treatments work as well as, or better than, conventional medicine or other methods?

"There's definitely a gap in the research there," says Michael Traub, N.D., head of scientific affairs for the AANP and a naturopathic physician practicing in Kailua Kona, Hawaii. "The naturopathic colleges are

help for AIDS

Some early research looks good. For example, one small study looked at 16 men infected with human immunodeficiency virus (HIV), the virus that causes AIDS.

All the men had developed an advanced form of an AIDS-related complex, though none had full-blown AIDS. The men were given a complete naturopathic regimen for the course of one year—including dietary supplements and nutritional counseling; homeopathic and herbal treatments; hyperthermic hydrotherapy, in which body temperatures are raised by immersing patients in very warm water; and psychological counseling.

The patients were evaluated during and after the one-year period. None of the patients died or even developed full-blown AIDS, and some showed improvements in blood chemistry and body functions. Further, the patients showed fewer adverse reactions to the treatment than patients taking a normal AIDS drug regimen. On the whole, the patients reported they felt better than they had before the treatment started. The treatments did nothing to eliminate AIDS in any of the patients, however, and the study was too small to be statistically significant.

The study, by the way, was conducted with help from Bastyr University in Seattle, a naturopathic medical school that since 1994 has been home to the national center for research into alternative treatments for AIDS. This program is funded in part by the National Institutes for Health.

starting to look at this question, but to date there's really nothing definitive."

Except for the study on AIDS (see above), most the evidence for naturopathic medicine is anecdotal. It comes from individual reports from naturopathic physicians who have been treating patients for various ailments. But even though the science remains scant, naturopathic treatments have been winning converts in both government and health-care circles nationwide. For example, King County in Washington has opened the nation's first tax-supported clinic that offers natural medical treatments to Seattle-area residents. And the American Dietetic Association has certified nutritional courses offered at Bastyr University in Seattle for the training of registered dietitians.

Although many remain skeptical, some medical doctors support the type of medicine practiced by naturopathic physicians. "We use these treatments regularly," says David Edelberg, M.D., founder of American WholeHealth Integrated Medicine Centers, a chain of eight clinics across the country. "We use herbal remedies, nutritional supplements, counseling, and other things that we feel will benefit our patients. There's a lot to be said for an approach that uses nontoxic, noninvasive treatments to improve the health of patients."

In fact, the more medical doctors learn about alternative treatments, the more likely they may be to embrace parts of it. A survey of Australian medical school students found that even a single lecture on complementary medicine made the students more positive about the field. "When the word about naturopathy reaches the public—and that includes doctors—we start looking pretty good," says Dr. Schoenbeck. "We're an eclectic bunch, but we're doing very good work."

Naturopathic Training

Dr. Schoenbeck speaks from personal experience about conventional medicine's reluctance to accept naturopathy. She comes from a family of M.D.s that spans four generations, but she's the first to venture into naturopathic medicine. "I was disowned by my father," she says. But the two have reconciled many of their differences, to the point that she has served as an operating room assistant to her dad, who is a surgeon. "When he saw the kind of training I got and the experience I have, I think it made him change his mind a little," she says.

In fact, naturopathic physicians must pass a rigorous, four-year program before they can be licensed to practice. This comes after they've completed four years of pre-med studies at the undergraduate level. The postgraduate curriculum includes about 4,500 hours of traditional science—including chemistry and biochemistry, physiology, anatomy, and pathology. This scientific grounding compares favorably with that of medical doctors, who take a similar number of classes in the same disciplines.

In the second half of their college training, students focus on specialty areas like pediatrics, cardiac care, gynecology, and other specialty fields of interest to them. While this study is not as extensive as that of medical students, it's supplemented by a number of additional programs. These include hundreds of hours of coursework in nutrition, bodywork, herbal medicines and other modalities that students will later use in their practices.

These courses will serve them well, Dr. Edelberg says. "Most M.D.s don't have enough background in these areas. It's not emphasized, or it's just plain left out," he says. "I think it's important that caregivers have as broad a background as possible, so that they can provide a thoughtful, integrated program for their patients."

There's one key training difference between naturopathic doctors and medical doctors. After they've finished their schooling, medical doctors must go through a residency program. This gives them several years of supervised training, during which they receive thousands of hours of hands-on training. N.D.s, on the other hand, are not required to complete residency programs, except for those who wish to practice in the state of Utah.

State Laws Vary

Currently, only 11 states license naturopathic physicians: Alaska, Arizona, Connecticut, Hawaii, Maine, Montana, New Hampshire, Oregon, Utah, Vermont, and Washington. The commonwealth of Puerto Rico also requires N.D.s to have a license.

To practice in these jurisdictions, candidates must graduate from an accredited school of naturopathic medicine (or one that's a candidate for accreditation) then pass the state's licensing examination. The exams focus on everything from basic anatomy to minor surgery and nutritional counseling. Once they have received licenses, N.D.s can function as primary care physicians—meaning that you can use them in place of, or in addition to, a medical doctor for everyday health care. A growing number of insurance companies offer coverage for naturopathic care as well.

Naturopathic physicians are banned from practicing altogether in two states: South Carolina and Tennessee.

Naturopathy Takes On Many Ailments

In addition to using natural treatments, N.D.s in licensing states are also permitted to perform a limited number of medical procedures. Though they vary from state to state, these usually include most of the following: taking and reading Xrays, performing pap smears and breast exams for women, ordering blood and urine tests, prescribing a limited number of drugs, and performing minor surgeries.

Because of their broad backgrounds, naturopathic physicians attract people with a variety of ailments. These include common problems like colds, allergies, digestive disorders, obesity, and chronic fatigue. N.D.s may also prescribe treatments for more serious conditions like arthritis and asthma. It's important to keep in mind, however, that naturopathic treatments have not always proved effective—although they're almost always viewed as safe.

In fact, conscientious N.D.s will refer patients to medical doctors in cases where naturopathy doesn't have the answers. "We're good at just about everything," Dr. Kruzel says. "But there are times when it's best to see an M.D. for a condition." These include irreversible conditions such as late-stage kidney disease and cancers. Even then, Dr. Kruzel says, naturopathic treatments may help improve the quality of life in patients who are also receiving conventional care.

Naturopathy is not just about treating disease, however. It's also about creating better health. "I can't stress prevention and wellness enough," Dr. Schoenbeck says. "Our goal is to make someone healthy, not just free of symptoms." Many patients visit naturopaths once or twice a year for checkups, just to see what they can do to make themselves feel even better through stress relief, diet, and other lifestyle changes.

Finding a Naturopath

If you live in an area covered by a license law, you can be fairly certain that the N.D. you plan to visit has completed the proper training and passed the state's licensing exam. Still, it doesn't hurt to ask. Before you go for your first visit, be sure to ask about credentials. Where did he or she go to school? Does he or she have a license, and can you see it? How long has he or she been in practice? It's also perfectly fine to ask for patient references, if you'd like a little extra peace of mind.

You'll also want to know if the naturopath specializes in treatments that you desire. All naturopaths use nutritional counseling and herbal medicine, for example, but not everyone is qualified to practice acupuncture. Also ask if the N.D. has experience in treating your particular ailment.

Unfortunately, things get a lot murkier in nonlicensing states. It doesn't take much to call yourself a naturopath—sometimes as little as a correspondence course or two. "Just about anyone can hang out a shingle in these places," says Dr. Crinnion. That's why it's essential that to do your homework before visiting the doctor's office.

Recommendations from friends or relatives are a good place to start, but they're not enough. You'll need to ask where the practitioner went to school; the only three schools in the United States that offer license-level educations are Bastyr University in Seattle, the National College of Naturopathic Medicine in Portland, Oregon, and Southwest College of Naturopathic Medicine in Scottsdale, Arizona. You'll also want to know whether he or she has passed any licensing or certification examinations for other states, and if he or she is a member of the AANP, which requires its members to meet minimum education standards.

If not, don't necessarily rule out the practitioner. "Many of these folks have a solid background and can really help," Dr. Schoenbeck says. But be aware that their practices may be limited in scope. The caregiver may not have experience in a broad range of treatments or with a variety of health conditions.

The AANP is pushing for licensing laws in all 50 states. "It's the only way to assure quality care," Dr. Kruzel says. "We want people to know that when they go to an N.D., they're going to someone with the background, knowledge, and skills to take care of them properly."

If you're looking for a naturopathic physician in your area, you can call AANP. They'll provide you with a list of members who have met the group's qualifications and are practicing in good standing. The number for the AANP is 206/298-0125.

One note of caution: Some naturopaths do fall into the more extreme end of alternative medicine—outside the realm of accepted science. Steer clear of any naturopath who seems "fringey" to you.

What to Expect

Once you've found a naturopathic physician who meets your criteria, it's time for your first office visit. Don't be surprised if the appointment takes a lot longer than most trips to the doctor. You and the N.D. are going to spend a lot of time exchanging information and sharing ideas about health care.

- **Expect it to take time.** "I tell patients to figure on at least an hour the first time," Dr. Schoenbeck says. "Remember that we're going to look way beyond trying to eliminate symptoms. We're going after the causes, and we're looking for what's going to make a person truly healthy."
- **Be prepared to answer questions.** You'll probably start by filling out some paperwork, as with any doctor. Expect to see questions about your health history, such as whether you have conditions like high blood pressure, diabetes, heart trouble, arthritis, past surgeries, and anything else that might affect your treatment. You'll also be asked about family history. Has anyone in your family had breast cancer, a stroke, or a condition that could be inherited?
- **Be ready to talk about your life.** Then comes the initial interview with the naturopathic physician. This is where things differ the most from conventional medical visits. The N.D. will certainly ask you what problem has brought you to the office—and what symptoms you'd like to have relieved. But you'll also get some questions that may seem downright shocking in their simplicity: How do you feel? What's your home life like? How are the kids? Are you under a lot of stress? What's life like at work—and how do you cope when problems arise? What do you typically eat for lunch?

"Physical health isn't just about genetics," Dr. Schoenbeck says. "It's about emotions, stresses, the environment, and spirituality. In short, a lot of health is about one's state of mind. That's why we need to know as much about a patient as possible."

- **Expect a multifaceted treatment.** Once the interview is over, the N.D. will get to work on developing a treatment plan for you. You may need some standard preliminary tests—an N.D. may do anything from checking your ears and lungs to taking Xrays or doing blood work—to help define the state of your health. Because of their broad background in natural medicine, naturopathic physicians can draw on a great number of options. A typical prescription may call for a combination of relaxation techniques, dietary changes, massage therapy, homeopathy, acupuncture, and other natural methods.

The key is integration, taking the strengths of one type of treatment and adding the strengths of another. "I'm going to try any number of things," Dr. Schoenbeck says. "The combination of treatments will differ from person to person, depending on their needs and their bodies."

- **Be open to other options.** Sometimes, the treatment plan will include things that the naturopath is not always qualified to perform—such as acupuncture or conventional medical procedures. In these cases, you'll be referred to a specialist or medical doctor.

Treatment Can Take Commitment

Individuals should expect more than just a list of things to do from an N.D. A good naturopathic physician will always take the time to explain why certain treatments are called for. Remember, teaching is a hallmark of naturopathy. "The better a person understands why we're doing something, the more likely he or she is to follow the instructions and help themselves," Dr. Crinnion says.

After the initial visit, the doctor will schedule a follow-up appointment to see how you're doing. How quickly you'll go back depends on the types of treatments you're getting and how serious your illness and symptoms are. It could be a couple of days or a few weeks. In any case, expect the second appointment to last for at least one-half hour, as you and the N.D. discuss how the initial round of treatments went.

Don't ever be afraid to ask questions. After all, it's your health that's at stake. If you have fears or concerns, tell your doctor. Doctors can only help you as much as you're willing to help yourself.

resources

Organizations

American Association of Naturopathic Physicians
601 Valley St., Suite 105
Seattle, WA 98109
206/298-0126
Referral line: 206/298-0125

Colleges

These are the three American colleges that teach naturopathic medicine. Each can provide you with general information and can direct you to a naturopathic physician:

Bastyr University
14500 Juanita Dr., NE
Kenmore, WA 98028
425/823-1300
www.bastyr.edu

National College of Naturopathic Medicine
Referral line: 503/499-4343, Ext. 103
www.ncnm.edu

Southwest College of Naturopathic Medicine and Health Sciences
2140 E. Broadway Rd.
Tempe, AZ 85282
602/858-9100
www.scnm.edu

Books

Alternative Medicine: The Definitive Guide (Future Medicine Publishing, 1993)
This is a comprehensive manual of alternative therapies and includes a sizable section on naturopathy.

American Holistic Health Association Complete Guide to Alternative Medicine by William Collinge (Warner Books, 1997)
Another book that looks at naturopathy among many other alternative treatments.

Alternative Medicine: What Works by Adriane Fugh-Berman, M.D. (Williams & Wilkins, 1997)

chapter 17

osteopathy

A MANIPULATIVE OPTION

> The human body is a machine run by the unseen force called life.
> —*Andrew Taylor Still, founder of osteopathy*

You've been bothered by a nagging pain in your hips and lower back, and now you're having severe muscle spasms in one leg. In succession, you visit a general practitioner, a physical medicine specialist, and a physical therapist. As you trudge from appointment to appointment, you can't help but feel that something is missing in this fragmented approach to health care.

One person is tending to diagnostic tests and dispensing medication, another is in charge of making sure your body is working right, and seemingly no one is trying to determine what caused the problem in the first place—or ensure that it doesn't happen again.

A visit to an osteopathic doctor may be the solution for you. Osteopathy melds "conventional" medical care such as medication and diagnostic tests with manipulative techniques designed to relieve pain and help your body heal.

"As a doctor of osteopathy, I can do manipulation, prescribe medications, or do surgery, whichever is the best treatment for that patient," says Kitturah B. Schomberg-Klaiss, D.O., who specializes in family practice at the West Blocton Family Health Center in Blocton, Alabama. "In one light, it's one-stop shopping to get the health care you need."

What It Is: How It Works

An osteopathic doctor, or D.O., is a trained physician and can treat any condition an M.D. can. An osteopath can dispense drugs and do surgery. In addition, D.O.s are trained in manipulative techniques, using their hands to diagnose problems and "encourage your body's natural tendency toward good health," according to the American Osteopathic Association (AOA). But perhaps the most important distinguishing characteristic of osteopathy is that osteopathic doctors consider the whole patient and focus on preventive care.

The late George W. Northrup, D.O., the longtime editor of the *Journal of the American Osteopathic Association*, once wrote: "Our physicians do take a different attitude toward the patient, his illness, and his various physical, emotional, and even spiritual responses to it."

Multifaceted Therapy

For the troublesome back and hip, the osteopathic doctor could prescribe medications to help reduce inflammation. But the osteopath might also perform manipulative techniques and massage, much as a physical therapist would.

A D.O. will also likely consider how the injury occurred and strive to determine the cause, whether it be a discrepancy in leg length or too many hours working in an awkward position.

Muscle or joint problems are common reasons for seeking an osteopathic doctor, but a D.O. can treat any condition. For sinusitis, for example, an osteopathic doctor might prescribe an antibiotic for the infection and use manipulative techniques to relieve pain and help the sinuses drain.

"Osteopathy is an attitude from which the physician starts that says the patient is a whole unified being, not a collection of systems," says Dr. Schomberg-Klaiss. Osteopathy also teaches that given the appropriate encouragement—whether medications, surgery, or manipulation—your body has the ability to heal itself.

The College of Osteopathic Medicine of the Pacific in Pomona, California, touts these four principles of osteopathy:

- Your body has a tendency to be self-healing. It has an elaborate communication network that includes the circulatory and neuromusculoskeletal systems.
- Structure and function of the body are intimately related.
- In most diseases, there are abnormalities of your neuromusculoskeletal system that can be corrected by manipulation.
- Maintaining a state of health requires constant biological adjustment, including manipulation and other means of diagnosis and treatment.

Manipulative Techniques: Using Hands to Heal

Your body is an intricate, well-designed system of bones, joints, muscles, nerves, and connective tissues. The osteopathic premise is that if there's a problem in your musculoskeletal system, the rest of your body won't work right. Osteopathic doctors are trained in the musculoskeletal system, training that helps them understand how an injury or illness in one part of the body can affect another. This gives them what the AOA calls "a therapeutic and diagnostic advantage."

The manipulative techniques that osteopaths use are known as either Osteopathic Manual Medicine (OMM) or Osteopathic Manipulative Treatment

in the beginning

When Andrew Taylor Still was a youth, he had a bad headache one afternoon. Instinctively he felt that he could relieve the pain by suspending his head. He laid flat on the ground with his head pillowed in a dangling loop of rope, cushioned by a blanket. He'd stumbled across one of the principles of osteopathy that he would later develop.

Dr. Still trained as a medical doctor, like his father, but became vastly disillusioned with conventional medicine in 1864 when he watched three of his young children die from spinal meningitis, despite the best medical attention. He devoted himself to finding a better way and spent many hours dissecting corpses and exploring other healing techniques.

By 1872, he had developed his new and controversial philosophy of medicine. He believed the smooth functioning of the musculoskeletal system was crucial to good health and that the body could help heal itself. He named his new philosophy after *osteon*, meaning bone, and *pathos*, meaning to suffer, intending it to reflect a science "founded on the knowledge of bones."

"The human body is a machine run by the unseen force called life, and that it may be run harmoniously it is necessary that there be liberty of blood, nerves, and arteries from the generating-point to destination," he wrote. "Learn that you are a machine, your heart an engine, your lungs a fanning machine and a sieve, your brain with its two lobes an electric battery."

In 1892, Dr. Still founded a school of osteopathy and began teaching his methods to others. Although he initially decried the use of all drugs, he soon modified his theories to include some drugs, including antiseptics, antidotes, and anesthetics. Some of his followers, however, argued that more drugs and other treatments should be accepted.

By 1929, osteopathic schools included courses on medications. So students could pass state medical licensing exams, schools continued to include more and more mainstream courses, although they retained instruction in manipulative techniques and the "whole body" concept. Today osteopathy still embraces the healing powers of manipulation but encompasses modern medicine as well.

(OMT). They are hands-on treatments that involve working with ligaments and muscles. Some are similar to techniques used by chiropractors and physical therapists.

"OMT is a tool to be used to help people to heal themselves, just like drugs or surgery, and needs to be thought of in the same category," says Dr. Schomberg-Klaiss. "It's not some mystical process. It's a tool to help put things back the way they should be."

There are more than two dozen types of manipulations, and which ones are used depends on the problem involved as well as the person's age and physical conditions.

Some osteopathic doctors, such as Bradley Klock, D.O., of Phoenix, specialize in manipulative techniques. For example, Dr. Klock has worked extensively on hospital patients who've had severe injuries or open-heart surgery. He has also helped people recovering from pneumonia.

"The treatments improve the motion of the rib cage," he explains. "This allows the lungs to expand more fully, which helps them recover."

osteopathy helps heal

- Asthma
- Carpal tunnel syndrome
- Low back pain
- Menstrual pain
- Migraines
- Sinus problems
- Sports injuries

In children, cranial osteopathy may help:

- Colic
- Distortions of cranial bones caused from birth
- Ear problems

Training an Osteopathic Doctor

A D.O., like an M.D., has a four-year undergraduate degree, usually emphasizing science, and must complete four years of medical school. An osteopathic doctor, however, attends one of 19 osteopathic medical colleges.

Some of the educational differences are subtle. The osteopathic curriculum involves preventive care and treating the person as a whole. In addition, a D.O. degree requires 300 to 500 hours in the study of the musculoskeletal system.

After medical school, osteopathic doctors complete a one-year internship, rotating through specialties such as family practice, internal medicine, obstetrics/gynecology, pediatrics, and surgery. Most then select a specialty, such as surgery or radiology, which requires two to six more years of training.

Like an M.D., osteopathic doctors must pass a state licensing exam. They can practice in hospitals and medical centers, as well as in private practice.

Like M.D.s, osteopathic physicians can specialize in any area of medicine. These include cardiology, family practice, general surgery, obstetrics/gynecology, internal medicine, neurology, neurosurgery, pediatrics, sports medicine, otorhinolaryngology (ear, nose, and throat), and psychiatry.

The Great Debate

It is possible to visit a D.O. who uses no manipulative treatment whatsoever and, in fact, seems no different than any M.D. you've ever encountered. What gives? Here's the fly in the ointment: After years of fighting to be regarded as much a "real" doctor as an M.D., some osteopathic doctors fear that the distinction between allopaths (M.D.s) and osteopaths is becoming blurred.

Charles Truthan, D.O., of Grand Rapids, Michigan, suggests in a letter to the *Journal of the American Osteopathic Association*: "We've come dangerously close to the elimination of our reasons to be separate from allopathic physicians."

The philosophy and practices distinctive to osteopathic medicine seem to be disappearing from medical schools, says Norman Gevitz, Ph.D., a professor at Ohio University College of Osteopathic Medicine in Athens, and author of *The D.O.s: Osteopathic Medicine in America*.

At a 1995 symposium on osteopathic medicine, Edward O'Neil, Ph.D., spoke of osteopathic doctors' "sometimes anemic commitment to manipulative therapy." In one study of 506 second-year students at 11 osteopathic universities, most were unconvinced of the effectiveness of osteopathic manipulative therapy—and weren't even sure that enough difference existed between D.O.s and M.D.s to warrant distinct professions.

And two-thirds of osteopathic doctors who are training in primary care are in allopathic residency programs, perhaps because fewer M.D.s are interested in primary care and because of a lack of osteopathic hospitals.

Jack Tuber, D.O., an internal medicine respiratory specialist at the Sun Valley Arthritis Center in Phoenix is a firm believer in manipulative techniques. He once used them in the treatment of people with asthma and restrictive lung disease, but he stopped because of time constraints.

He now refers patients to osteopathic doctors who primarily do manipulations. What remains of the osteopathic principle in his practice is his holistic treatment of patients.

"I think a lot of nonosteopathic subspecialists concentrate on their small area, while my consults reflect the whole system," he says. "There's no such thing as your lungs working independently from the rest of your body."

Scientific Rationale

Osteopathic medicine has come a long, long way since the early days when osteopaths were consider little better than quacks or charlatans. In 1925, for instance, Morris Fishbein, M.D., then editor of the *JAMA* referred scathingly to osteopathy as "an attempt to enter the practice of medicine by the back door."

These days you can rest assured that your D.O. is likely just as qualified as a comparable M.D. In a 1971 study published in the *JAMA*, 9.3 percent of graduates of U.S. medical schools failed their medical board exam. In contrast, only 1.6 percent of graduates of U.S. osteopathic medical schools failed.

And osteopathic manipulative techniques have certainly shown their value in one scientific study after another.

osteopathic treatments

In addition to simple movement of the joints to improve range of motion or to move past a restriction, treatment may include these techniques:

- **Counterstrain.** This technique reduces restriction by placing the affected joint or muscle in a position of comfort and at the same time applying a counterstretch to the tight muscles, directly opposite to the strain.
- **Cranial treatment.** This technique involves palpating bones of the cranium and spine, and may help people with headaches and many other problems.
- **High velocity low amplitude thrusting (HVLA).** Better known as "popping," this technique involves fast, short thrusts. It's usually used on people who are generally healthy to quickly realign joints that are out of place, says Kitturah B. Schomberg-Klaiss, D.O., who specializes in family practice at the West Blocton Family Health Center in Blocton, Alabama. Any time you pop your knuckles or stretch and pop your neck, you're doing much the same thing as when a doctor does HVLA, just in a less controlled fashion.
- **Lymphatic technique.** The aim here is to encourage the circulation of lymphatic fluids. While the patient is lying on his or her back, pressure may be applied with the hands to the upper chest wall then removed suddenly.
- **Muscle energy.** In this technique contracted muscles are released by alternately being stretched then made to work against resistance supplied by the doctor. This is an isometric stretching technique done to relax muscle spasms. To get some pelvic muscles to relax, for example, there is a technique called Fabre's maneuvers, in which the patient pushes with his or her legs on the practitioner, while the practitioner resists the motion. The patient then relaxes, and the practitioner pushes the leg back farther. It's done three times in each of three positions on both legs, then one position involves both legs. It causes the muscles to stretch out and relax and is good for low back and pelvic pain.
- **Range of motion.** Joints are taken through their range of motion.
- **Visceral techniques.** These involve gentle and rhythmic stretching of the visceral areas to improve the health of internal organs.

Which techniques will your doctor use? It depends on you, your age, your condition, your problem, and even on your doctor. Some osteopaths are more skilled and hence more comfortable with certain techniques than others.

What's the difference between visiting a physical therapist or a chiropractor and visiting an osteopath? Unlike either of those two professions, an osteopathic doctor can order lab tests, prescribe medication, and do surgery.

"While there can be some overlap with different therapies like chiropractic and physical therapy, neither has the depth or scope of osteopathic medicine," says Dr. Schomberg-Klaiss.

Osteopathy Shows Its Stuff

Researchers at the New York College of Osteopathic Medicine in Old Westbury, New York, suggests that the best treatment of osteoarthritis may be a combination of osteopathic manipulative therapy and moderate exercise.

In one study at the Philadelphia College of Osteopathic Medicine, osteopathic manipulative treatment helped to relieve headache pain, regardless of what kind of headache it was.

It turned out that treatment with more than one pain-relieving technique was more effective than one technique. The kind known as myofascial release was the most effective.

Osteopathic manipulation apparently can help relieve the pressure on the median nerve that causes carpal tunnel syndrome, according to a study done at the Center for Carpal Tunnel Studies in Paradise Valley, Arizona.

Benjamin Sucher, D.O., a specialist in physical medicine and rehabilitation, says that manipulation can lengthen the transverse carpal ligament, which compresses the nerve in the carpal tunnel. (The carpal tunnel is an opening in the wrist bones through which nerves to the hand must pass. Compression of these nerves causes the pain and numbing associated with carpal tunnel syndrome.)

How to Find the Best Practitioner

Osteopathic doctors are outnumbered by their M.D. colleagues: There are roughly 600,000 M.D.s in the United States, and around 37,000 D.O.s. Half of these osteopathic doctors practice in family practice, internal medicine, obstetrics/gynecology, and pediatrics; and they make up just 5.5 percent of the total number of doctors in the U.S.

You can find an osteopathic doctor by opening your telephone directory to the Physicians section and finding ones with D.O. after their names.

Remember that not every osteopathic physician uses manipulative techniques, points out Richard A. Feely, D.O., senior clinician at American WholeHealth and adjunct associate professor of osteopathic medicine at the Chicago College of Osteopathic Medicine at Midwestern University in Downers Grove, Illinois. In a 1998 survey by the AOA, 85 percent of the 523 osteopathic doctors surveyed did use manipulative treatments. Doctors living in the West were more likely to use OMT, as were family practitioners. Many osteopathic family physicians do OMT or OMM regularly.

If you specifically want a doctor that does manipulative techniques, call a D.O.'s office and ask, says Dr. Schomberg-Klaiss. Or your current doctor may be able to refer you. You also can contact your state's osteopathic association, says Dr. Feely. It offers a list of members who do manipulation.

the osteopathic oath

I do hereby affirm my loyalty to the profession I am about to enter. I will be mindful always of my great responsibility to preserve the health and the life of my patients, to retain their confidence and respect, both as a physician and a friend who will guard their secrets with scrupulous honor and fidelity, to perform faithfully my professional duties, to employ only those recognized methods of treatment consistent with good judgment and with my skill and ability, keeping in mind always nature's laws and the body's inherent capacity for recovery.

I will be ever vigilant in aiding in the general welfare of the community, sustaining its laws and institutions, not engaging in those practices which will in any way bring shame or discredit upon myself or my profession. I will give no drugs for deadly purposes to any person, though it may be asked of me.

I will endeavor to work in accord with my colleagues in a spirit of progressive cooperation and never by word or by act cast imputations upon them or their rightful practices.

I will look with respect and esteem upon all those who have taught me my art. To my college I will be loyal and strive always for its best interests and for the interests of the students who will come after me. I will be ever alert to further the application of basic biologic truths to the healing arts and to develop the principles of osteopathy which were first enunciated by Andrew Taylor Still.

Using Osteopathy

So you're making your first visit to an osteopathic doctor. What should you expect? Will anything be different? First, the doctor will ask you to fill out a complete medical history form. "Then I ask everything I feel I need to know about what may have caused their problem," says osteopath Dr. Klock.

An osteopath may ask if you've been coughing or if you've had digestive problems, for instance, to try to determine if something other than a mechanical problem may be causing your pain.

The osteopathic doctor will do a physical exam, manually examining and moving your joints and checking the curves of your spine, how your chest moves, and the symmetry of both sides of your body. He or she may check your posture and your balance and look for areas of tenderness in your muscles or tendons.

The osteopath is investigating to determine which muscles may be holding your bones in odd positions, and your treatment will be aimed at stretching the muscles, repositioning the bones, and establishing body symmetry by relieving joint misalignments.

Your doctor may also check your blood pressure or test your reflexes, or perhaps order lab tests or Xrays if warranted. Your doctor may give you advice on how to help correct your posture, change your diet, or alter your exercise or work habits.

When treatment begins, your doctor may use heat packs to help relieve muscle spasm or to improve your blood flow. Both of these things can help you relax and make manipulation easier.

What to Expect

Your initial visit to an osteopathic doctor may take up to an hour. Future visits for manipulative treatments will not take as long, but the time will vary. And there's no way to accurately predict how long or how often your doctor will want to see you, because it will vary greatly depending on your problem. In some cases, however, your doctor may need to see you as often as two or three times a week for a few weeks.

Costs vary greatly. But on average, osteopathic treatment may cost less than treatment by an M.D. In a 1996 study of 1,000 worker compensation claims in Colorado, the average cost per claim for an osteopathic doctor was $1,007, compared to $2,895 for a nonsurgical M.D., $2,775 for a chiropractor, and $2,457 for a physical therapist.

Insurance pays for visits to D.O.s just as it does for M.D. visits. Some plans, however, don't cover manipulative treatments. According to a 1998 survey by the AOA, half of managed-care providers did not reimburse for OMT, but 80 percent of other health plans did.

Safety and Warnings

Just as every M.D. isn't the right doctor for every condition, neither is every D.O. "The osteopathic physician is licensed and trained in the diagnosis of and treatment of all diseases, like M.D.s, and likewise, all doctors might not be expert enough or the right fit to effectively diagnose and treat your condition," says Dr. Feely.

Here are some tips for making the most of osteopathic resources:

- **See a specialist when necessary.** If you have a condition that needs specialized treatment—such as the services of a surgeon or a cancer specialist, for instance, your osteopathic doctor will refer you, just as an M.D. would. (It's possible that your specialist could be a D.O. as well.)

- **Don't expect to use osteopathy for everything.** For certain conditions osteopathic manipulation wouldn't be an appropriate treatment. Acute appendicitis, for instance, will require emergency surgery, and a heart attack will likely need clot-busting drugs.

"Which is not to say OMT can't help in these circumstances," says Dr. Schomberg-Klaiss. "For example, I will do some OMT on a patient having acute asthma while I wait for the inhaling apparatus to be set up to deliver the breathing treatment to the patient, to buy a little time. It's not a definitive treatment, and nowhere near as effective as the breathing treatment, but it can buy me a little time to get it set up."

Some manipulative techniques should not be used in other cases, notes Dr. Klock, such as in people with significant osteoporosis, bone cancer, a bone or joint infection, or severe slipped disks.

- **Change treatments if you're not satisfied.** And, just as with any doctor, your doctor must fit your needs, which sometimes can be a matter of personality or simply communications. "If you are uncomfortable or unhappy with any physician or the treatment, you should either look for another doctor or another form of treatment," says Dr. Schomberg-Klaiss.

- **Appreciate what osteopathy has to offer.** In some cases OMT may not affect the outcome, but can make a person more comfortable, says Dr. Schomberg-Klaiss. She cites the case of her father who was hospitalized with a severe infection, a kind that is frequently fatal. His temperature was 104 degrees and not responding to conventional treatment. He was red and flushed. She performed several osteopathic techniques, including effleurage (a kind of stroking of the face designed to improve circulation), lymphatic pump techniques (designed to improve function of the lymphatic system, which is involved in the immune functions), and foot massage (to improve their circulation).

Within 90 minutes, his temperature dropped to 101 degrees, the flushed quality of his face improved, his heart rate dropped by about 10 beats per minute, and they were able to decrease the amount of sedation he was under while still maintaining his comfort.

"The next day, my father died," says Dr. Schomberg-Klaiss. "By that measure, what I did wasn't helpful. But he was more comfortable in his last hours, and most people would consider that a big benefit."

osteopathy for your head

You may be surprised to learn that your skull isn't a solid piece of bone. It consists of plates connected by joints called sutures. If all is well, the fluid that flows around your brain, spinal cord, and tailbone (sacrum) pulses at a rate of eight to 14 times a minutes, says Richard A. Feely, D.O., of Chicago College of Osteopathic Medicine at Midwestern University in Downer's Grove, Illinois.

Cranial osteopathy is a subspecialty of osteopathy that works with the bones of the cranium. "It involves freeing up the circulation, balancing the circulation of the spinal fluid," explains Bradley Klock, D.O., a Phoenix osteopath who specializes in osteopathic manipulation.

Pressure on your cranial or spinal bones can apparently affect the rate of flow, called the cranial rhythmic impulse. A trained cranial osteopath can detect problems in the flow rate by touch, then correct problems by gently manipulating the cranial and spinal bones. Cranial osteopathy, developed by William Garner Sutherland, D.O., in 1899, can help with asthma; sinusitis; ear, nose, and throat problems; and headaches, says Dr. Feely.

Many childhood problems emanate from cranial problems, according to Viola Frymann, D.O., founder of the Osteopathic Center for Children in San Diego and one of the founders of Western University in Pomona, California. Roughly 1 of 10 babies has a visible cranial problem at birth; another 1 of 10 has a perfectly adjusted cranium, says Dr. Frymann. The other 80 percent have minor misadjustments that may cause an irritation of the nerves involved in the sucking process or in digestion, for example, possibly resulting in eating problems.

Recurrent ear infections in children have also been linked to cranial problems. In a study of Missouri children in kindergarten through third grade, children born with abnormal head shapes had more inner ear infections. Injuries, as from a fall in which the back of the head is struck, says Dr. Frymann, may result in ear problems because of problems in the temporal bone (which holds the ear) or neck bones.

Another, somewhat similar technique called CranioSacral Therapy was developed by John Upledger, D.O., in the 1970s. A primary difference is that CranioSacral Therapy focuses on fluid and membranes rather than bones. The Upledger Institute in Palm Beach Gardens, Florida, offers classes and certification in CranioSacral Therapy, which the institute describes as using the rhythm of the craniosacral system to find restrictions and relieving these by "light touch therapy."

While a cranial osteopathist must have a medical degree (either a D.O. or M.D.), craniosacral therapists are not required to have medical training.

resources

Information

To locate a D.O. in your area, write to:
American Osteopathic Association
142 E. Ontario St.
Chicago, IL 60611
800/621-1773

For more information about osteopaths who are board-certified in osteopathic manipulative medicine or about Osteopathic Manipulative Treatment or D.O.s, contact:
American Academy of Osteopathy
3500 DePauw Blvd., Suite 1080
Indianapolis, IN 46268–1139

To find a D.O. who specializes in cranial osteopathy—an offshoot of osteopathy that involves manipulating cranial and spinal bones—contact:
Cranial Academy
8202 Clearvista Parkway, No. 9D
Indianapolis, IN 46256

Books

The D.O.s: Osteopathic Medicine in America by Norman Gevitz, Ph.D. (Johns Hopkins University Press, 1991)

Foundations for Osteopathic Medicine by Robert C. Ward, John A. Jerome, and John M. Jones III (Williams and Wilkins, 1997)

Discover Osteopathy by Peta Sneddon and Paolo Coseschi (Ulysses Press, 1997)

An Integrated Approach to Musculoskeletal Disorders Through Eastern & Western Methods by Alon Marcus (North Atlantic Books, 1999)

Your Inner Physician and You: CranioSacral Therapy and Somatoemotional Release, 2nd Ed., John E. Upledger (North Atlantic Books, 1997)

(Of Historical Interest)
CranioSacral Therapy by John Upledger and Jon Vredevoogd (Eastland Press, 1983)

Teaching in the Science of Osteopathy by William Garner Sutherland (Sutherland Cranial Teaching Foundation, 1990)

chapter 18

relaxation therapy

PURE STRESS RELIEF

You can think of spirit as the subtlest form of matter, or you can think of matter as the densest form of spirit. Physical bodies, emotions, thoughts, and spirit are all interpenetrating energy structures. —*Patricia Norris, Ph.D.*

"You need to relax!"

How often do you say this to the people around you or mutter it to yourself as you try to cope with the pressures of daily living? You're not alone. Almost everyone feels this way.

If you're feeling more stressed and overwhelmed than you were 15 or 20 years ago, it's not just that you've aged. "The world is more stressful," says L. John Mason, Ph.D., author of Guide to Stress Reduction. *"The pace of change has accelerated tremendously," and as a result, "more people are physically and emotionally overwhelmed today than ever before in human history."*

Modern Life Is Stressful

Shifting lifestyles and uncertain values, the incessant bombardment of information, economic demands, job insecurity, pollutants in our air, water, and food—all these and many other factors place constant stress on our fragile bodies. All of us feel the pressure to achieve goals, meet deadlines, organize our time, and live up to our many responsibilities at home and at work. As stress and pressure build up, the more urgent becomes the need to relax, to let go, to find a way to loosen tense muscles and reach a place of quiet within, a calm center in the midst of the storm. "As parents and as adults, we have to set an example for the younger generation, including our children, of actively caring for ourselves," says Dr. Mason. "The pace of change has accelerated, but our immune systems and survival mechanisms have not evolved. Unless we learn to relax, we simply can't keep up with the rate of change without suffering from stress-related health problems."

The practices and procedures in this chapter have been developed to help you slow down, release tension, and let go of stress. These techniques are among the safest, easiest, most widely researched, and enthusiastically prescribed of the healing modalities in this book. Some have come from ancient traditions of the East. Others have been created by Western physicians and psychologists. They are used in hospitals, clinics, and wellness centers around the country, and are an inseparable part of the Eastern approaches to health discussed in this book, including ayurveda and Chinese medicine.

These techniques have proved effective, and they have this added advantage: They are all relatively easy to learn. Once learned, they are entirely suitable for practice on your own.

Our Innate Stress Response

Just after the turn of the century, a Harvard scientist, the physiologist Walter B. Cannon, was documenting the stress reaction known as the "fight or flight" response. This spectrum of physiological events erupts instantaneously in our bodies whenever we become frightened, threatened, or otherwise agitated.

Whether the cause is a sudden loud noise, an angry remark, an impending deadline at work, or a near miss on the freeway, your entire system becomes primed for physical exertion. Adrenaline pours into your bloodstream to increase available energy, and your heart speeds up and pumps more blood with each beat, preparing you to fight or run. Your breathing also speeds up and becomes deeper, as more oxygen is taken in. Your muscles contract and tense up, and your hands and feet become cold, as blood vessels constrict to prevent blood loss in case of injury. Your blood pressure soars.

These reactions are entirely natural and eminently useful—if you really do need to fight or run. But if you have to keep on driving or continue working at your desk without a chance to release the built-up energy, and if this happens day after day, it takes a tremendous toll on the body.

Indeed, experts estimate that from 75 to 90 percent of all illnesses are caused or complicated by stress. According to Harold H. Bloomfield, M.D., one of the nation's leading health educators: "Stress weakens the immune system and adversely affects heart function, hormone levels, the nervous system, memory, thinking ability, and mind-body coordination. It raises blood cholesterol and blood pressure, and increases the risk of many, many diseases, including heart disease and cancer. Stress has even been found to kill brain cells and appears to prematurely age the adult brain."

In everyday terms, stress makes us feel tired, tense, rushed, and cranky. We become more susceptible to anger and impatience, more liable to make mistakes.

preparing the way

In 1904 Harvard psychologist William James addressed a class of young women about to graduate from a nearby college. In his talk, James spoke of "those absurd feelings of hurry and having no time, that breathlessness and tension ... that lack of inner harmony and ease ... the tension in our faces and in our unused muscles" that seemed, even then, to characterize Americans.

Remember, this was before automobiles and airplanes, telephones and television, cell phones and beepers. Imagine how our stress levels have escalated since then.

Professor James pointed prophetically to the future of mind-body medicine, as well as to the need for relaxation techniques, when he told the assembled young women, "If you never wholly give yourself up to the chair you sit in, but always keep your leg and body muscles half contracted; if you breathe eighteen or nineteen instead of sixteen times per minute ... what mental mood can you be in but one of inner panting and expectancy, and how can the future and its worries possibly forsake your mind?" On the other hand, he said, how can those worries "gain admission to your mind if your brow be unruffled, your respiration calm and complete, and your muscles all relaxed?"

Discovering the Antidote to Stress

A few pioneer researchers began advocating relaxation as a medical tool early in the 20th century, but their ideas didn't really start to catch on until after the turbulent 60s. When Edmund Jacobson, creator of the technique of Progressive Relaxation, revised his popular book *You Must Relax* in 1957, he told his readers, "I had to contend with the fact that doctors and laymen alike were prone to think of amusement, recreation, or hobbies at the mention of the word 'relax.'" It took a good many more years for the word to take on its current meaning, to become, as Dr. Jacobson said, a "part and parcel of daily speech in the sense of 'let go' or 'take it easy.'"

In 1970 a landmark paper appeared in the prestigious journal *Science*. In it, Robert Keith Wallace described the results of his research at University of California in Los Angeles on Transcendental Meditation (TM). His studies uncovered a whole constellation of positive physical changes in response to meditation, precisely opposite to what happens during the stressful fight or flight response:

- Breathing becomes slower and shallower.
- Metabolic rate slows down, indicating deep rest.
- Heart rate slows.
- Muscles relax.
- Blood vessels apparently dilate, as the hands and feet warm up.
- Blood pressure is slightly reduced, especially in individuals with high blood pressure.
- Changes in blood chemistry, such as decreased concentrations of lactate and cortisol, indicate a reduction of stress and anxiety.
- Brain waves tend to shift to an alpha pattern, long associated with calm and relaxation.

The "Relaxation Response"

From UCLA, Dr. Wallace moved on to Harvard Medical School, where he teamed up with Herbert Benson, M.D., a cardiologist and associate professor who was studying high blood pressure. Dr. Benson later confessed that when the idea of studying the TM technique as a potential remedy for high blood pressure was first proposed to him, he rejected it "with a polite 'Thank you.' Why investigate anything so far-out as meditation?"

But he relented, and studies were begun. As the results came in, Dr. Benson was surprised to find not only a lowering of blood pressure but also the broad spectrum of physiological changes described above.

These pioneer researchers had discovered an innate mechanism of the body that could easily be activated by anyone. By sitting quietly with eyes closed and practicing a simple meditation technique, a person could enjoy a pleasant, relaxed state with the power to reverse or neutralize the effects of stress. Over the next few years Dr. Benson extended his research to other meditation and relaxation techniques, identifying what he felt were the core ingredients needed to elicit the "relaxation response."

Since then, hundreds of scientific studies done around the world have scrutinized meditation and relaxation. Jack Forem, former director of the International Meditation Society in New York, recalls that "even though the early scientific research was consistent and convincing, many people remained skeptical about meditation and relaxation."

"Times have really changed," says Forem. "Now just about everyone realizes how important it is to use our God-given ability to deeply relax and dissolve stress."

Different Strokes for Different Folks

Not all relaxation therapies use the same approach. Some (like Progressive Relaxation) are essentially physical techniques, while others (like meditation and visualization) are entirely mental.

Results also vary. One scientific comparison (known technically as a

benefits of
relaxation techniques

Because so many illnesses and conditions are stress-related, it's no surprise that a long list of ills—mental, emotional, and physical—can be helped, sometimes dramatically, by eliciting the stress-neutralizing relaxation response.

Here are some of the proven benefits:

Physical benefits:
- Alleviation of PMS symptoms
- Deep rest indicated by reduced metabolic rate, slower heart rate, slower breathing (This deep rest, in some studies shown to be deeper than sleep, is relaxing and healing.)
- Increased longevity
- Pain relief
- Reduced muscle tension
- Reduction of high blood pressure, especially in mild to moderate cases
- Reduction of asthma symptoms
- Relief from arthritis pain

Other benefits, some primarily subjective and others increasingly supported by research, include:
- Help with insomnia
- Increased energy
- Relief from tension headaches, backaches, and gastrointestinal disorders

Psychological and spiritual benefits:
- Equanimity and emotional balance
- Faster reaction time and improved mind-body coordination
- Growth of intelligence, learning ability, and improvement of memory
- Heightened perception
- Improved concentration and attention
- Increased alpha brain waves (This type of mental activity is associated with a calm, relaxed state of being.)
- Reduced anxiety
- Synchronization of brain waves between the right and left, and front and rear of the brain—indicative of increased creativity

Behavioral benefits:
- Decreased use of alcohol, cigarettes, and other addictive drugs
- Greater ability to recover from stress
- Increased empathy, compassion, and ability to love

"metanalysis") of 146 studies on various relaxation methods purporting to relieve anxiety found that the TM technique was nearly twice as effective as any other practice.

Because you are a unique individual, however, you will undoubtedly find some method or methods easier to learn, more enjoyable, and more effective than others. It's a good idea to try several to find what works best for you. In this chapter, you'll find the basics of several different techniques.

rate your level of tension

One way to gauge the effectiveness of your experiments with relaxation therapy is to rate your level of tension before and after each relaxation session. On a scale of 0 to 100, with 0 being totally relaxed and 100 being very tense, rate your tension level. Make yourself a chart like the one below. If you lower your tension level even a point or two, you have done something important for yourself.

Please note: If keeping score makes you anxious because you feel you have to do well, forget this suggestion. The goal is to relax.

Day	Session One:		Session Two:	
	Before	After	Before	After
Monday	65	55	60	45
Tuesday	70	50	75	40

Practical Considerations

Instruction in meditation and relaxation techniques is offered by thousands of individuals and institutions. For maximum results, it's best to learn with a qualified, experienced trainer. Take some time to investigate the qualifications of your potential teacher and remember that not everyone who has learned a technique is qualified to guide others in learning it.

Most teachers offer classes for groups as well as individual instruction. Costs range from a few dollars for a class at a local Y or community center to $50 to $75 or even more per session, especially in a clinical setting. Instruction often requires a series of eight to 12 sessions.

The technique that is probably the most extensively studied, Transcendental Meditation, also costs quite a lot as an initial outlay (currently about $600, with reduced rates for students and families) but offers unlimited free follow-ups with trained teachers at any TM center worldwide.

For most of these methods, experienced trainers say it usually takes at least four to six weeks for results to take hold. So be be patient!

If your physician prescribes relaxation therapy for pain management, high blood pressure, or another health problem, it may be covered by your health insurance. But most insurers still do not cover relaxation or meditation programs for preventive purposes.

What kind of results can you expect? Many wonderful benefits of relaxation and meditation techniques have been documented in thousands of studies, including pain relief, freedom from anxiety and stress, a deeper sense of emotional balance and well-being, and enhanced overall health.

Now let's take a look at some of these helpful practices.

Progressive Relaxation: Letting Go of Muscle Tension

In 1908 Dr. Jacobson began his studies of muscle relaxation. Long before the days of mind/body medicine, Dr. Jacobson understood the intimate connection between body and mind. He saw that there was a correspondence between muscle tension and many illnesses that we today would call psychosomatic. He also believed that releasing the tension would be healing. To help people free themselves of unwanted and unneeded tension, he devoted his entire career to the study of relaxation.

Dr. Jacobson also believed that whatever our external circumstances may be, we can deal with them more calmly and effectively if we are relaxed. His research corroborated this commonsense notion, showing that people who were tense were easily startled and upset, while more relaxed individuals were much less prone to irritation or distress.

Dr. Jacobson's main method, which he called Progressive Relaxation, involves the sequential tensing and relaxing of various muscle groups. If you want to try it, here is a simple version you can do at home. You may find it easier if you make a tape of these instructions and play it softly to yourself. (For more details, see "Make Your Own Relaxation Tape" on page 219.)

Practicing Progressive Relaxation

Begin by lying on your back with your eyes closed, head resting on a small pillow so it's raised only a few inches. Your feet should be slightly apart, your arms at your sides.

- **Leave distractions behind.** Give yourself permission to use this period of time for yourself—to forget about the things on your mind, and on your to-do list.
- **Take a deep breath.** Fill your abdomen first and then your chest. Breathe out, letting go of as much tension as you can.
- **Start by slightly tightening your right fist.** Tighten it just enough so you can feel the tension (the tensed muscles) in your hand, wrist, and arm. Hold a few seconds, paying full attention to the feeling of tension. Then release. Let go and relax.
- **Observe the relaxation.** Notice how different it feels from the tension. Without trying to do anything, continue for at least a minute to relax your right hand and arm.
- **Now slightly tighten your left fist.** Tighten it just enough that you can feel the tension in the muscles of your hand, wrist, and arm. Again, hold for a few seconds, paying full attention to the tension. Then open the fist. Let go and relax.
- **Observe the relaxation.** Notice the difference between "doing" and "not doing."

7 more keys to relaxation

Everyone has a way to relax. There are certainly more than the few detailed in this chapter. Here are seven more that have proved effective.

- **Music.** The relaxing effects of music are well documented. (See Music and Art Therapy on page 171 for more details.) So treat yourself to half an hour of quiet listening to soothe your soul! Sit or lie down, close your eyes, and just be with the flow of sounds. Musical tastes differ widely so it's hard to make recommendations, but for deep relaxation, slow movements of classical music, especially from the Baroque era (Bach, Handel, the famous *Canon in D* by Pachelbel) are considered excellent. You might also try one of the hundreds of "meditative" CDs or tapes now available, or some minimalist or New Age compositions by Steve Halpern, George Winston, and others.
- **Exercise.** Physical exertion—but not too much for your age and fitness level—is the most natural way to defuse the stressful "fight or flight" response and restore equilibrium. A vigorous half-hour walk is good for almost everyone.
- **Yoga.** Yoga stretching exercises are an effective, enjoyable way to relax. Your best bet is a local class with a properly trained instructor. (For more on the benefits of yoga, see page 297.)
- **Breathing.** There is an ancient saying that "the mind rides on the breath." Calming the breath through deep, rhythmic yogic breathing quiets the mind and soothes the emotions.
- **Carbohydrates.** Proteins make the mind and body alert and lively, carbohydrates settle you down. Eat proteins early in the day for productivity. Have a high carbohydrate dinner (whole grain cereal, pasta, potatoes) for relaxation and sleep.
- **Prayer.** Like meditation, prayer is generally not undertaken to induce relaxation but to contact a higher reality. But the inward process of prayer may take us to a deep, silent level of our own being. In *Varieties of Prayer,* sociologist Margaret Poloma, Ph.D., and pollster George Gallup report that 88 percent of Americans who pray say they sometimes experience a deep sense of peace and well-being.
- **Avoid caffeine.** The speed-up effects of caffeine are just the opposite of what you need if you want to relax. But cut down slowly. Caffeine is addictive, and going cold turkey can give rise to headaches.

Whatever you have done (or not done) to relax, continue, allowing yourself to relax your left arm more and more.

- **Move through your body.** Next slightly tighten then release the following parts of your body. Each time, tense the muscles just enough to become conscious of the tension, hold a few seconds, then relax and continue to observe the feeling as the relaxation deepens.
  - Tighten and release your right foot and toes. Be careful not to tighten too much or the muscles may cramp.
  - Tighten and release your left foot and toes.
  - Tighten and relax the muscles in your right leg.
  - Tighten and relax your left leg.
  - Tighten your buttocks and release.
  - Drawing the stomach muscles slightly in, tense your abdomen, then relax.
- **Focus on your chest.** Breathe in deeply and hold your breath for a few seconds. Notice the tension in your chest. Then exhale, letting the tension melt and release.
- **Focus on your shoulders.** Pull your shoulders upward (toward your head) and hold for a few seconds. Notice the tension in the neck and shoulders. Then drop your shoulders back down and observe the feelings of relaxation.
- **Wrinkle up your forehead and tighten your scalp.** Feel the tension for a few seconds, then completely release.
- **Now frown.** Tighten the muscles of your forehead. Release.
- **Squeeze your eyes tightly shut.** Hold for a few seconds, then release and relax.
- **Clench your jaw enough to feel the tension.** Then release it, letting the tension go.
- **Focus on your tongue.** Press your tongue against the roof of your mouth for a few seconds. You will feel tension at the back of the mouth. Hold, then release.
- **Press your lips together.** Then, without relaxing them, move them into an "O." Relax and notice the contrast.
- **Focus on your head.** Turn your head to the right and notice the tension in your neck. Then turn your head to the left. Then come back to a restful position and completely relax.
- **Lie quietly for a few more minutes.** Mentally scan your body for any places that remain tense and allow them to relax. Let all tension dissolve away, as you completely relax.

Autogenic Training

Stanford University professor of medicine Kenneth Pelletier, M.D., Ph.D., a longtime leader in the field of stress reduction, described autogenic therapy as "one of the most comprehensive and successful Western deep relaxation techniques." The word "autogenic" means "self-generated" or "generated from within."

The purpose of this therapy is to generate, from within the mind, a deeply relaxed state of body conducive to health and well-being. The principles of Autogenic Therapy (also known as Autogenic Training or AT) were developed in the 1920s and 30s by the German neurologist and psychiatrist, Dr. Johannes Schultz. His work was furthered over the succeeding decades in Canada by his pupil and later colleague,

Dr. Wolfgang Luthe. There are now more than 3,000 scientific papers documenting the effectiveness of AT.

AT is taught and practiced widely in Europe, the United Kingdom, Canada, and Japan, and is beginning to be used in stress-reduction and holistic health centers around the United States, often in conjunction with biofeedback. As with all the techniques in this chapter, you should learn AT from a qualified trainer.

However, you'll find the basics of the AT course in this chapter, so you can at least try it for yourself. Keep in mind that it is usually taught in eight to 10 weekly lessons. Trainers in AT say it normally takes at least a few weeks for results to take hold.

What kind of results can you expect? Proponents point to research showing this training as a way to gain freedom from anxiety and stress, find a deeper sense of emotional balance and well-being, and enhance overall health.

At the beginning, practice the AT exercises for just a few minutes, three or four times a day. Once you have mastered them, you can increase the time up to half an hour. It's fine to practice on a train or plane, in a waiting room, or for a few minutes at your desk to defuse stress.

One of the main features of AT—as well as biofeedback and some traditional practices like Buddhist "mindfulness" meditation—is the attitude of what's known as "passive volition" (sometimes called "passive concentration"). Rather than making an effort or trying to achieve a specific outcome, you simply become an alert, relaxed observer.

Trainers emphasize that there are no right or wrong results during the practice of AT. All you need to do is carry out the exercises with the right posture and mental attitude.

Practicing Autogenic Therapy

To practice AT, sit up comfortably, preferably in a nice soft armchair, or lie on your back with head supported and arms resting by your sides. Your eyes should be closed. The practice consists of repeating (silently and not too quickly) a series of phrases while gently focusing your attention on different areas of your body in the following six stages:

- **My right arm is very heavy.** (six times)
  I am completely calm. (once)
  My left arm is very heavy. (six times)
  I am completely calm. (once)
  My right leg is very heavy. (six times)
  I am completely calm. (once)
  My left leg is very heavy. (six times)
  I am completely calm. (once)
- **My right arm is very warm.** (six times)
  I am completely calm. (once)
  My left arm is very warm. (six times)
  I am completely calm. (once)
  My right leg is very warm. (six times)
  I am completely calm. (once)
  My left leg is very warm. (six times)
  I am completely calm. (once)
- **My heart beats calmly and regularly.** (six times)
  I am completely calm. (once)
- **My breathing is calm and regular.** (six times)

(If you have trouble with this and find yourself controlling or regulating your breathing, add "It breathes me.")

I am completely calm. (once)

- **My solar plexus (or abdomen) is warm.** (six times)

I am completely calm. (once)

- **My forehead is pleasantly cool.** (six times)

I am completely calm. (once)

After you have completed all these steps and are ready to finish your session, say, mentally, "Arms firm; breathe deeply; open eyes."

Then take a minute or so to stretch, move your hands and feet, and rotate your head gently. Only then should you open your eyes.

If you were learning Autogenic Training with a therapist, you would most likely learn only one phase at a time: heaviness in the first session or several sessions, followed by warmth, then calm heartbeat, and so on. You can try it that way at home, taking four to 10 months to master all six exercises.

Meditation and the Quiet Mind

Meditation comes in so many different varieties it is difficult to adequately define in a sentence or two. There are techniques involving concentration and focus, contemplative practices of quiet thought, visualizations, mindfulness practices, even meditations to be done while walking. To choose among them is a daunting task, but don't be discouraged. The benefits of an authentic meditation practice are potentially life-transforming. Here are some guidelines:

Broadly speaking, the goal of meditation is to fathom deeper levels of the mind. "Our mind can be compared to an ocean," says the International Meditation Society's Jack Forem. "The surface may be choppy and full of waves, but deep down, it's quiet and still. Meditation is a way to allow the waves to settle down, so you can experience the calm and peace—sometimes called the Kingdom of Heaven—that is traditionally said to lie within us all."

It's important to remember, says Forem, that all the great religions in the world advocate quiet meditation. "Meditation is traditionally a spiritual practice, a doorway to the infinite," he says, "not a relaxation practice. But because of the mind-body connection, when the mind settles down, the body also quiets down, and you feel relaxed. That's the reason science has been able to document all those physical changes."

Practicing Meditation

Here is a simple but very effective meditation practice:

- **Get comfortable.** Choose a place where you can be relatively undisturbed. Sit comfortably, in a chair, on the couch, or on the floor, with your spine comfortably erect. Close your eyes.
- **After a minute or so, begin to notice your breathing.** Notice the in-breath and the out-breath. You may notice the rise and fall of your chest or abdomen, or, if you are quite settled, how the air is cool as it enters your nostrils and warmer as you exhale.

- **Focus on the breath.** Quietly and gently, without trying to accomplish anything, without manipulating the breath in any way, simply "follow" the breath with your awareness. Don't make an effort to concentrate.
- **Notice the pauses between breaths.** If this becomes easy for you, you may add an advanced level to your practice. At the end of each in-breath, notice the natural "turn" that precedes the out-breath. Likewise, after the out-breath, you will notice a "pause" and "turn" before the next inhalation. Simply note these with your quiet awareness.
- **Stay tuned.** Each time you become aware that your attention has drifted away from the breath—and it will happen several times—simply come back. You may find yourself thinking, planning, making lists, fantasizing, listening to sounds in the room. It doesn't matter. Shift your attention—gently—back to your breath.
- **Continue for 15 to 20 minutes.** When you are ready to stop, take a minute or two to just sit quietly, keeping your eyes closed. Stretch and move your hands and feet a bit. Then open your eyes.
- **Be consistent.** Practice this meditation twice a day if you have the time, preferably in the morning and evening. You may be surprised how settled you become and how much more energy and focus you have during your day's activities.

Using Your Imagination to Relax

We all visualize. When we dream, replay images of a past event, or worry about what may happen in the future, we are visualizing. The images that come to mind may be visual, but much of the time they include feelings, sounds, or any combination of the five senses. For example, almost all of us sometimes hear a song playing inside our heads. Most of the time, we experience this natural faculty passively—images just drift into our minds—but we can learn to use it consciously and intentionally to relax and facilitate healing.

"Imagery is one of the quickest ways I know to relax, to induce a relaxation response," says Martin L. Rossman, M.D., codirector of The Academy for Guided Imagery in Mill Valley, California. "It's the opposite of a stress response. It can interrupt the physiological effects of ongoing stress."

Visualization connects the mind and emotions to the body. Research indicates that when people use their imaginations to see, hear, feel, or use any of the five senses, the brain becomes activated just as it does when we actually see, hear, or feel, and the body responds. Fear about public speaking (imagining yourself standing in front of the audience) can create a dry mouth, butterflies in your stomach, sweating, cold hands, and other symptoms of anxiety.

You may wake from a bad dream in a cold sweat, with your heart pounding. Thinking about a sexual encounter—remembered or anticipated—can easily make you feel aroused.

make your own relaxation tape

You pop a cassette into the recorder, flip the switch, and follow directions. Ahhhh, instant relaxation.

Commercial relaxation tapes are available in most bookstores or by mail order. Your local library may also have tapes you can check out to discover what works for you. These tapes usually include music as well as verbal instructions for relaxation, some spoken by male voices, others by females. Some employ sounds of nature, such as the ocean or birdsongs, to help induce a peaceful feeling. You may find some of these quite adequate and helpful.

On the other hand, you may find that the voice isn't pleasing, the type of music or background sound is not soothing to you, or the particular technique doesn't seem to be helpful. The solution? Make your own tape. Here's all you need to do:

- **Get set up.** Take a blank 60- or 90-minute audiotape.
- **Consider background sounds.** If you wish, choose some music or natural sound effects that you really like and you find relaxing and soothing. Play your chosen selections in the background on your CD player or another tape player while you are recording your relaxation tape.
- **Pick your technique.** Choose one of the exercises in this chapter that appeals to you and record the step-by-step instructions in your own voice.
- **Speak softly.** Be sure to speak in a calm and soothing manner, and pause often, leaving yourself plenty of time to follow each step of the instructions before moving to the next.
- **Do retakes.** One advantage of doing your own tape is that if it doesn't feel right, you can always try again. Once you're following your own set of instructions, you may find that you need to allow far more time for each step or that you prefer a different kind of background music.
- **Enjoy.** The great advantage of using a tape, whether it be a commercial tape or one you make yourself, is that you won't have to stop to read or check on what to do. You can just lie down or sit quietly with your eyes closed and do what you're setting out to do: relax.

"Mental images can have a tremendous influence on us, both emotionally and physically," says Dr. Mason, director of the Stress Education Center in Cotati, California. "If a person thinks about the worst case scenario, the dark side of things, they will often find themselves depressed, with their energy level reduced, maybe even their immune system compromised."

On the other hand, he suggests, "if we consciously picture ourselves as healthy and strong, full of energy and vitality, it's creating a blueprint, an image of health and happiness that will become a self-fulfilling prophecy." The body can translate the positive imagery into health and wellness, promoting a sense of joy and well-being.

"Some people do not have mental pictures or images in their minds, so they think visualization will not be effective for them," says Dr. Mason. "Actually, visualization can use mental memories or images of a variety of sensations besides sight. In fact, using more of the five senses tends to coordinate the central nervous system and can make the exercise more powerful."

Practicing Visualization

When you have time, try this relaxing visualization, suggested by Dr. Mason. Feel free to alter it, choosing your own images that promote relaxation and feelings of calm and peace.

- **Get comfortable.** Sit or lie down, loosen your clothing, and put yourself at ease. Close your eyes.
- **Let go of tension.** As much as you can, relax your muscles and release any tension you may be feeling in your body.
- **Breathe deeply.** Take two or three full and complete breaths, breathing in from your abdomen first then filling your chest.
- **Now begin to create mental sense impressions.** Imagine yourself in a favorite place, perhaps outdoors on a beautiful day, in a place that is calm and peaceful, where you feel safe.
- **Begin to notice the details of the spot.** Especially focus on the great beauty. Perhaps you will notice the blue of the sky above, the clouds, or other objects around you. You may see a grove of trees, mountain peaks, or a calm ocean. Without any strain, try to see the images in as much detail of color, shapes, and textures as you can.
- **Add other senses.** Now see if you can hear the sounds that would surround you in your chosen place.

It may be the sounds of running water, the songs of birds, leaves rustling in the warm breeze. Perhaps you hear the voices of children laughing and playing or those of special loved ones.

What does it feel like here? Can you feel the warm sunshine or the breezes that are blowing on your skin and in your hair, helping you feel warm and relaxed? Can you feel your blood flowing through wide-open blood vessels, freely pulsating into your hands and feet?

Can you smell the fragrance of salt air, spring flowers, and green grass, or the pungent smell of pine woods?

- **Create a safe haven.** Make your imagery as rich as you can and, as you do, allow yourself to feel peaceful and relaxed.

When you are ready, take a few minutes to come back to the place where you are resting.

Safety and Warnings

Relaxation therapies are almost as safe as falling asleep. You are simply letting go of tensions. But here are a few things you need to be aware of:

- **Learn from a pro.** You will get best results from working with an expert. Good results are certainly possible by trying these methods yourself, but for maximum benefit, work with a trained, experienced, and certified teacher, and in a situation in which follow-up is available.
- **Use caution while pregnant.** According to Autogenic Therapy trainers, if you are in your third trimester of pregnancy, don't send feelings of warmth into the abdomen. "My personal experience is that most people can benefit from sending warmth," says Dr. Mason, who has been teaching AT since 1977, "but it's said that it may bring on premature labor." Instead of sending warmth, you might choose to use a phrase such as, "My stomach region is calm," he suggests. This alteration is also suggested for anyone who has either diabetes or a bleeding ulcer.
- **Don't misinterpret pain.** If you have pain or discomfort and you begin to relax, your awareness is quite naturally drawn to the pain. It may seem to intensify "until you learn to get to the source and release and relax," says Dr. Mason. This may happen with neck and shoulder pain, and especially with headaches. Don't be alarmed or think you are doing something wrong. You are just tuning in to the pain. The relaxation will help relieve it.
- **Monitor your medications.** Relaxation techniques are often so effective that medication dosages for various conditions may need to be *reduced*. If you are currently under a physician's care for diabetes, high blood pressure, a thyroid disorder, or a serious depression, consult with your physician before beginning a relaxation program. Explain what you are going to be doing and ask him or her to monitor your progress.

  If you have high blood pressure, for example, relaxation or meditation exercises might successfully lower the pressure. If your prescription isn't reduced, you might develop symptoms of low blood pressure and feel dizzy or even faint when you stand up. Similarly, for a person taking medication for diabetes, the blood sugar level may change and the need for insulin may be reduced.
- **Deal with disturbing thoughts.** Occasionally, the experience of deep relaxation may allow some disturbing memories, feelings, or images to come to mind. "I've worked with thousands of people, and it's been very rare," says Dr. Mason. "When I work with people, I tell them, 'If something disturbing comes to mind, great; it's a chance to just let go and release it.'"

resources

Organizations and Teaching Centers

The Transcendental Meditation Program
1000 N. Fourth St.
Fairfield, IA 52556
1-888-LEARNTM (532-7686) (This toll-free number will automatically connect you to the nearest TM center.)
www:tm.org

You'll find instruction and free introductory talks on TM in most cities in the United States and more than 100 countries worldwide.

Insight (Vipassana) Meditation
Insight Meditation Society
1230 Pleasant Street
Barre, MA 01005
(508) 355-4378

An effective and simple meditation method from the Buddhist tradition, taught in centers throughout the USA. (You do not have to be Buddhist or espouse Buddhist beliefs to do this form of meditation.)

SYDA Foundation
P.O. Box 600
South Fallsburg, NY 12779
914/434-2000

Offers talks and meditation instruction from the Siddha Yoga tradition in various centers around the country.

The Academy for Guided Imagery
P.O. Box 2070
Mill Valley, CA 94942
800/726-2070

Provides information, professional training, and a directory of imagery practitioners.

Mind-Body Medical Institute
Beth Israel Deaconess Medical Center
110 Francis St., Suite 1A
Boston, MA 02215
617/632-9530
www.med.harvard.edu/programs/mindbody

Uses yoga, meditation, and stress reduction in its treatment program. Cofounded by Herbert Benson, M.D., developer of the "relaxation response," and Joan Borysenko, Ph.D.

Stress Reduction and Relaxation Program
UMass Memorial Health Care
55 Lake Ave. N
Worcester, MA 01655
508/856-2656
E-mail:
stress.reduction@banyan.ummed.edu

The oldest hospital-based, outpatient stress-reduction clinic in the country uses mindfulness meditation and yoga to help patients work with their own stress, pain, and illnesses. Directed by Jon Kabat-Zinn, Ph.D.

Books

Meditation:

How to Meditate by Lawrence LeShan (Bantam, 1974)

Trancendental Meditation by Robert Roth (I. Fine, 1989)

A Path with Heart by Jack Kornfield (Bantam, 1993)

The Complete Guide to Buddhist America by Don Morreale (Shambala, 1998)

Lists more than 1,000 centers that teach Buddhist meditation techniques. (Again, you can use these techniques without being Buddhist. Discuss it with your minister, priest, or rabbi if you're not sure how your own religion views this kind of practice.)

Wherever You Go, There You Are: Mindfulness Meditation in Everyday Life by Jon Kabat-Zinn (Hyperion, 1995)

Relaxation and stress management:

The Relaxation and Stress Reduction Workbook, 4th Ed. by Martha Advise, Elizabeth Robbins Eshelman, and Matthew McKay (New Harbinger Publications, 1995)

Guide to Stress Reduction by L. John Mason (Celestial Arts, 1989)

Scientific Paper

For scientific research on meditation and relaxation techniques, read **"The Physical and Psychological Effects of Meditation: A Review of Contemporary Research with a Comprehensive Bibliography,"** available from:
Institute of Noetic Sciences
P.O. Box 909
Sausalito, CA 94966
415/331-5650

Internet

Perhaps the best source on the Internet for information on alternative health topics is **HealthWorld Online.** For information on stress reduction, relaxation exercises, and mind-body-spirit health, go to www.bodymindspirit.com

Mind-Body Medicine Center
www.mind-body.com

For relaxation, breathing, and other stress-reduction methods, go to www.healthy.net/sahem

For stress-reduction healing art and games, go to
Rainbow Stress Reduction
www.healthy.net/rainbowstress

However, if you are taking psychoactive medications for severe mental illness (such as major depression), talk to your physician before beginning any of these practices. If you get your doctor's approval, go ahead and practice. Later, if you find something disturbing coming to mind, discontinue the practice and talk to your physician.

How to Find Instruction

Instruction in relaxation and meditation techniques is widely available, but the quality of instruction varies greatly.

Unfortunately, there is no licensing or certifying organization for most modalities. Inquire of your instructor where, with whom, and for how long he or she studied. Ask whether the method has any scientific validation behind it.

Two of the most thoroughly researched programs are Transcendental Meditation (TM) and Autogenic Therapy (AT). Their teachers are well trained to guide you, not only through initial instruction but over months and years of experiences.

Insight meditation (also known as *vipassana*) also has been researched and proved to be helpful. Experienced teachers are available across the country.

Other places to learn include yoga classes, university counseling services and psychology departments, alternative health clinics, and from psychologists and other therapists.

You may also be eligible for instruction at work, through a company stress management program. Your local Y may offer classes, and the continuing education division of a local university or community college is likely to offer several alternatives.

Your church or synagogue may also offer classes. Many of the meditation techniques used in traditional religious practice have a profoundly relaxing and health-giving effect. By all means, check with your priest, minister, or rabbi about whether such instruction is available. If your motives have mainly to do with health, be frank about what you are looking for.

Be wary of notices on bulletin boards at the health food store and advertisements in New Age type magazines. Some may be quite legitimate, but you'll need to do some questioning and investigating about the trainer's expertise and the potential benefits of any practice being offered.

chapter 19

support groups

HELPING EACH OTHER

To me, it's God's blessing to see other people in the same situation that you're in. *Ellis Williamson, support group organizer*

It used to be that when a person developed a physical illness or emotional disorder, consultation with a doctor or psychotherapist was the only appropriate response. One's relationship with an expert was considered the be-all and end-all. No more.

Today, while obtaining professional treatment is still essential, millions of people suffering from everything from alcoholism to schizophrenia, from cancer to multiple sclerosis, are taking their treatment and recovery a step further. They are taking part in support groups—reaping the rewards of the firsthand experience, empathy, and practical wisdom that only other people in the exact same situation can provide.

Self-Help Movement Grows

"In support groups, the participants are the experts," says clinical psychologist Mitch Golant, Ph.D., vice president of research and development for The Wellness Community, a national organization dedicated to helping people with cancer and their families. "You know more about your life and what to do with it than anyone else in the world," says Dr. Golant, who has facilitated more than 1,500 cancer support groups. "Your group mates are there to help you look at the issues and make your own decisions."

Some support groups have been in existence for more than half a century. Alcoholics Anonymous, for instance, has been around since 1935, when two "hopeless alcoholics" teamed up to help each other stay sober.

In so doing, "Bill W." and "Dr. Bob" took addiction treatment out of the hands strictly of doctors and hospitals and instead put the responsibility for recovery into the lives of alcoholics themselves.

The switch in philosophy from passive patient to active participant took firm hold on the American psyche in the 1970s. "That's when the self-help movement in the U.S. swelled, responding to an immense unmet need for the application of experiential knowledge to problem solving, community interaction, and social advocacy," according to Linda Farris Kurtz, M.S.W., professor of social work at Eastern Michigan University in Ypsilanti and author of *Self-Help and Support Groups.*

No matter who you are or what problem you may be dealing with, there's probably a support group just for you. Generally the only requirement for participation is having the condition the group focuses on or being a family member or friend of such a person.

Approximately 7.6 million Americans were participating in a vast variety of groups coast to coast, according to surveys conducted in 1996. In the field of mental health alone, about 3,000 support groups meet on a regular basis nationwide, according to the National Mental Health Consumers' Self-Help Clearinghouse.

support groups help heal

Support groups have been organized to help members cope with a vast range of physical and psychological conditions. A sampling:

- Alcoholism
- Alzheimer's disease
- Anger management
- Anxiety and panic disorders
- Arthritis
- Asthma
- Autism
- Bereavement
- Bipolar disorder
- Blindness
- Burns
- Cancer
- Caregivers
- Cerebral palsy
- Child abuse
- Chronic pain
- Compulsive gambling
- Cystic fibrosis
- Deafness
- Depression
- Diabetes
- Down's syndrome
- Drug addiction
- Endometriosis
- Epilepsy
- Heart disease
- Hepatitis
- HIV/AIDS
- Job burnout
- Liver disease
- Miscarriage
- Multiple sclerosis
- Obsessive-compulsive disorder
- Pet death
- Schizophrenia
- Sickle cell anemia
- Single parenthood
- Smoking
- Spiritual crisis
- Stroke
- Suicide
- Unemployment
- Weight loss

Alcoholics Anonymous, the largest self-help organization in the world, reported 1,307,803 members and 58,084 groups in the United States and Canada as of January 1996. Thousands of people also take part in nearly 50 other "anonymous" groups based on the "12 Steps" of AA, including Narcotics Anonymous, Overeaters Anonymous, and Adult Children of Alcoholics.

Thanks to support groups, people struggling with challenges of every sort become "comrades in adversity," as one researcher described a support group for women suffering from postpartum depression.

"Support groups are absolutely paramount because they help people understand that they're not alone," says Susie Novis, director of the International Myeloma Foundation. "It's crucial to recognize that there are other people out there going through the same thing that you are."

Novis founded IMF 10 years ago with her now late-husband after he was diagnosed with multiple myeloma, a rare form of bone cancer.

Ellis Williamson of Galveston, Texas, organized a local support group shortly after he had a stroke at the age of 34. "To me, it's God's blessing to see other people in the same situation that you're in," says Williamson, who now runs a volunteer office for Stroke Clubs International. "A doctor can tell a patient that he understands what you're going through, but he doesn't, because he's never been down that road."

In the 44 years since his stroke, Williamson has married and raised two children. "I've become much more positive about things," he says. "Everybody has problems. It's just in how we cope with them. The more we can help each other, the better off we all are."

Support Groups Make a Difference

Support groups are much more than "feel good" get-togethers. Scientific studies have found that support groups can measurably improve participants' health and add years to their lives—even in the case of serious diseases like cancer.

In a groundbreaking 1989 study, David Spiegel, M.D., currently medical director of the Complementary Medicine Clinic at Stanford University School of Medicine in California, found that women with breast cancer who attended a weekly support group for a year lived twice as long as women who did not participate in the group. Support group women survived for 36.6 months, he found, while nonsupport group women lived for only 18.9 months.

Subsequent research by Dr. Spiegel and others continues to provide a growing body of evidence that one's social environment and cancer progression are closely linked. The connection, Dr. Spiegel hypothesizes, has to do with stress. "What it all seems to come down to is that stress does a number on one's immune system, " Dr. Spiegel notes. "Supportive social relationships may buffer the effects of cancer-related stress on immunity, and thereby facilitate the recovery of immune mechanisms that may be important for cancer resistance."

Studies of people who have suffered heart attacks have found that people who have social support live longer than those lacking in support. "Social support and networks may have a substantial influence on the speed and quality of recovery following myocardial infarction," noted a team of Canadian researchers who reviewed studies conducted over a 15-year period.

People with diabetes who are in support groups also showed improvements in health. In one study, researchers at Texas Tech University Health Sciences Center in Lubbock observed that groups that increased participants' knowledge of the disease and also offered social support led to increased glucose (blood sugar) control in adults with diabetes.

Doctors-Endorsed Support

The success of groups like Alcoholics Anonymous and Narcotics Anonymous is well documented. Such groups, say researchers, help participants deal better with problems that make commitment to abstinence difficult, including cravings, emotional distress, relationship and family problems, and financial difficulties.

So successful are groups like these that members of the American Society of Addiction Medicine, Inc., and the American Academy of Addiction Psychiatry routinely recommend participation to their patients.

Recovery from another kind of potentially life-threatening condition, severe obesity, has also been found to be well served by involvement in support groups. "People in our program have a lot of medical problems related to their weight, including hypertension, high cholesterol, and Type 2 diabetes," says psychologist and assistant professor of medicine Kevin R. Fontaine, Ph.D., who runs several such groups at Johns Hopkins Weight Management Center in Baltimore for participants on very low-calorie diets.

"Losing weight has miraculous effects on their health, but depriving oneself of food is extremely difficult," Dr. Fontaine says. "Being part of the support group is what helps them stay on the program."

"I'm absolutely convinced that self-help groups contribute to mental health," says Marie Verna, program director of the National Mental Health Consumers' Self-Help Clearinghouse, which oversees groups for people suffering from depression, bipolar disorder, schizophrenia, and other mental disorders. "Support groups give people something to fall back on rather than just getting into a downward spiral. The instability, the crisis, the hospitalizations can all be prevented. It's a miracle, actually, a very joyous thing."

Participating in a Support Group

It's the first Wednesday of the month, the evening the support group you've located in your community holds its meeting. You're getting close, driving down the street, looking for the right address. Finally you find it: a church social hall or perhaps a hospital meeting room or maybe even someone's living room. Wherever, the group is most likely located someplace where you and other participants can feel comfortable.

how support groups help

How exactly do support groups help their participants? Researcher Irving Yalom, M.D., of Stanford University Medical School in California identified a number of therapeutic factors common to support groups. These include:

- **Universality.** It is painful to believe that one's dilemma is unique and that one is alone with a seemingly unsolvable problem. Realizing that others in a support group are "in the same boat" comes as a welcome relief.
- **Hope.** Hope is the belief that the process of attending the group will help. In support groups, storytelling helps encourage hope. Newcomers listen to veteran members tell their stories of recovery. Realizing that the veteran was once in the same desperate state that the newcomer now experiences, the newcomer feels hope.
- **Information and advice.** Much that is learned in groups is implicit, but some groups have various forms of actual instruction, from speakers to written materials.
- **New coping methods.** Group members learn a wide range of techniques for coping with their situations through experiential sharing.
- **Improved relationship skills.** Group members interact with one another in much the same way that they would with their own families. In so doing, they often learn new and better ways of relating to others.
- **Altruism.** Support groups give members the opportunity to help others, a gift that is as beneficial to the giver as it is to the receiver.
- **Existential factors.** Together, group members face life's larger issues, from the reality that life may be unfair to the fact that every individual is ultimately responsible for his or her own life.

Someplace quiet. Someplace private. Someplace where after a short while you will no longer be consumed with newcomer nervousness but feel, instead, like you belong.

There are generally two types of support group meetings. "Closed" meetings are those that run for a specific number of weeks and for which you've probably had to sign up in advance. These groups are most often offered through a hospital, mental health facility, or similar organization. Cancer Care, Inc., in New York, for example, operates weekly groups that run from eight to 12 weeks. To participate, cancer patients and their families first meet with a social worker for evaluation and placement.

"Open-door" meetings, on the other hand, require no sign-up and meet on

getting the most from group membership

As convinced as you may be that attending a support group is a good idea, chances are that you're probably going to be nervous the first few times. "As a newcomer, it's perfectly normal to feel anxiety," says clinical psychologist Mitch Golant, Ph.D., of The Wellness Community. He offers these tips for cultivating a sense of comfort:

- **Be as interested as you can.** Be as interested and involved in the lives of your group mates as you can. The more interested you are in them, the more interested they will be in you. Friendship is built on shared intimacy. Even if you don't feel like it, consider taking a risk. The more involved you are, the better off you will be.
- **Be as open as you can.** Do your best to tell your group mates as much about yourself as you can. Self-revelation is an important way to build a feeling of intimacy and camaraderie. This is one place where you don't have to pretend or hold back. Be a part of the discussion. Ask questions. Give opinions. Make suggestions.
- **Participate at your own pace.** Warming up to strangers is easier for some people than for others. For some, it takes a long time. If simply getting through the door and listening to others works for you, then do just that. Remember that the group is there for you to use however you want.

a continuous basis. The large majority of support groups operate as open-door meetings, providing participants with maximum flexibility. The Y-ME National Breast Cancer Organization, for example, has been running open-door support group meetings for several consecutive years.

"There's no sign-up, no reservations," says Judy Perotti, Y-ME's director of patient services. "If you're available, you attend. If not, you don't, but you're always welcome the next time." Some AA groups have been running for decades, with participants coming and going as they desire.

How Often, How Long

Support groups may meet monthly, bimonthly, or even weekly. Meetings of the International Myeloma Foundation, for example, meet once a month. Most 12 Step meetings take place weekly. Participation is not necessarily limited, by the way, to one meeting. Most organizations welcome participants to as many meetings as they want to attend. It's not at all unusual, for example, for many 12-Step members to attend several such groups in the course of a single week.

The typical support group meets for about an hour. If the meeting is longer, a coffee break or other form of intermission will probably be scheduled in. Some groups reserve time before or after the meeting during which members are encouraged to socialize.

Most support groups are free of charge. However, a donation may be requested to pay for room rental, refreshments, and materials such as printed handouts.

Who's in Charge

Some support groups are led by a professional, such as a physician, psychologist, or social worker, particularly when the group is under the auspices of a hospital or similar institution. Groups for The Wellness Community, for example, are run by licensed psychotherapists who have been trained in support group techniques.

Professional support group leaders walk a fine line, says The Wellness Community's Dr. Golant, since the primary emphasis of support groups is to encourage participants to help themselves. "That's why we don't call our leaders 'therapists'; we call them 'facilitators,'" Dr. Golant says. "Their role is to facilitate communication and interaction among participants so that they build an extended family among themselves."

Leadership may also come in the form of trained peers. Y-ME groups are led by nonprofessional peer counselors, breast cancer survivors whose task it is to keep meetings focused and productive.

Similarly, support groups offered by the Chronic Pain Association are led by people who themselves are coping with chronic pain and who have been trained in teaching coping skills.

"We're much more likely to respond to someone who can say, 'I understand what you're going through' and can really mean it," says association founder and president Penny Cowan.

Finally, a large number of support groups are strictly nonprofessional, with participants taking turns in the leadership role. AA and other 12-Step groups have a long-standing and solid tradition of nonprofessionalism.

"These groups work just fine," says Dr. Fontaine, who has conducted research on support groups. "Some of the most effective people in terms of running groups are lay people with no formal background in mental health."

Who's There

Support group attendance varies widely. Six to 10 people attend Dr. Fontaine's weekly weight-loss support groups. An AA group can range from two or three participants to, in some major cities, hundreds.

Participants are frequently limited to people suffering from the condition, keeping the focus tight. "Anonymous" groups like

at-home support

You'd like to participate in a support group but can't get out of the house? Try a telephone or Internet support group.

A number of organizations offer support by phone. Cancer Care, Inc., for example, sponsors several hour-long monthly groups via telephone conference calls for homebound cancer patients and their families. Although a telephone support group is quite different from an in-person group, the results can be equally beneficial, say researchers who studied one 30-member Cancer Care group that had been meeting by phone for five years.

"Telephone support connects a group of people who cannot normally be together, allows patients to use a resource to which they would not have access otherwise, and helps them transcend physical limitations," the researchers noted. For people with access to the Internet, numerous support groups are available on line, from real-time chat lines to bulletin boards, where participants read and respond to messages at their convenience.

"The Internet is a valuable means of offering support in a nontraditional format," says support group researcher Paula Klemm, D.N.Sc., R.N., associate professor of nursing at the University of Delaware in Newark. "It offers the same wide range of communication as a live meeting, including personal experience and opinions, encouragement, and support. Considering that some 40 million American homes will have Internet access in the near future, electronic support groups will no doubt be an increasingly available option for vast numbers of people."

To find an at-home support group, contact organizations that offer referrals to more traditional support groups and ask if they know of any groups offered by phone or Internet. (For more suggestions, see "Finding a Support Group" on page 236.) On the Internet, you may also find a group by looking up a key search term such as "cancer" or "mental health" via your search engine.

AA and NA are often adamant about limiting attendance to "fellow sufferers," who feel most comfortable sharing with their peers alone.

Many support groups, however, are very welcoming to people close to those with the condition, in the recognition that family and friends are also deeply affected by serious problems and may need help of their own in dealing with stresses such as family disruptions, financial worries, and changing roles within the family.

Once the clock strikes the designated hour and the meeting begins, what typically happens? The leader begins with a few initial remarks. Perhaps he or she begins by reading a statement of purpose. The leader may go over ground rules, making suggestions such as "Please allow everyone an equal chance to share," or "What is discussed here is confidential."

Participants may be invited to introduce themselves. Going around the room, people give their names, perhaps first names only. The leader may invite everyone to add a few words about themselves and why they are attending.

Meeting Goals and Formats

Support groups have varied goals and formats. Here are several.

- **Become educated.** Many groups focus on educating and informing their participants about the condition they share, based on the assumption that this information will enable them to better deal with it.

Peter Tischler started a myeloma support group in Arlington, Texas, after being diagnosed with the disease three years ago. Tischler's group focuses on learning about the medical aspects of this rare disease.

"Everyone attending shares experiences of their medical treatment," he says. "I do research on clinical trials on the Internet. We bring things into the group that we can then ask our doctors about. It's all about choices. It all comes down to being able to sit down with your physician and become an advocate for your health."

Other support groups educate participants by bringing in professional speakers, holding question-and-answer sessions, or going through an official workbook, one lesson per meeting.

- **Learn to cope.** One of the most valuable aspects of support groups is helping members learn to cope with situations that are always going to be a challenge. Examples include chronic arthritis pain, migraine headaches, and chronic backaches. Participants in Chronic Pain Association support groups are taught pain management skills such as biofeedback and guided imagery—skills that redirect their attention away from pain and onto self-reliance.

Participants in Weight Watchers support groups trade ideas for getting through ongoing food-related challenges, discussing a different topic every meeting. "We share ways to find time in a busy day to plan a healthy meal, how to get through everyday stresses without bingeing, eating healthily on vacation," says member Connie Lee. "You realize that whatever the problem you're going through, everyone else in that room is going through it, too."

Coping techniques are a topic of continual discussion among recovering alcoholics and addicts at 12-Step meetings. "The whole point is to stay sober no matter what life throws your way," says Kerry W., who quit drinking a dozen years ago. "Listening to what others have to say at meetings about how they cope, from dealing better with job stresses to calling someone when you're feeling down, keeps me on the right track."

- **Get emotional support.** Sometimes just having others understand what you're going through is the greatest benefit a support group can offer, says Tina Levin, a licensed clinical social worker who facilitates support groups for HIV patients at Warren Grant Magnuson Clinical Center at the National Institutes of Health in Baltimore.

"It's the 'all in the same boat' phenomenon," Levin says. "In our groups, issues that otherwise seem so individual turn out to be something that just about every gay man with AIDS can relate to. The kind of emotional support that group participants are able to give to each other is far more powerful than anything I could ever give. Someone else who has this illness understands it in a way than someone who doesn't have the disease never can."

"Emotional support helps people get their problems into perspective," says the Rev. Karen Morrow, chaplain at Warren Grant Magnuson Clinical Center in Baltimore, who leads Medicine for the Soul support groups for patients coping with a wide range of serious medical conditions.

"People have an opportunity to cry their tears, vent their anger, and share their fears," says the Rev. Morrow. "With other people hearing them and appreciating them, the problem becomes more manageable. They're able to say to themselves, 'If so and so, with what he or she has to deal with can face it, my problem, though it is large, is also manageable.'"

In the Long Term

Attending a support group meeting or two isn't going to solve all your problems. Making it to meetings regularly, getting to know fellow members, and learning to trust and fully participate in the process are key to reaping support groups' rewards.

"Go to at least three or four meetings to expose yourself to a variety of experiences and people, " advises Dr. Golant of The Wellness Community. "Remember that each time is different. Sometimes it might be boring, sometimes funny, sometimes sad. Support groups are, after all, a microcosm of real life."

"Keep coming back," members of groups like AA and NA urge one another at the end of each meeting. "I plan to go to meetings for the rest of my life," says AA member Kerry W. "Without them, I risk relapse, going back to a place I don't want to go to."

start your own
support group

Can't find a support group in your community for your particular condition or interest? Then consider starting your own.

A good place to begin is with a state or national self-help clearinghouse that can connect you with a larger organization already specializing in your condition. "Self-help clearinghouses recommend that if you want to start a group, you form an affiliate of a national organization," says Linda Farris Kurtz, M.S.W., a professor in the department of social work at Eastern Michigan University in Ypsilanti and author of *Self-Help and Support Groups*. "In other words, avoid reinventing the wheel. Most organizations will provide a starter kit and guidelines for the formation of new groups and offer telephone consultation."

Still, you may need to start from scratch. Peter Tischler, who organized a myeloma support group which he has run from his home with his wife Lucy for the past three years, recommends these steps:

- **Start small.** Find at least one or two other people who have the same idea or whom you can sell on the idea of starting a group. Ask your friends, doctor, clergy. Put an ad in the local newspaper. Post a notice on a local bulletin board.
- **Do a group-think.** Hold an initial planning meeting at your home, a restaurant, or some other convenient location. Discuss your goals and format and begin to set it down in writing.
- **Arrange for a regular meeting place.** Look for a comfortable, private room, where people aren't going to be constantly walking through. Possibilities include local churches, medical or mental health facilities, libraries, and schools.
- **Set a regular meeting time and date.** Should you meet weekly? Monthly? Or plan for meetings at regular intervals, such as the first and third Wednesdays?
- **Decide on a fee.** Most support groups are free, but you may decide to request donations for refreshments, room rental, and other costs.
- **Decide on leadership.** Hold your first meeting, facilitated by one of the initial planners. Be open to rotating the leadership.
- **Don't hog the show.** See that everyone gets a chance to introduce themselves.
- **Collect information.** Before the meeting ends, be sure to get everybody's name and phone number, and give out the name and number of a contact person.
- **Keep the door open.** On an ongoing basis, open up the thinking and planning process to all participants. "It's all too easy to get into a situation where the two or three people who have been involved from the beginning have some strong ideas about the group's goals," says Tischler. "The hope is to involve as many people in the work as possible."

Finding a Support Group

You may have to do some searching to find a support group that exactly suits your individual needs. It's worth making the effort to make a good match. You might try these avenues:

- **Ask friends and relatives.**
- **Ask your doctor or your doctor's nurse.**
- **Call a local hospital or mental health facility.**
- **Check your local newspaper's "events" section for listings.**
- **Check your library for books listing local support groups.**
- **Check your telephone directory for local self-help clearinghouses.**
- **Contact these national clearinghouses:**

American Self-Help Clearinghouse, Denville, New Jersey, 201/625-7101

National Self-Help Clearinghouse, New York City, 212/354-8525

National Mental Health Consumers Self-Help Clearinghouse, 800/553-4539

Safety and Warnings

Just because support groups are so good for so many doesn't mean they are completely without risk. Here are some tips on things to avoid from Eastern Michigan University's Linda Farris Kurtz:

- **Don't fall for fake experts.** Watch out for peer leaders or participants trying to act as medical professionals or psychotherapists, positions for which they are not trained. It's understandable that people feel enthusiasm for therapies that have worked for them. But that doesn't mean you need to feel pressured into getting the same treatment or thinking the same way.
- **Don't blame the victim.** Avoid group leaders that tell participants that they are at fault for the onset of their illness, including serious diseases like cancer, and that they alone are responsible for the course of the illness.
- **Don't get overwhelmed.** The expression of intense feelings and purely negative emotions can be too much for support group members who are struggling with pain and fear. While some negativity is inevitable and can even be helpful in releasing pent-up feelings, too much of it can be depressing and convey the message that the situation is hopeless. A support group should emphasize positive, concrete help. If you find yourself depressed at the end of every meeting, find another group.
- **Seek out true peers.** You might want to avoid groups that mix people in the end stages of a fatal medical condition with those in the early stages. This is very distressing to newcomers. Seek a group where others' situations closely match yours.
- **Don't fall into the cult trap.** It is possible to link up with support groups that encourage members to accept cultlike beliefs. If it doesn't sound right to you, head for the door.

chapter 20

tai chi & qigong

ANCIENT MOVEMENTS FOR MODERN MALADIES

Some people go through life not thinking about what they feel in their body, heart, soul, or mind. Tai chi and qigong will sensitize you to those things. —*Effie Poy Yew Chow, Ph.D.*

It's dawn. As the sun slowly rises over the cool lake waters, a lone figure steps out onto the dock. Dressed in a traditional black tai chi uniform, the petite woman slowly brings both palms together and bows to the huge expanse of nature before her.

She drops her hands to her sides and shakes off the tension, takes several deep breaths, then extends her arms out to her sides. Moving in slow motion, she bends her left arm at the elbow, slowly twists, and glides her left hand into position alongside her right arm. Sharon Harris, a 47-year-old artist from Macungie, Pennsylvania, has begun her morning tai chi routine.

Harris enrolled in a tai chi class at the local hospital as a gift to herself. "For once, I wanted to do something for myself, alone. It was a particularly stressful time in my life, and I heard that tai chi can be very relaxing," she explains. "I had always been fascinated with Eastern healing philosophies, and I saw it as a chance to explore something new.

"I tried joining the local gym, but it really turned me off. I took aerobics classes. The instructor was very demanding, and the music was extremely loud. I was looking for something to reduce my stress, not add to it!"

Did it work?

Apparently it did. "With tai chi," Harris says, "the exercises were very gentle, flowing, and slow, yet purposeful at the same time. As the classes went by, we all felt a camaraderie with each other that I didn't feel in the aerobics class. Tai chi teaches you that—how to be more aware of yourself and your surroundings."

Harris says she now practices tai chi at home and outdoors at her family's cabin. "It's become very important to me," she says. "It's helped me develop discipline, control, and a sense of calmness and peace with myself and the world around me."

tai chi and qigong help heal

- Conditions of old age: balance problems, falls, stiff muscles
- Depression
- Fatigue
- High blood pressure
- Heart disease
- Lack of mental clarity
- Poor vitality
- Poor circulation
- Stress-related conditions, such as anxiety and tension

Tai Chi: What's in a Name?

Tai chi (also known as *tai chi ch'uan* and *taiji*) is a noncombative martial art that enhances balance and body awareness through slow, graceful, and precise body movements. Tai chi, which comes from China, combines these movements with breathing techniques to improve the flow of what the Chinese call *qi* (pronounced chee).

According to traditional Chinese medicine, qi is life energy that flows in the body through pathways that are just below the surface of the skin. Practitioners of Chinese medicine believe that any disturbance or imbalance of qi can lead to illness. Therefore, they recommend tai chi more to prevent disease than as a treatment. But, it turns out, tai chi can also be used to treat or ameliorate a number of conditions.

According to Eastern medical practitioners, tai chi is used to achieve spiritual and mental clarity. The flowing movements are designed to focus body and mind in harmony and to encourage an even flow of energy throughout the body. These traditional experts maintain that practicing tai chi can promote flexibility and strength in the limbs and trunk and straighten out poor posture.

All of this has a romantic and exotic appeal. But do these claims hold up under the scrutiny of modern medical science?

Tai Chi: Medical Evidence

Western science is, in fact, lending credence to these traditional claims and finding other benefits from regular tai chi practice.

In one landmark study sponsored by the National Institute on Aging (NIA), an arm of the National Institutes of Health, tai chi reduced the risk of falling among older people by 47.5 percent. It is estimated that each year falls are responsible for medical costs of more than $12 billion in the United States, plus there is the profound impact they have on the person's quality of life.

Many is the elderly woman (or man) with osteoporosis whose independence ends following a hip fracture caused by a fall. Anything that can reduce the risk of falls by almost 50 percent deserves serious consideration.

The NIA study enrolled 200 people age 70 and older. The participants were divided into three groups. In the first group, participants attended 15 weekly tai chi sessions in which they progressed to more complex forms of the exercise. They were also asked to practice at home at least 15 minutes, twice daily.

The second group received balance training using a computer-operated balance platform in which participants tried to improve control of their body sway under increasingly difficult conditions. The third group was asked not to change any of its current exercise regimens and took part in weekly meetings on a variety of topics with a nurse/gerontologist.

"I think it's quite remarkable that tai chi significantly reduced their risk of falling," says study author Steven L. Wolf, Ph.D., director of research, department of rehabilitation medicine, Emory University School of Medicine, Atlanta, Georgia. "Tai chi is not an intense, strenuous physical activity. And they only practiced it for 15 weeks."

He adds, "Those in the tai chi group were also less afraid of falling than the other groups, and they had more confidence."

The study researchers also asked all groups to walk for 12 minutes after each intervention. "Blood pressure before and after the walk was much lower in the tai chi folks, so it had a cardiovascular effect," says Dr. Wolf.

Another interesting nugget the researchers discovered was that after the study was completed, about one-third of the people continued to practice tai chi.

"We followed them for over two years, and 35 percent of them still met twice a week," notes Dr. Wolf. "Many people told me they felt it kept them mentally alert and aware of their environment. However, I think a lot of it has to do with the socialization factor. Doing tai chi was their chance to get together and to move in unison as a group. It gave them a chance to participate in an activity that they enjoyed."

Better Balance, Greater Strength

In a second NIA study at the University of Connecticut in Farmington, researchers enrolled older people in a specific exercise program targeted to improve balance and strength. The positive results were twofold: First, their balance and strength improved. Second, after the study ended, they continued to do tai chi exercises for six months, which maintained these improvements.

Both studies were part of the NIA's Frailty and Injuries: Cooperative Studies of Intervention Techniques (FICSIT) initiative and the results were published in the *Journal of the American Geriatrics Society*. "The FICSIT studies have shown that we must look at every approach to help older people avoid frailty and falling," says Chhanda Dutta, Ph.D., of the NIA. "Tai chi is relatively inexpensive. People can do this at home and with friends once they have the proper training."

Other studies have shown that tai chi can improve cardiovascular endurance, breathing efficiency, and muscle flexibility.

Qigong—Movements to Rev Up Healing

Q*igong*—sometimes referred to as *chi kung* and always pronounced chee-gung—is a 5,000-year-old system of Chinese energy exercises for the body, mind, and spirit. This ancient discipline consists of movements, breathing techniques, and meditation, all designed to develop and improve the circulation of qi. It is a system for improving and maintaining health, as well as helping cure disease.

The basic aim is to bring the body into a state of balance and self-regulation. Qigong means "qi work" or "working with qi." It actually is a distillation of several ancient healing systems.

There are many forms of qigong. Tai chi is one of them. They all have the following theories in common:

- The energies that flow through the mind, body, and spirit can be regulated and cultivated through the relaxation and concentration that mental and physical exercises provide.
- Control of respiration (breathing) plays a central role.
- Bringing the body into a state of maximum repose and self-regulation can help an individual realize full physical potential, resist illness, heal the damage caused by diseases, and balance mind/body interaction.
- It is of primary importance to harmonize the human body with nature. Qigong theorists maintain that the human body and nature exist as an interrelated and inseparable unity. They believe that imbalances in this unity are a key cause of illness. Therefore, people should strive for the conscious awareness of their relationship with nature.

Medical Evidence for Qigong

The First World Conference for Academic Exchange of Medical Qigong was held in Beijing, China, in 1988. The meeting was attended by hundreds of researchers from around the world. Of nearly 140 papers presented, only three were from the United States, and one was from Canada. Almost all papers presenting hard clinical data on qigong originated from China.

Unfortunately, few of these studies have been translated into English, and some are incomplete. But those studies that are available in the West show qigong to be a

qigong can help heal

According to scientific research done in China, qigong can:

- Improve memory, attention span, and thinking processes
- Lessen paralysis
- Stop ringing in the ear (tinnitus)
- Improve nearsightedness (myopia)
- Increase blood flow to the brain
- Slow the aging process

Individual qigong instructors in the United States have their own lists of conditions that this ancient discipline can help. For example, San Francisco qigong master Effie Poy Yew Chow, Ph.D., coauthor of *Miracle Healing From China: Qigong*, says her clients have seen the following conditions improve:

- Allergies
- Arthritis
- Asthma
- Back pain
- Colds and flu
- Depression
- Low self-esteem
- Menstrual problems and other female disorders
- Multiple sclerosis
- Paralysis
- Parkinson's disease
- Sexual dysfunction
- Stroke

promising area for future research and for potential healing.

In one long-term study done at the Shanghai Institute of Hypertension in Shanghai, China, for example, a group of 204 people with high blood pressure was randomly divided into two groups. The first group took low doses of high blood pressure medicine, but did not practice qigong. The second group also took low doses of high blood pressure medicine but did practice qigong.

Both groups were followed for 20 years. The group that practiced qigong maintained better control of their blood pressure and experienced substantially lower overall death rates and stroke death rates than the other group that did not practice qigong.

Qigong is not as well known in the United States as tai chi. It will be interesting to note in the future whether the claims for qigong hold up as well under the scrutiny of Western medical research.

How to Find the Best Practitioner

Although instructional videotapes are available for both tai chi and qigong, it's better to learn these disciplines from a qualified teacher. A teacher can explain the philosophy of tai chi and qigong and make sure you are doing the

qi power

Doing either tai chi or qigong exercises can help you heal. And scientific research backs up that statement.

According to traditional Chinese medicine principles, qi (pronounced chee) is the vital life force present in all living things. Many traditional practitioners of qigong believe that qi not only flows through our bodies, but that through long practice and discipline, an individual can learn how to make qi flow from their bodies to another person in order to heal them.

"When a practitioner emits qi, he or she corrects the imbalance of the vital life force in the client's body," explains San Francisco qigong master Effie Poy Yew Chow, Ph.D., who maintains that she has healed many clients with emitted qi. "It's the imbalance of the vital life force that creates illness. Emitted qi brings the client's body into harmony and good health."

This process boosts the immune system and creates chemical and cellular changes in the body, she maintains.

In a typical session, the client lies on a table. "The hands are the vehicle for emitting qi, so I hold them over the body or place them on the skin," says Dr. Chow. The exact positioning of the hands is determined by the spot on the energy pathways, or meridians, where the practitioner suspects an imbalance.

"My qi then connects with the vital life force of the client, which creates change in their body, mind, and spirit," says Dr. Chow.

And what does science say about this form of healing? In America, not much. In China, however, research on emitted qi suggest that it has benefits on asthma, allergies, cancer, diabetes, paralysis, urinary problems, menstrual problems, depression, and stroke. There is no medical evidence for emitted qi or its purported healing effects in this country.

poses correctly. It's easy to think you're doing the poses exactly as you should, but still have aspects of the poses that need correction. Once you've attended classes, however, videotapes can help you maintain what you've learned.

The first step in finding a suitable teacher is to determine what you would like to get out of the class, says David Molony, tai chi instructor and executive director of the American Association of Oriental Medicine in Catasaqua, Pennsylvania. "If you're looking for a more intense form of exercise, tell the teacher your goal and ask if his classes are geared for that," says Molony. "But if you are an older person, ask if the instructor specializes in the more geriatric form of tai chi and qigong."

There are no national associations that regulate or certify tai chi and qigong, but several are in the works. In the meantime, here are Molony's tips for finding a good instructor:

- **Get a referral.** Ask your doctor if he or she can recommend a tai chi or qigong instructor. (This is your best way of finding an instructor.)
- **Check reliable sources.** Call local hospitals, community centers, colleges, and universities and inquire about classes.
- **Look in the phone directory under Acupuncture.** Many acupuncturists teach tai chi and qigong. And if they don't, they can usually refer you to someone who does. Interview the teacher. When you find an instructor, ask if you can take a free class. If you can, go to classes with at least three different instructors before you decide who you're going to pick. Find the one who fits most with your goals, and the one you're most comfortable with.
- **Inquire about how large the classes are.** Some people prefer a smaller class with more personal instruction; yet others like the social aspect of exercising with a large group.
- **Avoid classes with a strong sales pitch.** Does the practitioner give the impression of running the classes merely as a money-making exercise? Are you required to sign a contract? If you do sign up, and you find you don't like the classes, can you cancel and get a refund?

Taking That First Class

Tai chi and qigong classes range from one on one to larger classes of 15 to 30. It's a good idea to be prepared and have some idea of what to expect.

- **Dress the part.** Wear loose, comfortable clothing and flat-soled shoes. "Look for clothes that won't interfere with your body moving," advises Molony. "If you're interested, there are specific uniforms for the form of tai chi or qigong that you're practicing. Your instructor can guide you in choosing the right one."

If your class is held outdoors, notice the temperature and dress accordingly. The additional benefits of practicing outdoors can be negated if you're uncomfortable. You want to be at one with your surroundings. When you dress appropriately for the environment, you obtain the harmony that is key to Chinese medicine.

Realize and accept nature for what it is, not what you want it to be. For example, if it's chilly outside, dress in layers so that as you begin moving and feel warm, you can remove an outer layer.

- **Center yourself.** When you first enter the room, take a few minutes just to "be" in the room, or outdoor space, before you begin your practice.

quick stress buster

You're stuck in your car in a traffic jam, and the anxiety and stress start to well up. Think some ancient Chinese medicine can help you now? You bet! To relax in no time, follow this simple breathing exercise from San Francisco qigong master Effie Poy Yew Chow, Ph.D.

- **Adjust your posture.** "Proper posture is important to proper breathing, so sit up straight. Visualize that a thread extends from the car seat up through your spine, to the top of your head. Move your shoulders back and down. Keep your body still and calm. Tilt your pelvis forward slightly. Just below the lower end of your sternum, or breast bone, is the diaphragm area, or upper abdomen. Move this area out and in, out and in, slowly as you breathe.
- **Inhale deeply.** "To inhale, extend the upper abdomen and move the chest walls outward to expand the chest cavity. This should allow room for the lungs to expand. Inhale through your nostrils, keeping your mouth closed."
- **Exhale deeply.** "To exhale, move the upper abdomen in, and force air out through the lips."
- **Focus on the breath.** Repeat this deep breathing for several minutes until you begin to feel calmer.

"When you get anxious, your blood vessels get constricted, and oxygen isn't getting through to the cells," says Dr. Chow. "Deep breathing through the diaphragm helps relieve this constriction, moving oxygen to the blood. You get a sense of relaxation. Your stressful situation hasn't changed, but you're able to cope better."

- **Start slowly.** In the beginning, the teacher will instruct you on proper breathing techniques. This will be followed by gentle warm-up exercises, then the tai chi and qigong poses. At the heart and soul of the exercises are gentle, flowing movements, so the key here is to take your time and enjoy yourself. Sessions will be calm and unhurried, focusing on breathing and creating a calm, meditative state of mind.

- **Expect to learn about your body.** "In the first class, the students will begin to learn how to be more aware of any new sensations in their bodies," says qigong master Effie Poy Yew Chow, Ph.D., coauthor of *Miracle Healing from China: Qigong* and president of the East West Academy of Healing Arts in San Francisco. "They will learn how to feel their qi, and to be more cognitive of their feelings. Some people go through life not thinking about what they feel in their body, heart, soul, or mind. Tai chi and qigong will sensitize you to those things."

- **Be patient.** "In the beginning, it can seem like there are a lot of postures," says Molony. "It can seem very complex and intimidating. But stick with it; it will all flow together soon for you."

Time to See Results

How long will you have to practice tai chi and qigong before you start seeing results? That depends on the individual. In some of the studies cited earlier in this chapter, many experienced significant physical improvements after just 15 weeks of practice.

"My students tell me that they feel a difference almost immediately," says Molony. "Quickened reflexes are an automatic reaction. After one or two months, they feel they can move smoother and easier, and their immune system is better. Other benefits they tell me about include recovering faster from sprains, strains, and falls, and better coordination. They are generally happier people, and like the camaraderie of spending time with other people in the class."

"Learning qigong and tai chi takes time, work, and patience," explains Dr. Chow. "Some people notice energy sensations in the body almost immediately. Others may require weeks or even a year or two to notice any changes. It depends on the sensitivity and openness of the individual."

Safety and Warnings

One of the many benefits of tai chi and qigong is that they are not physically taxing on the body. Unlike other forms of more strenuous physical exercise, such as running or playing tennis, you generally don't run a high risk of injury when moving through these milder exercises.

"Even with yoga, another gentle form of exercise, you can stretch too far," says Molony. "But with tai chi and qigong, it's very difficult to hurt yourself."

As with any new physical exercise program, however, it's wise to tell your physician before beginning the classes. Here are some more tips:

- **Let your instructor know about medical problems.** Tell your instructor about any prescription medications you're taking and any serious medical conditions, such as back pain, osteoporosis, high blood pressure, or heart disease. Also tell your instructor if you are pregnant.
- **Keep up your regular medical regime.** Both tai chi and qigong (especially) have reputations for helping heal a number of different medical conditions. Do not attempt to replace conventional medication or treatment with tai chi or qigong. These exercises should be considered in addition to your regular medical care.

If you notice a condition getting better, discuss possible changes in medications or treatment with your doctor. Don't discontinue medications on your own.

Bone Marrow Cleansing

The following series of movements combined with visualization is a qigong exercise known as bone marrow cleansing. It is recommended by Ken Cohen, author of *The Way of Qigong: The Art and Science of Chinese Energy Healing.* Practiced daily, this ancient practice is said to help boost the immune system and promote healing.

Meditating Buddha: Stand with your feet parallel and about shoulder width apart and with your knees slightly bent. Put your hands in front of your tummy, as though you're holding an invisible ball of energy. Use your imagination to "see" and feel that ball of energy. Slowly bring your hands together and raise them up in prayer position in front of your breastbone. Stand like this for 2 to 3 minutes. Breathe slowly and deeply and calm your mind. Let your hands drop slowly and gently down to your sides and relax.

Cosmic being: Slowly raise your arms out to the sides with your palms facing forward. When your hands reach shoulder height, stop and turn your palms outward. Your fingers should be pointing upwards. Now, as you hold this position for at least 2 minutes, see yourself filled with the energy of the Cosmos. Imagine that qi, that universal life energy, is flowing through you, out your hands to the right and left. Use your inner vision to see yourself filled with healing energy, life, and light. Then slowly lower your arms and feel the energy concentrated in your lower belly.

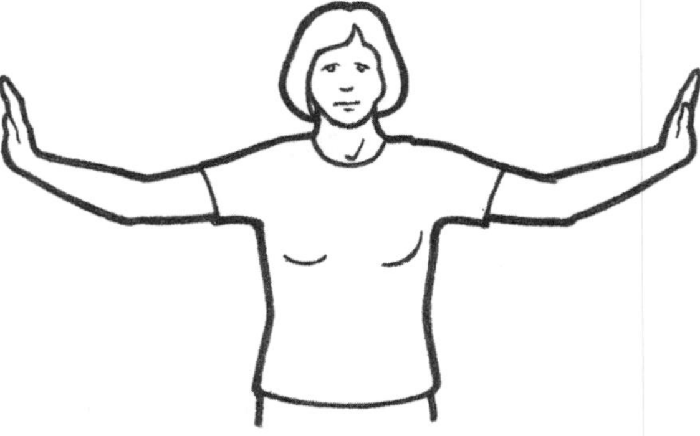

Wash marrow with one hand: Move your left hand slowly up the back of your body until the back of the hand is right at the small of your back, just behind the navel. Your palm will be facing outwards. At the same time, move your right hand up the right side of your body until the palm of your hand is about 6 inches over the crown of your head, facing downwards. Imagine that there's a connection between the center of your right palm and the top of your head. This is said to "balance your energy." Hold this position for a few seconds. It should feel pleasant.

Now slowly, ever so slowly, sweep your right hand down the front of your body. Your palm should be facing down and should be a few inches from your body. Use your imagination as the hand sweeps down the body and see in your mind's eye that the hand is helping qi move down through your body, sweeping it clean and bringing in healing energy. Envision that qi is moving through the bones of your body. As your hand drops to your side, envision anything impure leaving through your feet. (It's interesting to note here that while this exercise is really ancient, modern science now knows that the bone marrow is the birth place of white blood cells—an important component of your immune system.)

Now switch sides, placing your right hand behind your back and using your left hand to sweep qi through your bone marrow. Keep alternating hands for as long as it feels good—3 to 5 times is fine. Drop your hands to your sides and pause for a few seconds, breathing normally.

Wash marrow with both hands: You'll do this next movement just once. Slowly bring both hands up the front of your body, a few inches from your body, with palms facing up. When the palms reach the breasts turn your palms outwards and slowly raise them over your head. Your fingers should point inwards and your palms should face the sky. Imagine that you are a tree, with your feet rooted to the earth and your hands and fingers drinking energy from the sky.

Now turn your palms to face the top of your head and bring them down to about 6 inches from the top of your head. Your hands should not touch each other, and your fingers should be slightly separated. Now, with palms facing down, sweep both hands down the front of your body and imagine healing qi washing through your bones, pushing anything impure out through your feet.

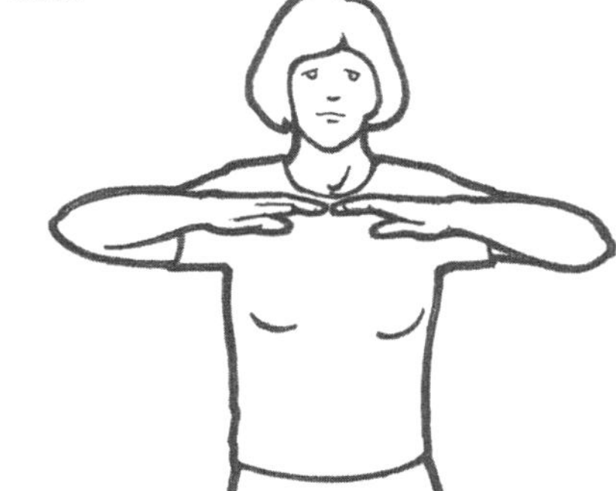

resources

Organizations

East West Academy of Healing Arts
450 Sutter St., Suite 2104
San Francisco, CA 94108
415/788-2227
e-mail: eastwestqi@aol.com

American Association of Oriental Medicine
433 Front Street
Catasaqua, PA 18032
888/500-7999

Patience Tai Chi Association
P.O. Box 350532
Brooklyn, NY 11235
718/332-3477
www.patiencetaichi.com

Magazine

Qi: The Journal of Traditional Eastern Health & Fitness
714/779-1796
www.qi-journal.com

Books

The Chinese Way to Healing: Many Paths to Wholeness by Misha Ruth Cohen, OMD (Perigree Books, 1996)

The Complete Illustrated Guide to Chinese Medicine by Tom Williams, Ph.D. (Element, 1996)

Miracle Healing from China: Qigong by Charles T. McGee, M.D., with qigong master Effie Poy Yew Chow, Ph.D. (Medipress, 1994)

The Way of Qigong: The Art and Science of Chinese Energy Healing by Ken Cohen (Ballantine, 1997)

Qigong Empowerment: A Guide to Medical Taoist Buddhist Wushu Energy Cultivation by Shou-Yu Liang and Wen-Ching Wu (The Way of the Dragon, 1997)

Videotapes

Tai Chi for Beginner, or ***Tai Chi for Seniors,*** both available in video stores

The Chow Qigong System, available by calling 800/824-2433

chapter 21

therapeutic touch

HEALING WITH THE HANDS

> Therapeutic touch helps relieve suffering. It really makes patients feel better and more comfortable. —*Susan Wager, M.D.*

When Susan Wager, M.D., was finishing her residency at New York University in the early 80s, she noticed that the patients of a particular nurse in the critical care unit always did better than the other patients in the unit. They were more comfortable, they rested better, and they improved faster. Dr. Wager learned that their nurse was using therapeutic touch. So began her own interest in this healing practice. Therapeutic touch, some might say, is a misnomer for this healing method, which often does not involve touching the body at all. Rather, the practitioner moves his or her hands over an individual at a distance of 3 to 5 inches in a process said to balance that person's energy flow to promote healing.

Manipulating Energy

Developed in 1972 by Dolores Krieger, Ph.D., R.N., and Dora Kunz at New York University, therapeutic touch is a descendant of the ancient practice of the laying on of hands. But practitioners emphasize that therapeutic touch is strictly a healing practice and not a religious one.

Therapeutic touch is based on the theory that a universal energy or life force flows through all living things and that the human body itself is an ordered, complex energy system combining our physical, emotional, and mental aspects.

This energy system is a highly organized one, say proponents of this form of therapy.

therapeutic touch
helps heal

Research shows that therapeutic touch induces deep relaxation, reduces anxiety, helps relieve pain, and accelerates the healing of wounds and infections. It is not a miracle cure for illness or disease. And practitioners recommend that it be used in addition to, not in place of conventional medicine to provide comfort and to help the body heal. Here are some specific ways therapeutic touch has reportedly been used successfully:

- Ease symptoms of PMS
- Heal wounds
- Lessen nausea and vomiting
- Reduce pain of osteoarthritis and rheumatoid arthritis
- Relieve depression
- Relieve fatigue
- Relieve headache
- Relieve pain of burns and speed healing
- Relieve stress
- Speed healing of fractures
- Treat asthma
- Treat colds and flu
- Treat pneumonia

During pregnancy:
- Induce relaxation
- Reduce discomfort
- Improve sleep
- Increase well-being

During labor and delivery:
- Provide relaxation and comfort

Postnatally:
- Lessen the pain of an episiotomy or Caesarean section
- Soothe a colicky infant

In the neonatal nursery:
- Reduce anxiety in premature babies and speed weight gain

In the emergency room:
- Reduce pain and anxiety
- Slow down heart rate
- Treat asthma

Prior to surgery:
- Nurses have administered therapeutic touch before anesthesia and have noticed that patients recover more quickly.

For people with cancer:
- Provide comfort
- Ease the side effects of those undergoing chemotherapy and radiation

For people with AIDS:
- Provide comfort
- Relieve pain and anxiety

For people with Alzheimer's disease:
- Improve sleep

For people who are dying:
- Ease anxiety
- Impart a sense of peace
- Increase overall well-being
- Provide comfort

When illness strikes, they say, our energy flow is disrupted in some way. Or, when our energy falls out of balance, we become ill.

Therapeutic touch is an attempt to restore proper energy flow so the body can heal itself.

This same principle guides acupuncture, which works by stimulating dozens of specific points along the lines of energy flow within the body.

Therapeutic touch relies on the belief that the body's energy field extends beyond the boundaries of skin and interacts with the universal life force or energy. That's why, proponents believe, it's not necessary to touch the body.

The practitioner becomes a conduit for the life force, the theory goes, directing that energy through his or her hands to the patient in a way that restores proper energy flow and enables healing to take place.

Since it was developed at NYU's school of nursing, therapeutic touch has been used primarily by nurses, but more doctors, psychiatrists, and other health professionals are showing interest in therapeutic touch and learning its practice, says Dr. Krieger, who has herself taught more than 47,000 health-care professionals. Currently therapeutic touch is used throughout the United States and in 73 countries around the world.

Controversial Science

Despite increasing interest, many scientists and physicians are skeptical. Though thousands of patients and practitioners of therapeutic touch report significant healing benefits, convincing research conducted by accepted scientific methods is not as extensive.

Small sample sizes of some studies and inconsistencies of methods and results in others indicate a need for more scientifically rigorous research before the American medical community will give therapeutic touch its official stamp of approval.

The highest standard for research—the double-blind controlled study, in which neither the patient nor the practitioner knows who is receiving the therapy, is impossible with therapeutic touch. Nonetheless, there have been several very good studies that show a significant healing effect when therapeutic touch is used.

Pat Winstead-Fry, Ph.D., R.N., professor and interim dean of the school of nursing at the University of Vermont in Burlington, and colleagues conducted a metanalysis—a rigorous review of the good available studies done on therapeutic touch. Their conclusion? It works!

"The studies showed that therapeutic touch reduced anxiety, pain, blood pressure, pulse, that it was soothing to premature babies, that it had a positive effect on CD4 cell counts in persons with AIDS, and that it helped to ease grief," reports Dr. Winstead-Fry. "There's fine research on therapeutic touch, but it needs to get more sophisticated." (CD4 cells are a type of body cells that serve as an important measure in people with AIDS—when these cell counts go up, it's an indication that an individual's condition is worsening.)

Relief from Pain and Anxiety

The largest and one of the best studies to date looked at the effect of therapeutic touch on burn patients. People with severe burn injuries suffer excruciating pain that can go on for months and create considerable anxiety. Medication alone cannot bring complete relief.

In 1997, Ann Clark, Ph.D., R.N., associate professor and director of the Center for Nursing Research at the University of Alabama, and colleagues tested 99 burn patients to see if therapeutic touch used in conjunction with medication would provide additional relief.

One group of burn patients received therapeutic touch and another received mimic therapeutic touch (it looks like therapeutic touch but isn't) over a period of five days.

"Those who received therapeutic touch showed a statistically significant reduction in pain as well as decreased anxiety," reports Dr. Clark.

"Also," she notes, "though we didn't test for this, the nurses noticed that the burn patients who received therapeutic touch were healing much faster than those who didn't receive therapeutic touch."

Science Supports Therapeutic Touch

While Dr. Clark's study is the biggest and best to date, several other studies also support the effectiveness of therapeutic touch in helping to alleviate pain and reduce anxiety.

In the fall of 1998, researchers explored the effect of therapeutic touch on 25 people with osteoarthritis of one or both knees. Some received therapeutic touch, others received mimic therapeutic touch, and the rest received standard treatment.

Results showed a significant decrease in pain and improved joint function in the group that received genuine therapeutic touch.

"Research has shown that therapeutic touch is effective alone in relieving minor to moderate pain, and in severe pain is best used along with medication," says Dr. Clark. "And, therapeutic touch is one of the most effective nonmedicinal methods of reducing anxiety. There's a very fast response to the therapy, and there's good evidence for it in the research."

Speeding Healing

Another way in which therapeutic touch seems to be effective is in speeding up wound healing. In the most convincing study thus far, researchers gathered 44 male university students and made an incision in their arms. The students and practitioners were separated by a door. Students were asked to place their wounded arms through the doorway for 5 minutes at a time. Twenty-three of the students received therapeutic touch just on the arm, and the rest were given no treatment.

Results showed significantly accelerated healing among those who received therapeutic touch, and of that group, 13

finding a practitioner

Do you think therapeutic touch might benefit you? Seek a practitioner with at least three years of experience, advises Susan Wager, M.D. But first, be aware that there is also a discipline called healing touch, which combines many techniques and is not the same as therapeutic touch. Therapeutic touch specifically refers to the practice developed by Dolores Krieger, Ph.D., R.N., and Dora Kunz.

To find a well-qualified practitioner, turn to the Nurse Healers Professional Associates (NHPA), the official organization of therapeutic touch. This organization will give you the names of NHPA members in your area. Contact this organization at:

1211 Locust St.
Philadelphia, PA 19107
215/545-8079
www.familyforum.com/nhpa

Currently there is no certification for therapeutic touch practitioners, but those who are members of the NHPA must fill out a lengthy application showing rigorous training in therapeutic touch before they are accepted into membership. The cost of a therapeutic touch treatment ranges from nothing up to $75 a session.

Note: If you or a loved one becomes hospitalized and would like to receive therapeutic touch *in addition* to your medical treatment, ask your nurse or doctor. They may be able to locate a practitioner within the hospital.

were completely healed by the 16th day of the study compared with none from the nontreatment group.

While these findings are startling, researchers are divided on their significance since true therapeutic touch, which treats the entire body to affect the whole energy field, was not performed.

Dr. Wager, who feels the study makes a good case for the validity of therapeutic touch, gives other examples where therapeutic touch has accelerated healing: "We've observed clinically that patients with fractures heal in two-thirds the time when treated with therapeutic touch. And people with skin infections tend to do better when treated with therapeutic touch."

Why It Works

How exactly does therapeutic touch alleviate pain, reduce anxiety, and accelerate healing? Experts don't really know. Some suggest that therapeutic touch may stimulate the release of endorphins—the body's natural painkillers.

But this hasn't been studied in the laboratory. There is some research showing a positive effect on the immune system of people who have undergone therapeutic touch, but again more studies need to be done.

What researchers do know, however, is that therapeutic touch produces a measurable relaxation response. The heart and breathing rate slow. Muscles relax. Metabolism slows. The skin becomes warmer and slightly flushed.

These physical changes connected with the relaxation response, first described in 1974 by Herbert Benson, M.D., a Harvard researcher and physician, have been measured in the laboratory in connection with therapeutic touch.

"With therapeutic touch, we can get a relaxation response very rapidly—in two to four minutes," says Dr. Krieger. "The next best thing is biofeedback, which takes five minutes."

Relaxation Makes For Better Healing

Experts suspect that this relaxation response may be at the heart of therapeutic touch's effectiveness. It does help reduce anxiety, which may also be linked to decreases in pain. And it may have a positive effect on the immune system.

There's strong scientific evidence that ongoing stress—emotional or physical—may depress the immune system, which is the body's illness-fighting resource. By reducing stress through deep relaxation, it's possible to boost the immune system. This may explain why therapeutic touch seems to speed the healing of wounds, fractures, and infections.

The Treatment

If you get a therapeutic touch treatment, the practitioner will ask you to sit, fully clothed, on a stool or on a chair turned sideways so your back is unobstructed.

First the practitioner "centers" herself or himself. Centering clears the mind and brings about a calm focus. It prepares the practitioner to be able to sense the disturbances in your energy field, clear those disturbances, then direct energy to you to assist healing.

To become centered, the therapist breathes deeply and focuses on an image that brings a sense of peace. This process may take anywhere from a few seconds to several minutes.

Next, the practitioner will do an assessment of your energy field. He or she places the hands 3 to 5 inches from your body and sweeps them in a smooth motion from your head to your toes. The practitioner may do this in one of two ways: with one hand in front of you and the other in back, or with hands side to side and palms facing you. The hands generally sweep down your front side then down your back.

"It's not that the hands can't be placed on the body, but when they are a few inches away, it's easier to feel the energy field," says Dr. Krieger.

If the hands are held too close to the body, the texture of clothing and heat from the body may interfere with the sensing of the energy field, explains Janet Macrae, Ph.D., R.N., who has practiced therapeutic touch since 1975.

Sensing Energy Disturbances

As the practitioner moves his or her hands over your body, the practitioner is evaluating your energy field. Therapists have difficulty describing the energy field, as everyone perceives it somewhat differently. There is a sense of pressure, they maintain, and different sensations, such as heat, cold, or tingling, may be felt. A healthy person's energy flows smoothly, and the field should feel even to the practitioner. With someone who is ill, the practitioner will feel disturbances in the flow.

In her book *Therapeutic Touch: A Practical Guide*, Dr. Macrae categorizes these disturbances as loose congestion, tight congestion, a deficit, and an imbalance.

Loose congestion feels to the practitioner like a cloud of heat, a thickness, or a pressure. It is often found in the area of a wound or infection but may also be "free-floating." Tight congestion indicates a blockage in the energy flow, and it will feel "cold" or empty, as though there is an absence of energy.

A deficit signals a true depletion of energy and is often found around the site of a wound or infection; it almost always occurs with congestion. The practitioner will feel a pulling sensation as his or her hands pass over a deficit.

Finally, an imbalance is an area of the energy field that flows differently from the whole. Often occurring around a malfunctioning organ, it may feel like static, pins and needles, or disordered vibrations to the therapist.

Depending on the individual's health, the practitioner may discover one or all of these types of disturbances. As complicated as this all sounds, the assessment takes only 15 to 20 seconds.

Clearing the Energy Field

Once the assessment is complete, any congestion or blockages in energy flow are cleared. The practitioner does this by gently sweeping his or her hands downward over your body from head to toe, which, proponents maintain, moves the congestion down and out through the feet.

Next, the practitioner moves on to the phase known as balancing the energy field and transferring energy. In this phase, the practitioner directs energy to you to help restore a balanced overall flow of energy.

The practitioner isn't transferring his or her own energy but is acting as a conduit for the universal energy to flow through him or her and into you.

one person's experience

Liz Smith, who'd been studying therapeutic touch and other complementary medicines, decided she wanted to learn firsthand what a therapeutic touch treatment felt like. So she made an appointment in New York City to meet with Janet Macrae, Ph.D., R.N., who has practiced therapeutic touch since 1975.

Liz didn't have any health problems but had been under a lot of stress from work and family demands and was feeling fatigued.

Dr. Macrae began the session by lightly massaging Liz's neck and shoulders. Almost immediately, Liz experienced a rushing sensation to her head that made her feel a bit woozy. "I wasn't expecting to feel anything so dramatic; it really took me by surprise," she says. "It was like a rush of energy to my head."

The feeling passed and soon Liz was feeling very relaxed. Dr. Macrae did a quick assessment, found tight energy congestion in Liz's lower back, cleared the congestion, then directed energy into Liz.

Liz noticed sensations of heat, first in her lower back and then later in her legs and feet. Several minutes into the treatment, though, Liz experienced something she hadn't anticipated. She felt a wonderful sense of clarity come to her head. "It was as though a breeze blew through my mind and cleared away all the fatigue and fogginess that had been lingering there," she says. "My head felt lighter."

At the end of the session, Dr. Macrae proclaimed Liz in good health, remarking only on the "tightness" she had felt over the area of Liz's kidneys, which she said was not unusual since the kidneys' function is to clear away toxins.

Liz left the treatment feeling refreshed and in a cheerful mood. The lightness and clarity of mind stayed with her throughout the day. "I felt surprisingly happy," she says. "I found myself smiling and cheerful toward everyone—and in the midst of New York City no less."

Often the practitioner will visualize the energy as a stream of light coming from above, traveling down through his or her body and hands and finally entering you, the patient.

Evaluation and Reassessment

The therapist will reassess your energy field to determine if all the congestion has been cleared and the energy is balanced and flowing smoothly.

Sometimes during treatment, congestion is moved from one area to another and more work is needed for it to clear completely. When the therapist feels that the energy field has become smooth and even, the treatment is complete.

The length of treatment varies, depending on an individual's condition, but generally a session lasts 20 to 30 minutes, says Dr. Macrae.

Acute health problems, such as a headache or upset stomach, can be cleared with only one treatment. A cold should be treated every day until symptoms are gone, and chronic conditions like osteoarthritis or asthma require several treatments.

Just as every individual responds differently to any given medication, each of us has a different response to therapeutic touch as well.

Dr. Macrae describes treating three boys who were admitted to the hospital with acute asthma attacks. One boy felt immediate relief. The second boy experienced some improvement. And the third boy wasn't helped at all by therapeutic touch.

The Experience

What does it feel like to have your energy field manipulated? Will you be zapped by the life force directed into your body?

The sensations reported by people who have undergone therapeutic touch vary and may include tingling, muscle twitches, and warmth traveling down the body as congestion is cleared.

In a small study that looked at people's experience of therapeutic touch, Melodie Olsen, Ph.D., R.N., and Nancee Sneed, Ph.D., R.N., of the Medical University of South Carolina in Charleston recorded the comments of 11 individuals on their first therapeutic touch treatment. Here are some of the physical sensations the patients noted:

- **Feeling lighter**
- **Goose bumps**
- **Heaviness**
- **Warmth**
- **Tingling**
- **Pressure around the head**
- **Something being drawn out of the body**

One individual reported, "I came in with a headache and left without one." All 11 of the people in this study reported that they felt calm and relaxed during and after the session, which is consistent with the experience of anyone who undergoes therapeutic touch.

Do-It-Yourself Therapeutic Touch

Though therapeutic touch is most often practiced by nurses, anyone can learn it and use it with family and friends. "This is what I hope the future of therapeutic touch will be," says Dr. Krieger. "I taught a couple who used it during pregnancy and continued to do it in their family and in the community. Many folks use therapeutic touch with their kids during the flu season, and it's used in nursing homes and with hospice patients."

Therapeutic touch can even be used on pets. "My Siberian husky is a therapeutic touch addict," confesses Dr. Winstead-Fry. "As soon as I walk in the door, she rolls over in anticipation of a treatment."

You can even use the healing power of therapeutic touch on yourself through visualization, as Dr. Macrae explains in her book. Here's how it works:

- **Center yourself.** Sit quietly and inhale and exhale deeply. Then focus on some image that brings you peace (perhaps some image from nature).
- **Open to energy.** When you feel calm and focused, visualize the universal energy coming down from above your head and flowing through you from head to toe. It may help to imagine this energy as light or water. Visualize this healing energy clearing away whatever pain or illness you are feeling.
- **Use your hands.** To enhance this self-treatment, place your hands over the area of your illness or pain (either directly on your body or a few inches away) and imagine the energy flowing through your hands, taking the pain away.
- **Stick with it.** Minor ailments such as a cut or upset stomach may clear up quickly, says Dr. Macrae, but for chronic problems, you need to practice this visualization regularly for several weeks, depending on the condition.

Safety and Warnings

"The worst that can happen," says Dr. Macrae, "is that the patient doesn't get better." There usually is no danger in using therapeutic touch unless you try to use it as a substitute for necessary medical treatment.

- **Watch for energy overload.** Therapeutic touch is a very safe practice; however, it is possible to take on an energy overload during treatment. Signs of excess energy include irritability or anxiety—the exact opposite of the calm relaxation that therapeutic touch usually induces. Experts emphasize that treatments should generally last no longer than 20 to 30 minutes and should be stopped sooner if symptoms of discomfort appear.
- **Show special care with children.** With children, who respond much more quickly to therapeutic touch than adults, treatments should be kept to only a few minutes. And for infants, several seconds should be sufficient.
- **Be aware of special needs.** Short sessions are also recommended for pregnant women, persons with head injuries, and individuals

touching the inner self

Often when we talk about healing and health practices, we slip into a discussion only of the specific ailments we can alleviate or cure. We lose sight of the whole. When we step back and look at therapeutic touch and its effects, what's finally so striking is not that it eases pain or helps mend fractures but that it raises patients *and* their practitioners to a greater sense of well-being. Nearly every practitioner of therapeutic touch holds this view.

"This hasn't been clinically tested or studied, but in my opinion, based on 19 years of practicing therapeutic touch and on the 3,500 carefully documented records of the patients I've worked with, therapeutic touch produces a great sense of well-being," says Ann Clark, Ph.D., R.N., associate professor and director of the Center for Nursing Research at the University of Alabama School of Nursing.

In fact, one study that recorded the experiences of 20 volunteers who had undergone therapeutic touch treatment reported that "therapeutic touch was described as intensifying and prolonging feelings of satisfaction, peace, and serenity." Susan Wager, M.D., echoes Dr. Clark's observations: "Many patients who are treated with therapeutic touch experience certain changes in their quality of life. They become more in touch with their inner selves and more intuitive." They begin to find solutions to problems they've been having.

"Through therapeutic touch, you become deeply connected to something greater than you," explains Janet Macrae, Ph.D., R.N., "to the flow of life, which is always creative."

experiencing trauma who may be in shock. It's better to repeat a treatment later than to overdo a single treatment.

Therapeutic touch should not be used with psychotic people, individuals who have a history of abuse, or persons whose sense of self is very vulnerable and who might be frightened or interpret therapeutic touch as an invasion of their space, warns Dr. Macrae.

But in most situations, therapeutic touch can be a valuable complement to conventional medicine. "Therapeutic touch helps relieve suffering. It really makes patients feel better and more comfortable," says Dr. Wager. "Anything we can do to those ends should be integrated into conventional medical care."

Apparently, a number of health-care professionals agree with her, as therapeutic touch is being used with ever-increasing frequency in hospitals across the nation.

resources

Seminars and workshops on therapeutic touch are taught throughout the country. For a referral to one near you, contact the **Nurse Healers Professional Associates,** the official organization of therapeutic touch, which has established criteria for workshops:

1211 Locust St.
Philadelphia, PA 19107
215/545-8079

Books

The Therapeutic Touch: How to Use Your Hands to Help or to Heal by Dolores Krieger, Ph.D., R.N. (Prentice Hall Press, 1979)

Accepting Your Power to Heal: The Personal Practice of Therapeutic Touch by Dolores Krieger, Ph.D., R.N. (Bear & Company, 1993)

Both books by Dr. Krieger offer detailed descriptions and illustrations of how to do a treatment, along with exercises to help you develop skills.

Therapeutic Touch: A Practical Guide by Janet Macrae, Ph.D., R.N. (Alfred A. Knopf, 1997)

This book provides clear and thorough instructions and explanations of the process of therapeutic touch and its effects.

Therapeutic Touch Inner Workbook by Dolores Krieger, Ph.D., R.N. (Bear & Company, 1996)

A Doctor's Guide to Therapeutic Touch by Susan Wager, M.D., and Dora Kunz (Perigree, 1996)

A Gift for Healing by Debora Cowens and Tom Monte (Crown, 1996)

Audiocassette

Therapeutic Touch: Practical Techniques for Healing Through the Vital Energy Field by Dolores Krieger, Ph.D., R.N (Sounds True, 1997)

chapter 22

vegetarianism
THE MEATLESS ADVANTAGE

A healthful vegetarian diet means much more than eating just vegetables. —*Suzanne Havala, R.D., nutrition adviser for the Vegetarian Resource Group*

Vegetarian. A few years ago, the word conjured up images of health-fanatic hippies munching sprouts, brown rice, and tofu. Today, going meatless is mainstream. More than 12 million American adults call themselves vegetarians, and meatless meals are common options on supermarket shelves and restaurant menus and in college cafeterias. Even tofu—once reviled—is gaining newfound respect from vegetarians and meat-eaters alike.

People become vegetarian for a number of reasons—religious beliefs and concerns about animals, the environment, and world hunger, for instance.

But the most compelling reason for many is the health benefits that being vegetarian is thought to offer.

Eating for Health And Well-Being

Compared to their carnivorous cousins, vegetarians are a healthier lot. They weigh less and enjoy lower blood pressure and blood cholesterol readings. Vegetarians also suffer less often from chronic diseases and conditions such as heart disease, high blood pressure, cancer, diabetes, kidney stones, gallstones, and diverticular disease.

Many findings about the link between vegetarianism and health come from studies of California Seventh-Day Adventists (SDAs). About half of this religious group are lacto-ovo vegetarians (meaning that they do eat both dairy products and eggs). Generally, SDAs follow health-promoting habits such as abstaining from alcohol, smoking, caffeine, and highly refined foods, and eating abundant amounts of grains, vegetables, fruits, and nuts.

Several studies among SDAs and other vegetarian populations show that vegetarians have about half the risk of death from heart disease than does the general population.

"One reason vegetarians are at lower risk for heart disease is because they eat less saturated fat and dietary cholesterol, which promotes lower blood cholesterol levels," says Mark Messina, Ph.D., associate professor of nutrition at Loma Linda University in California and former program director of the National Cancer Institute's Diet and Cancer branch.

"Another possible reason is that they consume more of the disease-fighting phytochemicals found in plant foods," he says. Dr. Messina also notes that the protective effect on the heart is strongest among vegetarian men.

Vegetarians Get More Vitamins

Vegetarians' higher intakes of some vitamins compared to those of meat-eaters may also contribute to better heart health. Vegetarians consume more of the antioxidant vitamins E and C and beta-carotene, which may protect against harmful changes in "bad" LDL cholesterol. (Antioxidants are substances that neutralize free radicals. These are naturally occurring molecules that damage the body's cells.)

Vegetarians also consume more of the B-vitamin folic acid. Getting enough of this vitamin helps lower blood levels of the amino acid homocysteine. High blood levels of homocysteine are a newly recognized risk factor for heart disease.

Vegetarianism Pays Off

What vegetarians don't eat may also play a role in heart disease risk. In SDAs, studies found that the risk of fatal heart disease among men who ate beef up to three times each week was nearly double that of men who did not eat beef at all. For men who ate beef more than three times each week that risk was more than double.

Several studies also show that vegetarians suffer from high blood pressure less often than meat-eaters. A review of clinical trials in which meat-eaters adopted a lacto-ovo vegetarian diet concluded that a vegetarian diet helps lower systolic (top number) blood pressure between five and 10 points.

Vegetarians' lower incidence of high blood pressure isn't explained by differences in body weight or fat, sodium, fiber, potassium, or meat intake. "It's possible that lower blood pressure in vegetarians results from a unique combination of foods or nutrients they commonly eat," says Dr. Messina.

Eating to Beat Cancer

Vegetarians are also at less risk of dying from cancer. A study of German vegetarians showed deaths from all types of cancer were reduced by 52 percent in vegetarian men and 26 percent in vegetarian women. SDAs show a similar pattern.

Regarding colorectal cancer, Dr. Messina says, "Vegetarians are at less risk because they don't eat red meat and possibly because they eat more fiber from grains, fruits, and vegetables." This pattern reflects the American Cancer Society's conclusion

vegetarian
daily food guide

For the most nutrients and fiber, select a wide and colorful variety of grains, legumes, vegetables, and fruits in their whole, unrefined state. To minimize saturated fat and cholesterol, choose protein and fiber-packed plant foods such as dry beans, peas, lentils, and tofu, and low-fat varieties of milk, cheese, and yogurt. Keep egg yolks down to four or fewer per week. Go easy on "extras" such as fats and oils, sweets, and snack foods.

Food Group	Suggested Daily Servings	Serving Sizes
Breads, cereals, rice, and pasta	6 or more	1 slice whole-grain or enriched bread, ½ bun, ½ bagel, or ½ English muffin 1 tortilla ½ cup cooked cereal, such as oatmeal, bulgur, barley, quinoa, or millet ½ cup cooked rice or pasta 1 ounce dry cereal
Vegetables	4 or more	½ cup cooked vegetables ¾ cup vegetable juice
Fruit	3 or more	1 whole apple, peach, banana, or other similar-size fruit
Legumes and other meat alternatives	2 to 3	½ cup cooked beans or peas 4 ounces tofu or tempeh 8 ounces soy-protein patties 2 Tbsp. peanut butter 2 Tbsp. nuts or seeds
Eggs (optional)	not more than 4 yolks a week	1 egg or 2 egg whites or ¼ cup egg substitute
Milk, cheese, and yogurt (optional)	2 to 3 servings	1 cup milk or yogurt 1½ ounces natural cheese or 2 ounces processed cheese
Fats, oils, and sweets	Eat sparingly	Oil, margarine, mayonnaise, salad dressing Candy and sugars

that a diet high in animal fats from foods such as red meat increases the risk for colorectal cancer, while a diet high in vegetables and fruits is protective.

Many questions are as yet unanswered about how and why vegetarianism seems to confer health benefits, and researchers are working to answer these questions. But you don't have to wait to "go veg," if you're so inclined. Existing evidence is compelling that a well-planned vegetarian diet contributes powerfully to good health.

Going Meatless Is Not Enough

Enjoying the health benefits of being vegetarian takes more than just nudging the meat off your plate. You need to pay careful attention to the foods that replace it. Vegetarians who load up on high-fat dairy products, fast foods, and snack items, and skimp on grains, fruits, and vegetables, negate the advantages of vegetarian eating.

A vegetarian diet takes some planning to make sure it's healthful and nutritious, says Suzanne Havala, R.D., nutrition adviser for the Baltimore-based Vegetarian Resource Group and author of *The Complete Idiot's Guide to Being Vegetarian*.

"Many people become what I call 'iceberg lettuce eaters,'" says Havala. "They unnecessarily cut out many foods, and vegetarian eating becomes an unpleasant experience. A healthful vegetarian diet means much more than eating just vegetables."

Havala also cautions against the "cheese and eggs" rut. "I see people relying on cheese and eggs at every meal to get protein. That's really not necessary and they're getting way too much saturated fat," says Havala.

Just like everyone else, vegetarians need to pay attention to eating well-balanced nutritious meals. The Vegetarian Daily Food Guide, based on the government's Dietary Guidelines for Americans, should help. It suggests the best balance from each food group.

Nutrients That Need Special Attention

Giving up meat, poultry, and fish (and dairy and eggs in the case of vegans) means vegetarians must keep tabs on some important nutrients supplied by these animal foods.

- **Calcium.** This mineral is important for strong bones and proper muscle function. Healthy adults ages 19 to 50 need 1,000 milligrams of calcium daily and 1,200 milligrams after the age of 50.

Vegetarians who include dairy products can easily meet their calcium needs by eating milk, yogurt, and cheese. Vegans must take special care to get enough calcium from plant sources. Good food sources for calcium include:

- Calcium-fortified soy milk and orange juice
- Dry beans
- Many green leafy vegetables
- Nuts and seeds

plant calcium counts

Even if you don't eat dairy products—and some vegetarians don't—it's still possible to get calcium from your food. You need to be aware, however, of which foods contain calcium.

Food	Calcium (milligrams)
Leafy greens, such as kale, bok choy, and turnip, collard, mustard, and dandelion greens, ½ cup cooked	75–100
Broccoli, ½ cup cooked	35
Legumes, such as chickpeas and pinto, navy, and great northern beans, ½ cup cooked	40–65
Almonds, ¼ cup	80
Soybeans and tempeh, ½ cup cooked	75–85
Tofu (calcium set), ½ cup	260
Soy milk (calcium fortified), 1 cup	200–500
Soy cheese, 1 ounce	200–300
Blackstrap molasses, 1 tablespoon	170
Orange juice, calcium fortified, 6 ounces	200
Orange, 1 medium	50
Figs, 5 dried	135

- Tofu processed with calcium
- "Plant Calcium Counts" above, shows the calcium counts in a variety of plant foods. Although spinach, beet greens, and Swiss chard contain calcium, don't count on them for your calcium. Calcium from these vegetables is not absorbed well. If you can't meet your calcium needs with food, take a calcium supplement to make up the difference.

- **Vitamin D.** This vitamin helps your body absorb calcium and phosphorus and deposit them in bones and teeth. Your body makes vitamin D when it's exposed to sunlight. Very few foods are naturally high in vitamin D, but in the United States, dairy products are fortified with this vitamin.

Vegans who don't get regular sun (20 to 30 minutes of summer sun on hands and face two to three times per week) may need a supplement that contains 100 percent of the Daily Value for vitamin D. Don't exceed this level. Vitamin D can be toxic in large amounts.

vegetarian varieties

- **Lacto-ovo vegetarians** don't eat meat, poultry, or fish, but may eat dairy products and eggs. Most vegetarians in the United States follow this type of eating plan.
- **Lacto vegetarians** don't eat meat, poultry, fish, or eggs, but do eat dairy products.
- **Semivegetarians** mostly follow a vegetarian eating pattern, but occasionally eat meat, poultry, or fish. A lot of Americans are now listing themselves in this category or at least aiming for it as a goal.
- **Vegans (VEE-guns)** are the strictest vegetarians. They avoid all animal products such as meat, poultry, fish, eggs, and dairy products.

• **Iron.** The mineral iron is important for healthy red blood cells and to prevent anemia. Good vegetarian sources of iron include:

- Blackstrap molasses
- Dried fruits
- Dry beans
- Fortified breads and cereals
- Nuts and seeds
- Tofu
- Turnip greens

The iron in plant foods is more difficult to absorb than the iron in meat, poultry, or fish, but you can boost the amount you absorb by pairing them with a vitamin C-rich food such as:

- Broccoli
- Citrus fruits and juices
- Tomatoes

• **Zinc.** This mineral is essential for proper growth, tissue repair, immune system function, and energy production. Vegetarians must keep tabs on their zinc intake because this mineral is most plentiful in animal foods such as meat, seafood, and liver. Good sources of zinc for lacto-ovo vegetarians include low-fat dairy products, such as:

- Cheese
- Milk
- Yogurt

Other foods supply this valuable nutrient in smaller amounts:

- Dry beans
- Nut and seeds
- Tofu
- Whole grains
- Whole wheat bread
- Wheat germ

Zinc from these foods may be more difficult to absorb. Studies show, however, that vegetarians usually get enough zinc.

• **Vitamin B12.** This vitamin plays a role in making red blood cells. It is found in foods from animal sources, so getting enough is generally not a problem for vegetarians who eat plenty of dairy products and eggs.

Vegetarians who choose to limit these foods and vegans should select a fortified breakfast cereal or take a supplement that provides 100 percent of the Daily Value for vitamin B12. Some older people (vegetarian or not) have difficulty absorbing the B12 found naturally in foods.

The National Academy of Sciences recommends people older than 50 choose fortified foods or a supplement to ensure they get enough B12.

- **Protein.** Forget the old rule about combining "complementary proteins" at each meal to build complete proteins from plant foods. Vegetarians used to worry about pairing the right foods in order to get top-quality protein.

Researchers have always been aware that most plant foods contain protein, but they thought that plant proteins needed to be eaten in certain combinations in order for the body to make the best of it.

Research now shows that the body makes its own complete proteins when a variety of foods and enough calories are eaten throughout the day.

Tips for Making The Transition

If you decide to go vegetarian—or even to begin adding a few more meatless meals to your recipe repertoire—experts say a gradual approach is easiest. Here's a four-step plan for making the transition:

- **Take stock.** Chances are you already enjoy many meatless dishes. A few examples:
  - Bean soup
  - Grilled cheese sandwiches
  - Pasta with tomato sauce
  - Peanut butter sandwiches
  - Vegetarian lasagna

Start by planning a few meals a week around these trusted favorites.

- **Make an adjustment.** Use tofu, nuts, or seeds in place of meat or poultry in your favorite stir-fry dish. Prepare your usual recipes for taco filling, spaghetti sauce, and chili with textured vegetable protein, a soy-based substitute for ground beef. Order pizza loaded with veggies instead of sausage and pepperoni.
- **Branch out.** Invest in a great vegetarian cookbook to learn some new recipes. Explore ethnic cuisines such as Italian, Indian, Middle Eastern, and Chinese that feature many vegetables and grain-based dishes. Shop for new options such as tofu, tempeh, hummus (chickpea dip), and veggie burgers.
- **Get support.** Check out the Vegetarian Resource Group website at www.vrg.org. You'll find excellent nutrition advice for planning a well-balanced vegetarian diet, plus loads of delicious recipes.

Sorting Out Soy

Reduce cholesterol! Prevent breast cancer! Keep bones strong! Stop hot flashes cold! With all the health benefits we've heard about the humble soybean, you might as well dub it "The Wonder Bean."

Soybeans and soy foods such as tofu, tempeh, miso, and soy milk have long been protein-rich staples in the vegetarian diet. But does soy really follow through on its health-protective promises? Here's the soy scoop from Clare Hasler, Ph.D., soy researcher and executive director of the Functional Foods for Health Program at the University of Illinois in Urbana.

- **Heart disease.** The research here is solid, says Dr. Hasler. More than 50 clinical trials

finding guidance

A well-balanced vegetarian diet can be healthful for anyone. But vegetarian diets for infants, children, teens, and pregnant and breastfeeding women need special planning to make sure they include enough calories and nutrients such as calcium, iron, zinc, vitamin B12, and vitamin D. Registered dietitians (R.D.s) are nutrition experts who can devise a healthful and delicious vegetarian diet for all ages and stages. To find an R.D. near you, contact The American Dietetic Association at 800/366-1655 or www.eatright.org. Look for an R.D. who specializes in vegetarian diets and meal planning.

show that eating soy protein helps prevent heart disease by lowering blood cholesterol levels.

You'll need to get at least 25 grams of soy protein each day from foods such as tofu, soy-based veggie burgers, baked goods made with soy flour, and soy milk. "But it won't work if you don't also eat a low-fat diet and exercise regularly," says Dr. Hasler.

• **Breast cancer.** The evidence here is not so clear. "The data showing that soy reduces breast cancer risk looks at large groups of women in soy-eating populations such as Asians," says Dr. Hasler. "There are no published clinical studies."

Another question mark: Researchers don't know whether soy only exerts a protective effect if it's eaten throughout life as it is in Asian populations.

If you have been diagnosed with what's known as estrogen receptor positive breast cancer, steer clear of soy foods and supplements for now. Researchers simply don't know whether soy stimulates the development of the disease. It's possible that it inhibits it, but they just don't know for sure.

• **Osteoporosis.** Researchers are investigating whether the phytoestrogens (estrogen-like plant chemicals) in soy help reduce bone loss in postmenopausal women. Results in studies using lab animals are promising but only preliminary.

"You can't say you should replace a proven osteoporosis treatment such as hormone replacement therapy with soy," says Dr. Hasler.

You can count on calcium-containing soy products such as calcium-fortified soy milk and tofu processed with calcium to contribute to the 1,200 milligrams of daily calcium recommended for postmenopausal women.

• **Menopause symptoms.** Dr. Hasler is "intrigued" by research showing that the phytoestrogens in soy can relieve hot flashes. One study, for example, found that postmenopausal women who ate 45 grams of soy flour per day had a 40 percent reduction in hot flashes.

Mind over matter was working here, too. Another group who received wheat flour also experienced fewer hot flashes, but the difference between the two groups was still significant.

There aren't clear-cut answers here, but Dr. Hasler says it's fine to try a serving or two of soy each day to see whether your hot flashes fade.

• **The bottom line.** As soy researchers continue to seek answers, Dr. Hasler offers some advice. "It's the pattern of what you eat that's most important, not any one food," she maintains. "Eat a low-fat, plant-based diet, get five to nine servings of fruits and vegetables each day, and then, yes, soy can be a healthful part of that plan."

Vegetarian Q and A

Q Can a vegetarian diet reverse heart disease?

A Yes, when it's very low in fat and one of many intensive lifestyle changes, according to research by Dean Ornish, M.D., head of the Preventive Medicine Research Institute (PMRI) in Sausalito, California.

The Ornish program for heart disease reversal combines a strict vegetarian diet containing less than 10 percent of daily calories from fat and almost no saturated fat, with a moderate aerobic exercise program, daily stress management techniques, group psychosocial support, and smoking cessation.

A recent study by Ornish published in the *Journal of the American Medical Association* reported on 20 heart patients who followed this regime for five years.

Their heart disease progression was compared to 15 control patients who followed the American Heart Association's (AHA) Step II diet for heart patients (30 percent or fewer of daily calories from fat, less than 7 percent of daily calories from saturated fat, and no more than 200 milligrams of cholesterol) and were asked to follow their personal physician's advice about lifestyle changes.

The Ornish group did not take cholesterol-lowering drugs, although 60 percent of the control group took medication.

After five years, the coronary arteries of the Ornish followers were slightly wider, while arteries in the control group were more blocked than when the study began.

During the study, people in the control group also experienced more than twice as many cardiac problems and treatments, such as heart attacks, angioplasties, bypass surgeries, and hospitalizations, than did the Ornish group.

The Ornish program is not without its critics, though. The AHA says the study was too small to call for a change in diet recommendations for the healthy, general public, and that only a select, highly motivated group can follow the intensive lifestyle regimen long term.

Vegetarian nutrition expert Dr. Havala, who is a PMRI staff member, acknowledges that adopting the program is a challenge that requires a solid support system, but says the excellent results are well worth the effort.

Extremely low-fat diets are not recommended for very young children, pregnant or breastfeeding women, and the elderly because it's difficult to get enough calories and essential fatty acids on this kind of diet.

Q **Does a vegetarian diet help sufferers of rheumatoid arthritis?**

A **With rheumatoid arthritis, the body's immune system for unknown reasons attacks healthy tissue in the joints, leading to painful inflammation.**

Some limited research shows that people with arthritis who followed a closely monitored low-fat vegetarian diet experienced some relief from symptoms such as tender and swollen joints, pain, and morning stiffness. But, says Dr. Havala, "more studies are needed before researchers can reach a consensus. A carefully planned vegetarian diet can be a healthful choice for people with rheumatoid arthritis, but should definitely not substitute for their prescribed treatment."

For now, the Arthritis Foundation recommends a well-balanced diet with adequate protein and extra folic acid to counteract losses of this vitamin caused by the anti-arthritis medication methotrexate. Vegetarian or not, it's wise for people with arthritis to seek nutrition counseling and meal-planning advice from a registered dietitian.

Q **What is a macrobiotic diet? Does it cure cancer?**

A **Macrobiotics is a way of life based on an Oriental principle of balance throughout the universe.** Followers believe incorporating spiritual and social aspects of macrobiotics, including diet, into one's life will promote health and healing.

The diet is near-vegetarian, mostly made up of whole grains and vegetables, and small amounts of beans, nuts, and seeds, seaweed, miso soup, and herbal teas. A small amount of fish or chicken is allowed once or twice a week.

A carefully planned macrobiotic diet can provide adequate nutrition for a person in peak health and, because it is low in fat and high in plant foods, may reduce the risk for heart disease and certain cancers.

However, the macrobiotic diet will not cure cancer or any other illness, says the American Cancer Society (ACS). Because the diet excludes many foods, it can place all but the most vigilant followers at risk for nutritional deficiency. The ACS says children, pregnant or breastfeeding women, and the elderly, frail, or ill should not follow this diet.

Q **I don't eat fish. What plant foods contain omega-3 fatty acids?**

A **The omega-3 fatty acids found in fatty fish such as tuna, salmon, and mackerel are linked to reduced risk for heart disease**. Ground flax seed, walnuts, soybeans, and canola oil are sources of omega-3s for vegetarians.

fascinating phytochemicals

The tongue-twisting phytochemicals in plant foods are a mouthful to pronounce, but they get much of the credit for the health benefits vegetarian diets appear to offer. One fruit, vegetable, or grain may contain hundreds of different phytochemicals. Here's a lineup of just a few that are being studied, the foods they're found in, and their potential health benefits:

Phytochemical	Food Sources	May Protect Against
Allyl sulfides	Garlic, onions, leeks, chives, and shallots	Heart disease and cancer May stimulate the immune system
Beta-carotene	Carrots, sweet potatoes, broccoli, spinach, mangoes, cantaloupe, and apricots	Cancer and heart disease May boost the immune system and help maintain healthy vision
Flavonoids	Fruits, vegetables, red wine, grape juice, and green and black tea	Cancer and heart disease
Genistein	Soybeans, soy milk, tofu, tempeh, and other soy-based foods	Heart disease and hormone-related cancers such as breast cancer May also reduce menopausal symptoms and protect against osteoporosis
Lignans	Flax seed and flour, whole grains, and some berries	Heart disease and hormone-related cancers
Limonene	Citrus fruits such as oranges, lemons, and limes	Cancer
Lutein	Spinach and collard greens	Age-related macular degeneration (an eye disease)
Lycopene	Cooked tomato products, such as tomato sauce or paste; pink grapefruit, and watermelon	Prostate cancer
Sulforaphane	Cruciferous vegetables such as broccoli, cabbage, and cauliflower	Cancer

resources

Books

Better Homes and Gardens® Low-Fat & Luscious Vegetarian (Better Homes and Gardens, 1997)

The Complete Idiot's Guide to Being Vegetarian by Suzanne Havala, R.D. (Chronimed, 1998)

Being Vegetarian by Suzanne Havala, R.D. (Chronimed, 1996)

The Vegetarian Way: Total Health for You and Your Family by Virginia Messina, R.D., M.P.H., and Mark Messina, Ph.D. (Crown, 1996)

Simply Vegan by Debra Wasserman and Reed Mangels, Ph.D., R.D. (Vegetarian Resource Group, 1995)

Eat More, Weigh Less by Dean Ornish, M.D. (Harperperennial, 1994)

Newsletter

Loma Linda University Vegetarian Nutrition and Health Letter:
888/558-8703

Websites

Vegetarian Resource Group:
www.vrg.org

Vegetarian Pages:
www.veg.org/veg/

chapter 23

vision therapy

EXERCISE FOR THE EYES

The visual system is an outgrowth of the brain.
We're not treating eyeballs, we're treating human beings.
—Anne Barber, Optometric Extension Program Foundation

Vision is a complicated process that involves taking in information and processing it. Our eyes must work together smoothly and in cooperation with each other. We must focus far away and close up, judge depth, see peripherally as well as straight ahead, remember images, and do all these things in rapid succession, often simultaneously.

But sometimes things go wrong. We may have blurred or double vision, eyes turned in or out, focusing problems, or reading and writing difficulties. These problems may begin in childhood or not become apparent until adulthood. They can even result from an injury such as whiplash.

What It Is: How It Works

Enter vision therapy, a host of techniques that coax your brain into sending the right messages to your eye muscles. It does this through specific exercises, such as following a moving object, focusing on beads on a string, or working with lenses, prisms, and filters.

vision therapy helps heal

The American Optometric Association and College of Optometrists in Vision Development consider vision therapy approved treatment for:

- Eye movement control problems (oculomotor dysfunction)
- Focusing problems (accommodative disorders)
- Inefficiency and lack of coordination using both eyes together (vergence dysfunction)
- Lazy eye (amblyopia, or poor acuity or muscle control in one eye)
- Misaligned eyes, such as crossed eyes or turned-in eyes (strabismus)
- Visual sensory and motor integration

Training may help visual skills such as:

- Acuity, both near and distant
- Binocularity (ability to use both eyes together)
- Depth perception
- Fixation (locating and inspecting a series of stationary objects)
- Focus change
- Maintaining attention on a skill or activity
- Peripheral vision
- Tracking
- Visualization, forming mental images in your mind

Visual therapy also is used after a brain injury or stroke that causes a problem in processing visual information.

"What we're really training is the visual processing system, how the brain processes information," says Barry Beck, a certified therapy technician and head of vision therapy at the Minnesota Vision Therapist Center in Minneapolis.

But the phrase "vision therapy" is a catchall, points out Stephen Miller, O.D., director of the College of Optometrists in Vision Development (COVD) in St. Louis, Missouri. It might describe progressive drills a child does to correct a turned-in eye; a program designed to improve how fast a person's eyes respond while participating in his or her favorite sport; or a do-at-home mix of yoga, relaxation techniques, and eye exercises.

It's important to note that not all vision therapy has the scientific stamp of approval. "There's lots of baloney out there," admits Bradley Coffey, O.D., a professor of optometry at the Pacific University College of Optometry in Portland, Oregon. "But in the middle there's a large body of good work, and in some cases, this approach to health care, applied properly to the proper patients, can be literally life changing." (O.D. stands for Doctor of Optometry.)

Controversial Beginnings

The father of vision therapy—some prefer to think of him as the black sheep—was William H. Bates, M.D., who in 1920 wrote an innovative and controversial book, *The Cure of Imperfect Sight by Treatment Without Glasses.*

Dr. Bates believed that glasses harm your eyes and that nearsightedness and farsightedness are caused by straining to see or by stress or fear. He believed that "rest or relaxation, first of the mind and then of the eyes" was essential to good vision.

He introduced focusing and relaxation exercises, and suggested memory involvement in vision.

Some still use his methods, modified in 1943 in *The Bates Method for Better Eyesight Without Glasses,* which is still in print.

Many vision therapists shudder at the mention of his name, however. "Bates is a minefield," says Dr. Coffey. "He did have a couple of good ideas, but the couple of good ideas were mixed in with some that were just dead wrong. He missed on a couple of the critical parts of his theory, not by a little but by a lot." Most mainstream practitioners completely dismiss him.

But from these early concepts of vision therapy, a diverse and promising field has developed, and scientific support is growing. Vision therapy is now used to correct or prevent vision problems, as well as to improve an individual's vision in sports performance.

"Unfortunately, the level of hype surrounding 'throw away your glasses' programs has overwhelmed the work that helps people overcome problems that relate to how their eyes focus or coordinate," notes Dr. Miller. "This may make you think that everyone can go through vision therapy and expect to throw away their glasses, and that's not going to happen."

Here's a look at conditions vision therapy is currently and legitimately used for.

Helping Your Eyes Work Together

Close first one eye, then the other: It's obvious that each has a different field of vision. Optimally, we blend those images seamlessly and use both eyes as a well-coordinated team.

When things go wrong, the result can be lazy eye (amblyopia), crossed eyes or turned-in eyes (strabismus), lack of depth perception, or problems in moving and using the eyes together (convergence) and focusing (accommodation). For these conditions, vision therapy often provides some relief.

Vision therapy is most commonly used for problems focusing and using the eyes together, according to Jeffrey Cooper, O.D., professor of clinical optometry at the State University of New York at Stony Brook. Up to 15 percent of the population has convergence problems, he says, and studies show that vision therapy is the preferred treatment for these conditions.

There's plenty of scientific support for using vision therapy for tracking, focusing, and binocular problems (ability to use the eyes together). It's also effective for many physiological and information-processing vision problems, according to the American Optometric Association (AOA).

A review of treatments for lazy eye found that scientific literature strongly supports vision therapy. And in a 1992 article, Dr. Coffey reviewed 59 studies that involved more than 3,500 people, evaluating the effectiveness of five treatments for intermittent exotropia, a wandering-eye problem.

Vision therapy, with a 59 percent success rate, was the most successful. Surgery was the next most effective of the treatments, at 46 percent.

When it comes to crossed eyes and other forms of strabismus, evidence suggests that vision therapy should be the first treatment—it's less invasive than surgery, and as successful, according to the authors of a 1994 review of literature in the *Journal of the American Optometric Association.*

"We can straighten eyes without surgery, in a nine- to 12-month program," declares Beck. And surgery is often not the best choice for another reason. While surgery may mechanically change the eyes' orientation, it doesn't help the brain adapt to this new position.

"The eyes are not where the brain expects them to be," Beck explains. "What often happens is that the brain doesn't like seeing double. Either the brain ends up ignoring one eye and just using one, or it gradually works the eyes back into the position they were before."

He often works with people whose eyes have drifted back into misalignment following surgery. "If you're going to straighten the eyes, you have to change the visual adaptation in the brain," he says. And that involves vision therapy.

Helping with Learning Problems

The Optometric Extension Program (OEP) Foundation, formed to provide postgraduate behavioral optometry education, maintains that visual problems account for many learning difficulties and should be nipped in the bud.

"Every child should be seen by a behavioral optometrist by six months of age," says Anne Barber, director of OEP program services in Santa Ana, California. "The visual system is an outgrowth of the brain. We're not treating eyeballs, we're treating human beings."

Developmental vision therapy related to learning and classroom performance is widely practiced but still touched with controversy.

Some reading problems are amenable to vision therapy, Dr. Coffey says, while others are not. The American Academy of Optometry and the AOA agree that vision therapy doesn't directly treat learning disabilities or dyslexia, but it does improve visual efficiency and processing.

True dyslexia, an inability to read or write words despite recognizing letters, is not specifically a vision problem.

Deficiencies in focusing, tracking, using the eyes together, plus having problems with perception, such as poor hand-eye coordination and poor visual memory, can all affect schoolwork, however.

"I look at graphs of kids' eye movements, and they're reading from left to right, right to left, then down and back," says Beck. "I can't see how anyone can say that ineffective eye movement skills don't lead to reading problems when someone can't even stay on the same line."

Robert Simon, O.D., works primarily with children in his practice in Brentwood, Tennessee. "What I tell parents is that 85 percent of everything you learn comes through your eyes," he says. "If the eyes don't function properly, when the eyes are not working together as a team, a child can't learn properly."

Being a Better Athlete

Much of vision therapy is remedial—getting the eyes to function normally—but sports optometry or vision therapy takes things one step further and uses the concepts of vision therapy to take people from normal to supernormal.

Ironically, this can make vision therapy more appealing for a number of people. "One of the things that helps parents decide to do a vision therapy program is not that their child will be able to read better," says Beck, "but that the child might be a better softball player."

The therapist determines what visual aspects of the sport are the most important and works on those, and some athletes claim dramatic benefits. Greg Vaughn, a Major League Baseball player, after struggling for two seasons and sinking to a .206 average, soared after vision therapy in 1998, hitting 50 home runs and helping the San Diego Padres to the World Series.

Behavioral optometrist Donald J. Getz, O.D., of Van Nuys, California, has worked with the U.S. volleyball team to improve response time.

Vision training can improve depth perception, visual acuity, field of recognition, motion perception, and simultaneous vision, according to a review of studies on vision and sports.

In a study done at Acadia University in Nova Scotia, students who participated in a visual skills program involving depth perception and reaction time improved their balance significantly after four weeks.

Another study reported that after three hours of training, students markedly improved their performance on spatial tasks. Volleyball players at San Jose State University in California who participated in visual skills training could better diagnose errors in three volleyball skills than players who didn't have visual training—even a full year later.

But not all studies are so promising. Researchers at the Centre for Eye Research at the Queensland University of Technology in Brisbane, Australia, for example, found no evidence that four weeks of visual training improved visual or motor performance.

Controversial: Improving Vision

Programs or therapy aimed at improving how well you see—rather than resolving recognized disorders—have even vision therapists disagreeing.

"I remember telling patients that it wasn't possible that their vision improved," says David W. Muris, O.D., in private practice at the Sacramento Vision Care Optometric Center, and coauthor of *Improve Your Vision Without Glasses or Contact Lenses.* "I've found that some people can be helped little to none, some moderately, but some can be helped tremendously."

A study dating to 1968 suggests that some vision problems are "learned." Psychologist Francis A. Young, Ph.D., led a research team to Alaska to study Inuits, and found that of 130 parents who were illiterate only two were nearsighted. But 60 percent of the children were, suggesting that close schoolwork had caused the problem.

Some eye-care professionals say a person may see better following vision therapy, although the eye itself is no more powerful than it was before the therapy.

"You can get improvements with visual acuity. I've documented it myself in patients," says Dr. Coffey. "What's not going to happen is actual change in the optical power of the eye. But the neurological and perceptual components of vision are quite amenable to training."

Other research offers some evidence of improvement with visual training. In a 1996 study at the Institute of Ophthalmology in Italy, 33 mildly nearsighted high school students had a type of biofeedback visual training for 12 months, and 22 similar students did not. Afterward, the treated students showed improved acuity when measured conventionally (but not when measured by computer). The training apparently helped acuity but didn't slow the nearsightedness.

And one small study reported in the *Journal of Behavioral Medicine* in 1986 found that 20 nearsighted adults improved in several ways after visual acuity training.

How to Find the Best Practitioner

Just about anybody can tell you they do vision therapy. There are no university classes on the subject, says Beck, who's certified as a therapy technician and works with a behavioral optometrist.

So how do you go about finding a qualified therapist?

A good first step is to contact the College of Optometrists in Vision Development (COVD), which certifies optometrists in behavioral, developmental, and rehabilitative optometry.

Becoming a COVD fellow requires submitting case reports to an internal exam board, passing written and oral exams, and taking a number of postgraduate class hours each year. An associate member hasn't gone through the certification process, but must take courses. The COVD will refer you to a fellow or associate in your area, or you could ask your optometrist or ophthalmologist for a referral, says Dr. Miller.

but can you really throw away your glasses?

Kip Bryan started wearing glasses when he was 10 years old. At age 42 he began to experiment with vision therapy. After a month he noticed his vision seemed to have improved. His ophthalmologist gave him a weaker prescription, and six months later he got a still weaker prescription. Over a period of three years, he says, he's continued to experience improvements.

"I've been measured by three distinct vision professionals, all of whom were quick to dismiss the possibility of vision improvement through my efforts," says Bryan, a computer consultant in Winchester, Massachusetts. "But I see my visual acuity improving every month." Now, he says, he can see license plates several car lengths ahead without glasses and can read overhead menus at fast food places.

Can vision therapy *really* improve your vision?

"There is a tantalizing little bit of research in that area," says Bradley Coffey, O.D., professor of optometry at Pacific University in Portland, Oregon. He points out that the power of your prescription doesn't always measure precisely how well you see. For example, he explains, two nearsighted people with exactly the same lens prescription may see quite differently without their glasses. Think of it this way: If you see a fuzzy letter B on the eye chart, but still identify it as a B, your vision may measure the same as if you see a clear, crisp B.

"There is no scientifically acceptable evidence that you can actually change the power of your eye, reducing the amount of nearsightedness that is measurable," says Dr. Coffey. "There is, however, a pretty solid body of evidence that it is possible to improve your clarity of sight or visual acuity, as measured on the letter chart, without changing refraction of eye or power of prescription."

Your acuity without glasses could be 20/100, fairly blurry. Visual acuity training could boost your acuity to 20/40 or so—you're in effect training your eye to see the image more sharply. Dr. Coffey compares it to sending a fuzzy photo through an enhancing process that makes it clearer.

"People can do that at some level of their visual system," he says. "They learn to see detail on an imperfect retinal image, without changing the power of their eyes."

The outcome is that you may be comfortable with less powerful glasses, or may not always need to wear them.

Even devout advocates of vision therapy for improvement promise no more: Steven M. Beresford, Ph.D., coauthor of *Improve Your Vision Without Glasses or Contact Lenses,* doesn't promise you can toss away your glasses. "Most people who wear glasses can certainly reduce their dependency on them," he says, "but will still need them for some activity."

For information, contact:
College of Optometrists in Vision Development
243 N. Lindbergh Blvd., Suite 310
St. Louis, MO 63141
Phone: 888/COVD-770 (268-3770)
Web site: www.covd.org.

There is a great deal of diversity among eye-care professionals. Ophthalmologists, who perform surgery, may be more likely than optometrists to consider the field of visual therapy medical voodoo, but some do use components of it in their practice.

"One doctor will be enthusiastic about vision therapy, and another will tell you not even to consider it," says Dr. Miller. Some therapists specialize in working with children. Some work one-on-one or in groups. Others rely on at-home exercises.

What about do-it-yourself programs? "Some individuals who aren't eye-care professionals offer simple eye exercises for simple eye strain and coordination problems," says Dr. Miller. "Just as general health care can be helpful, if you do these simple eye exercises, they may be helpful. But many individuals have a more involved process that requires professional care." When in doubt, ask an optometrist who does vision therapy.

Using the Therapy

How do you know if you might benefit from vision therapy? Obvious conditions such as crossed eyes, turned or drifting eyes, or lazy eye are prime candidates for therapy. A child struggling in school with problems reading or writing may benefit, depending on the specific problem. Symptoms such as headaches, blurred vision, eye discomfort while reading, and being tired after using a computer or reading may suggest a need for vision therapy.

The first step is an exam by an optometrist, according to Lori Mowbray, O.D., of the Minnesota Vision Therapy Center in Minneapolis. It should evaluate:

- **Acuity.** How sharply you see at a certain distance, such as on an eye chart
- **Optics.** Whether you are nearsighted, farsighted, or astigmatic (refractive status)
- **Eye tracking.** How well you track a moving target or move your eyes from one object to another (oculomotor skills)
- **Focusing.** Shifting clearly from one distance to another (accommodation)
- **Eye teaming.** How well your eyes work together (binocular vision)

Other tests may evaluate:

- **Visual analysis skills.** (including visual memory, which helps with reading comprehension and spelling)
- **Visual motor skills.** (such as eye-hand coordination, which can influence handwriting)
- **Visual spatial skills.** (such as reading in one direction)

If needed, the optometrist will devise a treatment plan. You may work with your optometrist or a technician trained in vision therapy.

The specific exercises will depend on the problem. They could include eye tracking by keeping your eyes on a moving pencil or working on hand-eye coordination by hitting at a swinging ball that has letters written on it.

To improve focusing problems, you may read from a book, using different lenses so you constantly switch focus. You may use a long string with beads attached to it at specific distances, holding one end to your nose and looking at different beads.

Often people with reading problems have problems with tracking. "Usually their eye movements, or ability to follow words across a page, are very jerky and almost uncontrollable," explains Beck. "We may also find a problem in the way they aim and position their eyes. They either undercut or overshoot the plane of the paper, as if looking through it, and words tend to run together."

Some children manage with the large print in beginner books, and problems only become apparent as the print in their books gets smaller.

"Normally people start struggling when they go from that learning-to-read stage to reading to learn, in the late second to third grade," says Beck.

But there are adult patients as well. Some have struggled throughout school, but others have managed with well-developed listening skills.

"We've had patients who were in a lot of study groups," says Beck. "They could hear people talk about the topic but couldn't read the material."

The first step of therapy may be working to improve eye movement then focusing. At some facilities, therapists work one on one, once a week, while others work with two or more people. Sometimes therapists advise a home computer program or other at-home exercises, particularly if you live too far away to come in for weekly visits or your insurance only covers a certain number of visits.

What You Can Do at Home

If you stumble across a shelf of eye-care books at your favorite bookstore or library—or type in the words "vision therapy" in an Internet search of online bookstores—you'll likely be overwhelmed. You'll find literally dozens of books touting ways to improve your eyesight, some promising that you'll never need glasses again. You may also notice ads in your Sunday newspaper for at-home computer programs.

Many of these advertisements and books may be tempting. And a program that grabs your attention may be well founded and just might help you—but then again, it might not. In vision therapy, one size *doesn't* fit all.

"It probably won't hurt you, but it may not significantly help you, either," says Dr. Miller. "With a diagnosis, a doctor can direct a very specific program for your problem. That's the advantage of working with a professional." And for disorders such as crossed eyes, lazy eye, or wandering eye, you must have professional help.

There's also an inherent disadvantage in a self-help eye program. "It really helps to have someone guide you," explains vision therapy technician Beck. "If you're the one moving the object you're tracking, for example, you know what you're going to do. If someone else is moving it, the motion isn't predictable." And unpredictable motion is a big plus in this particular technique.

What about home computer programs? Vision therapists say some are helpful, although the benefits are not as great as one-on-one therapy. But if the program isn't offered through or recommended by an eye-care professional experienced in vision therapy, forget it.

Dr. Muris promotes at-home exercises, but adds, "I believe everyone who does these should be under the care of an optometrist." Some home exercises he uses include:

- **Pumping.** Change your focus back and forth from something 6 inches from you, such as a pen or your finger, to something more than 15 feet away. Change focus every two seconds.
- **Tromboning.** Hold your finger or a pencil at arm's length. As you breathe in, bring it slowly toward you, touching the tip of your nose. As you breathe out, move the object out to arm's length. Look at the smallest detail you can see on the object.
- **Slow blinking.** Breathe deeply and slowly, and as you breathe in, blink a few times. When you breathe out, close your eyes, relax, and repeat to yourself, "Relax. Relax."

The following procedure was first recommended for relaxing the eyes by founder Dr. Bates in his 1920 book:

- **Palming.** Simply close your eyes and cup your palms over your eyes so that all light is shut out, but don't press on your eyeballs. Rest this way for a few minutes, letting the darkness and warmth soothe your eyes.

For those who want to improve their sports skills, the AOA suggests:

- **Eye tracking.** To help learn to watch things without moving your head, balance a book on your head and watch an item thrown through the air. You also can follow the path of a ball as it rolls around inside a Frisbee.
- **Peripheral vision.** To improve what you can see out of the corner of your eyes, try watching television or a live sport with your head turned to one side and your eyes focused straight ahead, not turned toward the screen.
- **Dynamic visual acuity.** To help yourself see objects while both you and the object are moving (as in tennis or soccer), cut letters of varying sizes out of a magazine. Lay them on a stereo turntable and try to identify them from arm's length at different speeds. When you improve, use smaller letters.

What to Expect

For conditions such as strabismus and lazy eye, there are no quick fixes. Treatment programs may run six to 12 months, and longer when a brain injury is involved. Specialized sports vision drills, however, apparently can offer some benefit within weeks or months. And advocates of vision improvement programs say you can see some results in a week or two, but more dramatic improvement takes much longer.

Does insurance cover vision therapy? Sometimes yes, sometimes no. Some plans cover 80 percent of your costs. Managed care programs, however, may limit the number of visits. Mitchell Scheiman, O.D., chief of the Pediatric Binocular Vision Service at The Eye Institute at the Pennsylvania College of Optometry in Philadelphia, says some insurers cover only 12 or 16 visits a year.

Some optometrists have turned to home-based programs, such as Home Therapy System and Computer-Aided Vision Therapy, to supplement office-based therapy.

If your insurance declines payment, Dr. Scheiman suggests that you ask the optometrist to appeal the decision. Appeal it a second time, if you have to. Some plans, he says, won't pay unless an M.D. refers the patient or does the therapy, but freedom of choice laws in many states allow you to use an optometrist.

"We do find that the more our patients fight, the more likely they are to get covered," says Beck, adding that HMOs are the least likely to cover therapy.

Costs range greatly, depending on the facility, the diagnosis, and how long treatment is required. At the Minnesota Vision Therapy Center, costs for weekly visits, plus follow-up care, can run from $2,000 to $6,000 for problems such as crossed eyes or wandering eye. Problems from brain injuries generally take longer and cost more.

Nationwide, a one-on-one session with a therapist might cost $100 an hour or more. Conversely, focusing and convergence problems treated with home computer therapy and two office visits can run as little as $500.

Safety and Warnings

For eye disorders such as turned eyes or tracking or focusing problems, turn to a professional eye-care provider without delay.

In general, steer clear of programs offered by nonprofessionals. Home programs that concentrate on relaxation techniques won't harm you, but they may not help your specific problem.

The disadvantage occurs if working with a home program keeps you from seeking the help you need. "If someone goes through one of these programs and wasn't helped, they may say, 'Oh, vision therapy doesn't work,'" says Dr. Miller.

Some forms of self-therapy suggest using gradually weaker corrective lenses to "train" the eyes to see better. "Sometimes I get calls from patients asking if I'll prescribe a reduced prescription," says Dr. Coffey.

If you choose to try this, don't suddenly abandon your glasses or switch to a greatly reduced prescription. With a large change, you'll have so much blur that your eyes cannot adapt, he warns, and there are obvious safety risks.

The downside of weaker lenses is that you'll be giving up crisp, detailed distance sight. Critics point out that your reaction time while driving may be slower if your vision is even slightly blurry.

Dr. Coffey cautions against "patching" (covering one eye), unless prescribed and monitored by an eye-care professional. He also advises against prolonged looking at something up close, within 6 inches.

resources

These organizations can either help with referrals or supply helpful information:

Organizations

College of Optometrists in Vision Development
243 N. Lindbergh Blvd., Suite 310
St. Louis, MO 63141
888/COVD-770 (268-3770)
www.covd.org

Parents Active for Vision Education
Phone: 800/PAVE-988 (728-3988)
Web site: www.pave-eye.com/vision
This is a nonprofit resource and support organization.

Optometric Extension Program Foundation
1921 E. Carnegie Ave., Suite 3L
Santa Ana, CA 92705
www.oep.org
This organization will refer you to behavioral optometrists and can supply informational pamphlets.

Books

20/20 Is Not Enough: The New World of Vision by Arthur S. Seiderman, O.D., and Steven E. Marcus, O.D. (Crest, 1991)
Good explanations of common vision problems that can greatly affect children's performance in school.

Improve Your Vision Without Glasses or Contact Lenses by Steven M. Beresford, David W. Muris, Merrill J. Allen, Francis A. Young (Fireside, 1996)
Offers lots of home exercises.

The Bates Method for Better Eyesight Without Glasses, William H. Bates, M.D. (First published in 1943, now available from Henry Holt, 1986)
Interesting from the historical perspective; controversial.

Web sites

www.vision3d.com
www.children-special-needs.org

chapter 24

walking & other exercise

THE RIGHT MOVES

Increasing physical activity, even a small amount, is the best way to stay healthy.
—C. Everett Koop, M.D., former U.S. Surgeon General

"Before I started walking, everything ached," Debbie Cooper recalls. "Sitting at my desk at work, my neck and shoulders were constantly sore. My back hurt. My legs felt achy or would go numb. Plus I was always tired, and I felt depressed a lot, too."

Debbie started exercising by walking before work, first just a few blocks, gradually building to 3 miles three times a week and shorter walks in between. In the dozen years since, during which she's also fit in some swimming, aerobics classes, and weight training, she has been largely relieved of her aches and pains. She also lost 15 pounds and stayed strong and energetic through two pregnancies.

"I'm not a fanatic about it, but I do try to do something just about every day," she says. "I just know that if I don't, I feel bad physically, I start putting on weight, and I get cranky and depressed. Sometimes it's a real effort just to walk around the block, but it's worth it."

You've heard it before—from your doctor, perhaps, or a friend or in the news: Exercise is good for you. A regular program of physical activity can make your heart stronger, help you lose weight, and give you muscular definition where you haven't seen muscles in years.

But exercise is much more than a healthy addition to your lifestyle. According to C. Everett Koop, M.D., former U.S. Surgeon General and founder of Shape Up America!, exercise is the most important health habit you can have. (Shape Up America! is a national coalition of health and fitness organizations that promotes the importance of getting regular exercise and maintaining a healthy weight.)

exercise helps heal

Is there anything that exercise doesn't help? Once you start looking into the various conditions that exercise is good for, it can sure seem like the list is infinite. Here are the conditions that regular exercise seems to help the most:

- Anxiety
- Arthritis
- Back pain
- Colon cancer
- Depression
- Diabetes
- Heart disease
- High blood pressure
- High cholesterol
- Hot flashes
- Osteoporosis
- Overweight
- Stress

Regular physical activity can substantially reduce the risk of developing or dying from heart disease, diabetes, colon cancer, and high blood pressure, according to a report by the nation's Centers for Disease Control and Prevention. Exercise can help relieve arthritis pain, reduce menopausal hot flashes, and help you get a better night's sleep. It can also reduce symptoms of depression and anxiety, improve your mood, and make it easier and more enjoyable to perform daily tasks.

Every Bit Helps

A well-rounded exercise program combines an aerobic activity such as walking with strength training and stretching exercises. But it isn't necessary to exercise for hours or at vigorous levels to enjoy what experts call "health-related fitness."

"Many people think they need to have sweat running down their brow and be out of breath in order to get health benefits," says James M. Rippe, M.D., associate professor of medicine at Tufts University School of Medicine in Medford, Massachusetts, and a member of the Shape Up America! advisory committee.

Not so, say Dr. Rippe and other experts. By becoming even moderately active on a regular basis, people who are currently inactive can significantly improve their health and well-being, according to a report from the U.S. Surgeon General that summarizes decades of research on physical activity and health.

What qualifies as moderate activity? Going for a walk. Taking a bike ride. Swimming. Even doing moderately challenging household tasks like vacuuming your carpet and carrying laundry up and down stairs can contribute to your fitness and health.

What does medical science have to say about all this? How exactly is exercise good for you?

• **Increasing immunity.** Regular exercise can boost your immune system, better protecting you against infection and disease, according to Richard Cotton, an exercise physiologist and spokesperson for the American Council on Exercise (ACE).

"Fitness enthusiasts have frequently reported that they experience less sickness than their sedentary peers," Cotton says. "One survey revealed that 61 percent of 700 recreational runners reported fewer colds since they began running, while only 4 percent felt they had experienced more."

Even during moderate exercise, research has shown, various immune cells circulate through the body more quickly and are better able to kill bacteria and viruses.

• **Adding to life expectancy.** Life isn't just healthier but may indeed be longer for those who walk regularly. Researchers in a 12-year study at the Honolulu Heart Program found that walking 2 miles a day cut the mortality rates by one-half of people in their 60s, 70s, and 80s.

In another study, researchers from the University of Virginia in Charlottesville calculated that every mile older people walk on a daily basis lowers their death rate. And in a study in Finland, researchers found that even heredity may be overcome by exercise. Tracking 16,000 male and female twins for 19 years, the researchers found during the study that people who took at least six brisk half-hour walks or more per month were 44 percent less likely to die in a given year than their sedentary twins.

• **Strengthening the heart.** "Walking just three times a week for 20 minutes at a brisk pace can lower your risk for coronary disease by as much as 40 percent," says Marianne Legato, M.D., professor of clinical medicine at Columbia University in New York. "Exercise also relieves the kind of internal pressure that causes blood pressure to go up, which is a risk factor for a heart attack."

• **Lowering high blood pressure.** Strength-training exercise—lifting weights or working out with Nautilus-type equipment—done in conjunction with aerobic exercise can lower high blood pressure, according to Wayne Westcott, Ph.D., national strength-training consultant for the YMCA and author of *Building Strength and Stamina: New Nautilus Training for Total Fitness*. In a study by Dr. Westcott, 785 men and women participated in a two-month strength and aerobic exercise program. The program significantly lowered the exercisers' resting blood pressure—a measure of blood pressure taken when they were not exercising.

• **Losing weight.** Being overweight increases your risk of a wide range of disorders, including high blood pressure, elevated cholesterol, heart disease, stroke, diabetes, gallstone formation, certain types of cancer, osteoarthritis of the knee, even infertility.

Studies also show an increased risk of death from excess weight. As many as 300,000 premature deaths occur each year due to obesity-related illness. One study showed that middle-age women who were just 30 to 40 pounds overweight increase their risk of premature death by 60 percent, and by more than 100 percent if they're even more overweight.

Even a relatively small weight loss can make a big difference health-wise. "A loss of 10 or even 15 pounds can improve your health significantly," says Barbara Moore, Ph.D., executive director of Shape Up America! For example, shedding even a little weight can lower blood levels of "bad" low-density lipoprotein (LDL) cholesterol and increase "good" high-density lipoprotein (HDL) cholesterol, which in turn reduces the risks associated with high blood pressure and coronary heart disease.

"Exercise is absolutely as critical to weight loss as a good diet is," Dr. Moore says. "Physical activity is the part of the equation that can really make the long-term difference."

Exercise gives fat cells the double whammy. "A person not only burns calories while exercising, but calories will continue to be burned at a higher rate for up to several hours afterward," says obesity expert Wayne Callaway, M.D., associate clinical professor of medicine at George Washington University in Washington, D.C.

Exercise also helps prevent middle-age spread. A study at NASA/Johnson Space Center in Houston of about 500 employees found that those who walked about 2 miles a day didn't put on a single pound over a 10-year period, even though they didn't cut calories in their diets.

• **Combating colon cancer.** A daily walk coupled with dietary changes such as eating less red meat may cut your risk of colon cancer in half, according to Graham Colditz, M.D., associate professor of medicine at Harvard Medical School in Cambridge, Massachusetts. In research he conducted—the Nurse's Health Study of 121,000 women—one hour of brisk walking a day was associated with a 26-percent reduction in colon cancer risk. Dr. Colditz hypothesizes that exercise speeds the passage of stool through the colon.

• **Coping with Type II diabetes.** People suffering from Type II diabetes have elevated levels of blood sugars (glucose). This occurs when the body produces too much insulin, throwing insulin/glucose balances out of kilter. A program of regular exercise such as walking, along with a modified diet, can help normalize glucose levels. This helps prevent serious complications of the disease, which can include heart disease, kidney failure, blindness, and nerve dysfunction.

• **Relieving arthritis and back pain.** The painful joint inflammation of arthritis can be relieved by a program of moderate physical activity. A well-rounded routine incorporating walking and other aerobic exercise, strength training, and stretching can improve the range of motion of joints and reduce joint stiffness.

Another painful condition, sporadic or chronic lower back pain, can be relieved and even prevented by regularly exercising the lower back muscles, according to Dr. Westcott. Extensive studies have shown, he says, that strong lower back muscles are less likely to be injured than weaker ones. In one study he did, people reported experiencing

managing menopause

With all the talk of hormone replacement therapy to help women deal with the discomforts of menopause, one important therapy often doesn't get mentioned. We're talking about exercise, of course. Physical activity has been found effective in helping women cope with many of the symptoms and potential problems of menopause. Here's a look at how exercise can help.

Osteoporosis. This disease, in which bone mass is lost over a period of many years, accelerates during menopause as levels of the female hormone estrogen decline. Exercise helps increase the density and strength of one's bones by stimulating them to retain the minerals that keep them dense and strong.

"The data are incontrovertible that weight-bearing exercises such as walking or strength training maintains and even improves bone strength," says Mary Jane Minkin, M.D., associate clinical professor of obstetrics and gynecology at Yale University School of Medicine and author of *Menopause and Beyond*.

In one study, women who walked at least 7 miles per week had higher bone density than women who walked less than a mile per week. In research conducted by Wayne Westcott, M.D., national strength-training consultant for the YMCA, just four months of strength training exercise measurably increased exercisers' bone mineral density content.

Hot flashes. Research has shown that exercise temporarily raises levels of estrogen, and this coincides with an overall decrease in the severity of hot flashes. "Most women who are physically fit tell me that hot flashes are less of a problem," says Dr. Minkin. "Exercise usually makes hot flashes much more tolerable in general."

Breast cancer. The risk for developing breast cancer increases after menopause. Women who engage in aerobic exercise during their childbearing years, research has shown, reduce their chances of developing breast cancer.

significantly less back pain after doing 10 weeks of strength exercise for the lower back muscles.

- **Promoting emotional well-being.** Exercise is good for your mind. Regular moderate physical activity has been found to reduce feelings of depression and anxiety and promote psychological well-being, according to a report by the U.S. Surgeon General.

"Any time you're moving your body and increasing your metabolic rate, you're going to have 'feel-good' hormones like endorphins released," says Barbara Ainsworth, Ph.D., associate professor of exercise physiology at the University of South Carolina in Columbia. Endorphins are a type of neurotransmitter chemical produced in the brain that is believed to play a part in our moods and emotions.

Research has demonstrated that exercise can help relieve anxiety. In one study, researchers found that people were less jittery and hyperactive after an exercise session.

"Exercise is definitely a stress-buster," says Joyce Nash, Ph.D., a clinical psychologist in San Francisco and Menlo Park, California, and author of *The New Maximize Your Body Potential.* "Exercise helps modulate your emotional reaction to everyday frustrations and even redirects your focus away from your problems overall."

Engaging in a regular program of exercise also boosts self-esteem, Dr. Nash says. "We notice that we're doing something good for ourselves," she says. "We're accomplishing our goals, and this feels really good."

Exercise Basics

"Health-related fitness has three major components: a healthy cardiorespiratory system—including the heart, lungs, and blood vessels—strong muscles, and flexibility," says exercise physiologist Thomas Martin, Ph.D., a fellow with the American College of Sports Medicine. "An effective exercise program should include something for all of these—aerobic exercise, strength training, and stretching."

Before you get overwhelmed thinking about all that exercise, consider this: You're much more likely to keep at it if you think "variety."

"Think of all the different things you can do to keep physically active," suggests exercise physiologist Richard Cotton. "Walking, bike riding, softball, some working out with weights, stretching—make your decisions based on your own needs and resources. The important thing is to choose things that are fun and that you're willing to do consistently."

Getting Started

There are plenty of ways to launch an exercise program.

- **Just do it.** Want to walk? Start by lacing up a good pair of walking shoes and simply putting one foot in front of the other. In the same way, for other activities you're already familiar with, such as riding a bike and taking a swim, just get moving.
- **Check out exercise videos.** Libraries and video stores carry a wide range of videotapes that take you through the basic moves of everything from aerobics to kick-boxing, from lifting weights to practicing yoga.
- **Sign up for a class.** Check your local YMCA, schools, and other community organizations for exercise classes that strike your fancy. Water aerobics? Line dancing? Start with a beginners' class, advises Lauri Reimer, coordinator of the aerobic instruction training division of the Aerobics and Fitness Association of America (AFAA). As you get comfortable with the moves, she says, you can go ahead and move on to a more advanced workout.

- **Join a gym or health club.** This kind of facility can offer you plentiful exercise options, as well as the motivating company of other exercisers. Prices range from a few dollars a month to thousands of dollars a year, so shop around. Some clubs allow you to pay per session or by the month, which is a good idea if you're not sure about making a long-term commitment. When considering a gym, take a tour and ask about the qualifications of the staff. Also make sure the club is convenient to your home or your workplace and that it's open during hours when you can realistically get there.
- **Hire a personal trainer.** If it's one-on-one instruction and encouragement you're looking for, and you can afford from $30 to more than $100 per session, hire a personal trainer. You can find one through a health club, a YMCA, or one of the major certifying bodies: the American Council on Exercise (ACE), the American College of Sports Medicine, or the Aerobics and Fitness Association of America (AFAA).

No matter what type of exercise you choose and what route you choose to get started, you will probably experience some of the positive rewards quickly, says ACE's Cotton. While your body isn't going to change shape overnight, you are likely to experience other positive benefits of exercise within just a few weeks—renewed energy, stronger muscles, an improved mood, and an overall sense of well-being.

Aerobic Exercise

Aerobic exercise engages large muscle groups such as your legs and arms in rhythmic movement. It challenges your heart and lungs to work hard and, in the process, get stronger.

A regular program of aerobics helps fight fat and tone your body, which improves your appearance, strength, and stamina. Aerobic exercise is closely linked to decreased feelings of anxiety and depression and increased feelings of well-being.

The best kind of aerobic exercise doesn't involve a lot of impact on the joints. Walking is one of the best because it's low-impact and is easy to do anywhere. Activities such as swimming or bicycling are great options, too, because they are virtually nonimpact forms of exercise.

Here are some basics for getting started on a regular program of aerobic exercise:

- **Warm up.** A five- to 10-minute warm-up will help your muscles work faster and more forcefully. It will also decrease the chance that you'll hurt yourself, because a warm-up improves muscle elasticity and prevents the buildup of pain-provoking lactic acid in the blood. On top of all that, warming up helps your body burn calories more efficiently by increasing your core body temperature. Focus on warming up the muscles you'll use in your exercise. Before a brisk walk, for example, walk around the house for a few minutes. Follow with a few gentle stretches of your legs, back, shoulders, and arms.
- **Take it easy to start.** If you're taking up walking, start by going just a short distance, Cotton advises. Even a five-minute stroll is fine. And forget about speed. Walk at a

comfortable pace. If you find you can't catch your breath, slow down. Focus on good posture, keeping your head lifted and shoulders relaxed. Swing your arms naturally and breathe deeply.

- **Increase your distance gradually.** Then, after you've reached a point where you can walk a few miles with relative ease, you can think about increasing intensity. Try walking hills, lengthening your stride, or increasing your speed.

The same guidelines go for other forms of aerobic exercise: Focus on duration first, then add intensity.

- **Aim for 30 minutes.** You may start out exercising only five or 10 minutes. That's fine, but make it your goal to work up to 20 to 30 minutes (or as long as 45 minutes if your aim is weight loss) at a moderate level of intensity for maximum health benefits.

You can also accumulate exercise time—10 minutes here, 10 minutes there, as long as it adds up to about 30 minutes a day. Recent studies have shown that the health benefits of exercise are cumulative.

- **Cool down.** Walk slowly for at least three minutes after a workout and do a few gentle stretches, AFAA's Reimer advises. This enables your muscles to pump blood out of your extremities and back to your heart and brain. And stretching helps remove lactic acid from your muscles, minimizing muscle soreness. (Lactic acid naturally builds up in muscles during demanding workouts and is responsible for some of the soreness you can feel afterward.)
- **Work out three to five times a week.** Three days are the minimum for improving health and fitness through exercise, according to the American College of Sports Physicians. If you're trying to lose weight, aim for more, says AFAA's Reimer.

Strength Training

Sometimes called "weight training" or "resistance training," strength training involves challenging your muscles to "resist" a force in order to grow stronger. Lifting weights, working out on Nautilus-type equipment, and doing calisthenics like push-ups all qualify as strength training.

An important component of a balanced fitness program, strength training builds the strength of muscles, bones, and connective tissue. This increase in strength enhances our quality of life by making the performance of everyday activities, from climbing stairs to lifting heavy grocery bags, easier.

Strength training also boosts our metabolism, a crucial issue as we age. Most American adults, due to decreased physical activity, lose about a half pound of muscle per year after the age of 20.

Because muscle tissue is partly responsible for the number of calories burned, the more muscle we have, the more efficiently we burn calories and fight fat. Every pound of new muscle tissue, in fact, burns another 35 calories a day.

Here's how to get started.

- **Get instruction.** If you've never lifted weights or used weight equipment, you'll do yourself a big favor by getting some instruction in types of exercises and proper form. If you belong to a gym, ask for instruction on how to use the equipment.

Or ask a friend who knows how to do it. At the very least, consult a videotape or book.

- **Warm up.** Five to 15 minutes of an aerobic warm-up like walking or riding a stationary bike helps get your muscles ready to handle the challenge of strength training.
- **Start small.** When using free weights or weight equipment, start light. You'll be less likely to injure yourself, and your muscles can always build from there. For each exercise, choose a weight that's light enough that you can perform 8 to 12 repetitions in good form to the point of fatigue without hurting yourself, but not so light that when you reach 12 repetitions you feel like you could do quite a few more. As you grow stronger, increase the amount of weight gradually, by 5 to 10 percent.
- **Train head to toe.** Even if it's your abdomen or your thighs that you consider your problem areas, don't exercise those areas alone. For optimal muscle strength and balance, strength-train all of your major muscle groups in a series of 10 to 15 exercises. The major muscle groups are: legs (calves, thighs, buttocks, and hips), back, chest, shoulders, arms (upper and lower), neck, and abdomen.
- **Work big muscles first, then small muscles.** Exercising your large muscles first allows your smaller muscles to warm up for more direct attention later. For example, do leg presses for your entire leg before even thinking about calf raises. Exercise your back and chest, which involves your arm muscles, before doing arm work. Save abdominal exercises like sit-ups for the very last, because your abdominal muscles are involved as "stabilizer muscles" for most other types of exercise. If you exercise them earlier in your routine, you'll tire them out before you get started.
- **Do one to three sets.** Research has shown that one set—eight to 12 repetitions—is sufficient for building strength and gaining health benefits. Adding sets helps build more strength but isn't necessary for basic benefits. Bear in mind that you're probably more likely to stick to a brief, efficient workout than you are to a lengthy one.
- **Train two or three times a week.** For best health and fitness benefits, you need to strength-train at least twice a week and three times at the most. Your muscles need about 48 hours to recover and repair, so take at least one day off in between strength-training workouts.
- **Be patient.** An encouraging aspect of strength training, says ACE's Cotton, is that you'll likely experience rapid improvements in strength and muscle tone right from the start of your program. "Don't be discouraged, however, if visible improvements begin to taper off after a few weeks," he says. "It's only natural that, as your fitness level improves, improvements in strength and appearance will follow at a slightly slower pace."

Stretching

Researchers have found that a regular program of stretching helps release muscle tension and soreness, increase physical and mental relaxation, improve posture, allow greater freedom of movement, and reduce risk of injury from a variety of physical activities.

Here's how to move into such a program.

- **Do it regularly.** Try to stretch for a few minutes every day. While some people are naturally more flexible than others, regular stretching improves anyone's flexibility. It's especially important to stretch regularly as we age. As we grow older, we tend to lose flexibility, usually as a result of inactivity rather than the aging process itself.

Ideally, at least 30 minutes three times per week should be spent on flexibility training. But even a mere five minutes of stretching at the end of an exercise session is better than nothing. And all aerobic activity should be followed by at least a few minutes of stretching. Yoga is a particularly beneficial form of stretching. For more details, see "Yoga" on page 297.

- **Take it easy.** Proper stretching involves slowly moving into and holding a mild stretch for 10 to 30 seconds while you breathe normally. Don't bounce while in a stretch. Holding a stretch is more effective and there is less risk of injury. Also don't strain or push a muscle too far. If a stretch hurts, ease up.
- **Stretch head to toe.** Like strength conditioning, flexibility exercises should include stretching for all the major muscle groups.

At Home with Exercise

You don't have to join a gym to get regular exercise. In fact, for some people, that just complicates things. "It's important to 'lower the barriers' to exercise," says psychologist Dr. Nash. "If you have to get in the car, drive to the gym, change clothes, exercise, shower, dress, drive home—by the time you're done it has taken hours. This is a significant barrier to motivation."

Instead, she advises, find a way to exercise near home or even at home. Try the following approaches:

- **Exercise to videos.** Choose tapes that spark your personal interests and offer effective but brief workouts.
- **Use home exercise equipment.** For indoor walking, a treadmill can't be beat. Shop around for a good-quality, motorized type. Or perhaps you prefer a stationary bike or stair-climber. When it comes to weight training, expensive, complicated equipment is unnecessary, says exercise physiologist Lisa Hoffman, author of *Better Than Ever.* "I have a set of 5-pound weights and a weight bench at home," Hoffman says. "That, added to some sit-ups and push-ups, is all you really need for a home workout."

Safety and Warnings

See your doctor. If you're 35 or older, or have heart disease or other medical conditions, you should check with your doctor before starting or increasing your exercise program.

Some conditions may require special exercise guidelines. Talk to your doctor if you have heart disease; breathing difficulties or conditions such as asthma; bone or joint problems, such as low back pain or arthritis;

target heart rate

How hard should your heart be working while you're doing aerobic exercise?

You don't need to guess. There's a simple formula: For maximum health and fitness benefits, exercise at a target heart rate (THR) of 50 to 80 percent of your maximum heart rate (MHR).

To figure your MHR, subtract your age from 220. For example, if you're 40, your MHR is 180 beats per minute, and you should aim to exercise at a THR between 90 and 144 beats per minute. Start at the lower end of the range.

As your body adjusts to exercise, your heart will grow stronger and it will take greater intensity levels to reach higher heart rates. Check your pulse five minutes into any kind of aerobics. You'll have to learn how to take your pulse while you're still moving.

you're pregnant; or you have any other condition that you think may affect an exercise program. In fact, if you have any concerns at all, talk to your doctor before getting started.

- **Monitor your intensity.** While exercising, especially during aerobic exercise, be sure to pay close attention to how hard your heart is working so as not to overdo it. One good measure is the "talk test." You should be able to talk at the same time you're exercising. If you can't, slow down.

  You can also monitor your heart rate. This helps ensure safety and also helps you exercise most effectively. When you exercise, your heart beats faster to meet the demand for more blood and oxygen by the muscles of the body. The more intense the activity, the faster your heart will beat.

- **Watch for danger signs.** If you experience any of these while exercising, stop immediately: unusual fatigue, dizziness, light-headedness, breathlessness, loss of muscle control, nausea, blurred vision, tightness in your chest, or any pain from your jaw to your waist. If the condition persists, seek medical attention.

- **Protect yourself.** Basic safety equipment is essential. For walking at night, wear light-colored clothes and add gear like adhesive reflectors. Don't ever wear a Walkman-type headset in or near heavy traffic.

  For skating, biking or similar activities, be sure to wear a helmet and other appropriate protective gear.

resources

Organizations
For more information on the importance of and instructions for regular exercise, contact:

American Council on Exercise
San Diego
619/535-8227

American Fitness Association of America
Los Angeles
800/446-2322

American College of Sports Medicine
Indianapolis
317/637-9200

Shape Up America!
6707 Democracy Blvd., Suite 306
Bethesda, MD 20817
E-mail: suainfo@shapeup.org

Books
Fitness for Dummies by Liz Neporent and Suzanne Schlosberg (IPG Books, 1996)

Better Than Ever: The 4-Week Workout for Women Over 40 by Lisa Hoffman (NTC/Contemporary)

Strong Women Stay Young by Miriam Nelson, M.D. (Bantam Doubleday Bell, 1997)

chapter 25

yoga

STRETCHING FOR HEALTH

Pain creates muscular tension, which in turn causes more pain. Yoga breaks up that vicious cycle. —*James Gordon, M.D.*

If the case hadn't been documented in a medical journal, it might have been dismissed as a farce. A pilot with the United States Air Force, grounded for six years because of high blood pressure, tries exercise, dietary changes, and even medication to no avail. When as a last straw he tries yoga, within six weeks his blood pressure is down, and he's back up in the air.

The director of the Center for Mind-Body Medicine in Washington, D.C., James S. Gordon, M.D., tells of another yoga "miracle" experienced by a person with rheumatoid arthritis. After 10 unsuccessful years of conventional medical treatment this individual finds dramatic relief within just two weeks of giving yoga a try. Not even the traditionally skeptical scientific journals have been able to ignore the healing power of this ancient discipline. The *Journal of the American Medical Association*, for example, in 1998 reported that an eight-week yoga class had a significant impact on both the pain and loss of strength associated with the wrist-crippling disorder known as carpal tunnel syndrome.

Medical journals from around the world have reported positive effects from yoga on more than a dozen physical or mental conditions in the past few years alone, and the list is likely to grow based on research currently under way. People suffering from heart disease; high blood pressure; fatigue; back pain; diabetes; asthma; menopause; epilepsy; and even psychological disorders such as anxiety, depression, drug addiction, and obsessive-compulsive disorder have been shown to benefit from the gentle rigors of this 5,000-year-old art.

In addition to what's been verified by scientific research, the list of yoga's alleged benefits is even longer. The Iyengar Yoga

National Association, for example, offers its certified instructors routines customized to treat more than 50 medical conditions including Alzheimer's disease, chronic fatigue, constipation, psoriasis, yeast infections, and even AIDS.

yoga can help heal

- Anxiety
- Arthritis
- Asthma
- Back pain
- Carpal tunnel syndrome
- Depression
- Diabetes
- Drug addiction
- Epilepsy
- Fatigue
- Heart disease
- High blood pressure
- Learning disabilities
- Menopausal discomfort
- Overweight
- Stress

Healing with Yoga

Scientific studies have shown, for example, that yoga affects how the body uses blood sugar, how the nervous system responds to pain, how the hormonal system reacts to stress, and how the brain increases its alpha wave activity in ways that can help us think more creatively and relax. These are important and fundamental changes attributable in part to the calmness produced by yoga, and possibly the way its movements and postures are thought to massage vital internal organs.

Certain postures are designed to target specific areas of the body to improve blood flow, free up the activity of the nerves, and facilitate hormonal activity in ways that reportedly have clear-cut therapeutic effects.

These widespread changes that yoga produces make it "fundamentally different from conventional medical practice," write the authors of *Yoga for Common Ailments*, Drs. H.R. Nagendra, R. Nagarathna, and Robin Monro: "Instead of trying to reduce the cause of disease to a single factor, yoga aims to treat illness by improving health on all levels and by restoring inner harmony."

The different components of a yoga program tend to complement one another, these authors explain. "When you do the asanas and stretch your muscles, muscular tension is released and you are more able to relax your mind. Likewise, when you relax your mind and release suppressed emotions, you tend to become less tense physically." One positive change produces another, in other words, and the body and mind benefit in unison with every twist and turn.

While researchers are finding that yoga does have an overall therapeutic effect, they are also documenting the powerful impact it can have on a number of specific diseases. Here's a brief roundup of the research (and expert endorsements) that back up yoga's ability to heal several common diseases and conditions.

Arthritis

Yoga has a reputation for being able to help ease the discomforts of both rheumatoid arthritis and osteoarthritis. In his book *Manifesto for a New Medicine*, Dr. Gordon calls yoga "wonderfully useful for people with the stiff joints and inflexible muscles of arthritis."

Even rheumatoid arthritis, the more serious type that can affect the entire body, responds well to yoga's combination of physically as well as mentally relaxing exercises, Dr. Gordon says. "On the purely physical side, yoga gives all the benefits of range-of-motion exercises," he explains. "It helps restore flexibility and improves circulation to the joints, allowing more healing nutrition to reach them. It also forces more oxygen into the joints and facilitates the release of endorphins, the body's own natural painkillers."

Yoga also helps relieve pain by reducing muscular tension. "Pain creates muscular tension, which in turn causes more pain," notes Dr. Gordon. "Yoga breaks up that vicious circle."

Then, too, yoga can help strengthen the muscles needed to protect joints from the undue stress that can cause osteoarthritis in the first place, says Karrie Demers, M.D., a board-certified internist who serves as the medical director of the Center for Health and Healing at the Himalayan Institute in Honesdale, Pennsylvania.

Asthma

As anyone with this dread condition can attest, the shortness of breath caused by the bronchial spasms of asthma can feel truly life threatening. (In some cases these spasms *are* life threatening.) Yoga appears to reduce both the frequency and severity of such spasms and can claim several well-done studies as proof. One done in 1993 looked at 46 people with asthma. It found that yoga improved their lung function and ability to exercise. It also reduced their need for medication. These effects lasted fully a year after the yoga sessions ended.

Other more recent studies have produced similar results. One done in 1996, found that people with asthma showed significant improvement following a yoga program that lasted just one week. Yoga appears to exert its benefits by helping to relax the entire respiratory system.

Diabetes

Diabetes is characterized by an inability to metabolize glucose—the simple sugar the body uses as its principal source of energy. As glucose levels in the blood rise too high, the excess glucose can damage blood vessel walls as well as other body tissues.

Yoga appears to help keep glucose levels in check, possibly by altering levels of stress-induced hormones known to affect glucose uptake. Yoga's ability to treat diabetes has been shown in at least two studies. One done in India in 1993 found that 104 of 149 people with diabetes were able to substantially reduce their oral medication levels after just 40 days of yoga therapy. The other study, done in 1995 in India, found that 40 days of yoga training helped 30 people with diabetes metabolize glucose more normally when their customary medications were stopped. In both studies the people had adult-onset (non-insulin-dependent) diabetes.

Research data suggest that yoga training along with diet and medical management can play a role in the prevention and treatment of this disease, researchers who conducted the second study say.

Fatigue

"The degree to which most people report feeling invigorated by yoga is remarkable," says Dr. Demers. And there's ample research to back her up. One 1993 British study found that a 30-minute yoga class "produced a significantly greater increase in perceptions of mental and physical energy and feelings of alertness and enthusiasm" than two other calming techniques (progressive relaxation and visualization). In another study with college students, a yoga class left its participants feeling more positive and energized than people who swam for an equal amount of time, participated in a fencing class, or lifted weights.

Peace Between Body and Mind

Why would there be such widespread effects from something that at first glance seems as simple as a few deep breaths, some gentle stretching, and an unusual posture or two?

Yoga, first of all, is not quite that simple. The word itself derives from the Sanskrit word *yug*, which means to bring together—a reference to yoga's venerable goal of achieving a healthful union between the body and the mind (and between the individual and God, but that is another story altogether).

Yoga is as much a mental discipline as a physical one in this regard, says Dr. Demers. "Yoga helps us find a peace between what our minds may want and what our bodies truly need," she says, "thus eliminating not just destructive behaviors but also a lot of stress-producing inner turmoil along the way."

Sometimes people lose sight of this more cerebral aspect of yoga, turning to it more for its physical benefits instead, but it is precisely this spiritual component of yoga that makes it unique, Dr. Demers says. "Yoga above all teaches us to relax, and this can have amazingly far-reaching effects physically and psychologically," she explains. "People who come to the Himalayan Institute for physical problems often leave with a much-improved sense of well-being overall, which is, after all, yoga's ultimate goal."

To approach yoga purely for its bodily benefits alone, therefore, is to miss much of what it has to give.

All is not in the mind with yoga, however, as a typical session—especially if it's the most popular type called *hatha* yoga—can be very physical, indeed. Sessions generally last from 30 to 90 minutes and include body-challenging postures (called

but is it good exercise?

Many people ask that question—especially those who advocate breaking a sweat by sustaining a target heart rate for at least 20 to 30 minutes at a stretch. The answer is an unqualified "yes."

In a 1997 study reported in the *Journal of Alternative and Complementary Medicine,* previously untrained women participated in twice-a-day yoga sessions for four weeks. During this time period, the women boosted their cardiovascular endurance (as measured by running on a treadmill) by an average of 21 percent. Studies have shown that yoga also can build strength and increase flexibility, both of which become progressively more important as muscles weaken and connective tissues (ligaments and tendons) shorten and tighten with age.

"Yoga's postures can be deceiving," Dr. Demers says. "They can appear quite easy, especially those that don't require much movement, but many of these postures can be very demanding and especially the longer they're held." As for flexibility, few other stretching routines require the range of motion for as many different parts of the body as yoga, she adds.

Still, if people are really serious about exercising for purposes of weight control or the health of their hearts, supplementing yoga sessions with more aerobic activities such as walking, cycling, swimming, or jogging can be a good idea, Dr. Demers says. "The two types of workouts tend to complement each other quite nicely, in fact, because yoga helps improve flexibility and strength while many aerobic routines do not."

asanas) that build strength and increase flexibility in addition to relaxing the mind. Sessions generally are less strenuous than standard aerobic exercise classes, and yet offer considerable benefits in terms of fitness and weight loss.

Something for Everybody

All of these healing benefits of yoga, along with its gentleness, make it especially well suited for older people, the mentally handicapped, and even people with specific medical conditions such as heart disease, arthritis, or disabilities due to stroke. Not for the feeble only, however, yoga has been shown to benefit even well-conditioned athletes, as evidenced by one study in which highly fit subjects were able to exercise more strenuously while consuming less oxygen in response to a yoga program. Another study showed that a yoga program improved both the fitness levels and the ability to relax in a group of 40 physical education teachers who had been exercising regularly for an average of nine years.

But perhaps yoga's ability to boost the spirits has been its most surprising benefit of all. In one study done with college students, yoga did a better job of producing an "exercise high" than an equal amount of time spent swimming, even though yoga required less expenditure of energy.

Studies with people experiencing depression have shown yoga to have a positive impact. Yoga has also been used successfully to help people break drug addictions. Even prison inmates, children with learning disabilities, and people suffering from obsessive-compulsive disorders (such as uncontrollable hand washing and irrational fears) have benefited from the relaxation produced by yoga's techniques.

Some experts credit yoga's ability to spur the body's production of natural mood-elevating chemicals called endorphins for much of its spirit-boosting as well as pain-quelling effects. We normally associate strenuous exercise with endorphin production, but certain pleasurable physical activities such as yoga (and sex) also can produce endorphins that send quieting signals to the pain center of the brain.

Good Instruction Means Everything

If you're interested in giving yoga a try, it's best to learn from a qualified instructor, says professor of medicine and clinical nutrition at the Oregon Health Sciences University in Portland, William E. Connor, M.D. Since taking up yoga on the advice of his daughter 20 years ago, Dr. Connor has been amazed at its effectiveness in reducing the pain of his own arthritic hip.

No certification is required to teach yoga, unfortunately, but you should be able to find a good instructor or class by checking with your local hospital, YMCA or YWCA, a reputable health club, or even by cruising the Yellow Pages under Yoga in your phone book. He also recommends a book entitled *Back Care Basics* by Mary Pullig Schatz, M.D., as a good source for beginners as well as *Yoga Journal*, a magazine that regularly features simple instructions for beginners.

As for which style of yoga to pursue—and there are several—you'll probably be most satisfied with hatha yoga, if you're looking to use yoga as a form of healing therapy. Hatha yoga, the most popular and readily available style, gives the best workout from a physical standpoint, while still emphasizing the importance of relaxation through proper breathing and meditative techniques, Dr. Connor says.

getting started

Prior to lifting as much as a finger in beginning a yoga session, be sure to prepare yourself as follows:

- **Dress the part.** Wear loose clothing that does not restrict your circulation, movement, or breathing.

- **Go on empty.** Wait at least two hours after eating, four hours if your meal has been large.

- **Make sure you're comfortable.** Do not practice in direct sunlight or in a room that's too cold.

There are also a couple of things to keep in mind during classes:

- **Do not hold your breath during the exercises.** Breathe deeply but smoothly and slowly, remaining as relaxed and focused as possible.

- **Go slow.** Your movements should be smooth, never jerky or abrupt.

There are several approaches to hatha yoga, but Dr. Connor recommends Iyengar yoga. (This is a type of hatha yoga developed by B.K.S. Iyengar of India. His schools now certify teachers throughout the world.) Dr. Connor favors this particular style. Its instructors generally are well-trained in addition to being well versed in working with beginners and people with medical problems or other special needs. If you find an Iyengar-certified teacher, you know you're dealing with someone who really knows how to teach yoga. A teacher seriously working toward this certification is also a good bet.

Other approaches to yoga are well worth pursuing, Dr. Demers adds. "The key is to find an instructor you like and whose approach seems to work for you. Try a class and see how it makes you feel. If you like the results, sign up and give it the best effort you can."

As for the differences that exist between the types of yoga, they are more subtle than substantive and have arisen over the years mainly to accommodate people's varying personalities as well as physical capabilities, Dr. Demers says. Some styles put a greater emphasis on yoga's meditative aspects, while basic hatha yoga concentrates mostly on postures that produce benefits in a physical sense. No styles are mutually

breathing:
the soul of yoga

If postures and stretching could be said to constitute the heart of yoga, its soul lies in proper breathing.
Yoga teaches that the breath is the most direct connection between the body and the mind. Yoga teaches *how* to breathe so both the mind and the body benefit as much as possible.

So what's the proper way to breathe? In a word, deeply.
The lower portions of the lungs are more efficient at exchanging oxygen and carbon dioxide because gravity causes more blood to reside there, explains Georgetown University clinical professor James S. Gordon, M.D.

Yet where do we breathe?
Most of us breathe from just the upper portions of our lungs. Shallow breathing is symptomatic of our upbringing. We're told to suck in our guts and puff out our chests, Dr. Gordon says. Shallow breathing is also the price we pay for constant low-level stress that comes from living in the modern world.

So what's a shallow breather to do?
Take time out each day to breathe right. By taking 10 to 15 minutes twice a day, or for just a few minutes more often, people can begin to reverse years of bad breathing habits, Dr. Gordon says. The key to deep breathing is just that—to inhale deeply enough and slowly enough so that even the lowest portions of your lungs fill with air. You'll be able to see for yourself once you begin to do it correctly: Your belly, not just your chest, will begin to swell with each inhalation.

Practice this type of breathing whenever you can, Dr. Gordon says. Take several seconds to inhale, then several more to exhale, paying attention to feeling your abdomen rise and fall with each breath. (To assist one patient in learning to breathe deeply, Dr. Gordon advised him to repeat the words "soft belly" while envisioning his midsection expanding accordingly.)

Its long-term health benefits aside, deep breathing can be useful during acute times of stress, such as pre-speech jitters, being cut off in traffic, or stepping to the plate with the bases loaded, yoga experts note.

exclusive, however, Dr. Demers points out. All styles of yoga should be viewed simply as different spokes of the same wheel headed in the common direction of helping people be as healthy and happy as they possibly can.

Yoga 101: What to Expect

If you decide to try hatha yoga, expect the sessions (which can last anywhere from 30 to 90 minutes) to include instructions on how to breathe properly. Breathing exercises will involve long, deep inhalations through the nose, designed to help you focus and relax. Yoga instructors maintain that proper breathing is fundamental to yoga because it's considered the most direct connection between the body and the brain.

The purpose of these breathing exercises is to teach you to more fully oxygenate your body by filling your entire lungs. (Most people breathe with only the upper part of their lungs.) Full, deep breaths help relieve stress and banish fatigue.

You'll also learn some gentle stretching exercises and some yoga asanas. Some are done while standing to improve balance and strength. Others, designed more for enhancing flexibility, are done sitting or lying down.

As a beginner, you won't be asked to stand on your head. But this and other inverted postures, which you will learn if you continue to practice yoga, bring better mental clarity by boosting blood flow to your brain.

You'll be asked to hold postures for anywhere from a few seconds to a few minutes, depending on your strength and level of expertise. Sometimes the postures will be presented in flowing sequences, so be prepared to improve your coordination as well as balance and strength.

Holding stationary postures might *look* easy enough. But be forewarned that it can be more difficult than your experienced instructor or fellow classmates make it appear. Expect to challenge yourself during these exercises, but never to a point of enduring sharp or sudden pain. You should always stop immediately if any posture causes you pain, and let your instructor know what happened. You may be asked to sit one out. But more likely, your instructor will be able to modify the posture to suit your body. Never push yourself to the point where you experience uncomfortable fatigue. "No pain, no gain" may still be the anthem of some misguided aerobics enthusiasts, but it has no place in the more gentle discipline of yoga.

The session will end, typically, with a period of relaxation in which you'll be asked to focus on your breathing while clearing your mind of all worldly concerns. While this might sound easy enough, it can be a formidable task, causing some people actually to become more tense. Simply continue to focus on your breathing if you do feel yourself tensing up.

How can you expect to feel following your first class?

In a word, "great," says Dr. Demers, "alert and yet relaxed, the best of both worlds." Research shows, in fact, that many people report feeling more positive and content after yoga than following a strenuous aerobic workout.

Safety and Warnings

Yoga is generally safe for most healthy people, but if you have any doubts, check first with your doctor.

- **Make sure you have competent instruction.** Yoga must be practiced properly to avoid injury, which is why a good instructor is paramount, Dr. Demers says. If you encounter an instructor who is pushy or insensitive to your particular restrictions or needs, find another instructor.
- **Get doctor's approval for certain conditions.** Most practitioners recommend against yoga during pregnancy, its later stages especially. Yoga should be approached with caution—and a doctor's approval—by anyone with back problems, cardiovascular disease, or high blood pressure. (Some doctors are recommending yoga for people with certain kinds of back problems.)
- **Don't put up with pain.** Also important for keeping yoga safe is to learn the difference between good pain and bad, Dr. Demers says. "Pain that's mild and passes quickly usually is nothing to worry about."

Stetching by its very nature sometimes causes moderate but tolerable discomfort. It's the pain that persists during a posture or stretch or that is sharp or makes you hold your breath that should be avoided.

"If such pain occurs, it means that you're doing a posture improperly or that you're simply pushing the posture too far," Dr. Demers says.

If this happens, simply ease your way out of the posture as comfortably as you can and perhaps try it again to a lesser degree. If pain still occurs, take it as a sign that the posture is simply one that you shouldn't do at the present time. Your instructor may be able to adjust a posture to eliminate pain for you, but if pain persists, simply stay away from that particular posture for a time.

"Yoga should be a pleasurable experience, not a painful one," says Dr. Demers.

- **Make sure you let your instructor know immediately if you experience pain.** It may be that you're doing the movement incorrectly and a minor adjustment will eliminate discomfort.
- **Don't practice while sick.** Do not do any yoga exercises if you have a fever or are in any other way feeling ill. And do stop if you start feeling dizzy or overly tired.

Yoga in a Pinch: Postures for Pain

Although yoga in the United States is used mostly for relaxation and fitness by people already in good health, doctors more and more are discovering its remarkable abilities to treat a wide range of health problems. To derive such benefits from yoga, it's best to learn in person from a qualified instructor and to perform yoga regularly, even daily, if you can afford the time, Dr. Demers says.

Yoga also can be used for acute conditions, such as daily stress and common aches and pains, Dr. Demers says. "Certain postures can be used whenever a particular need may arise, such as to relieve stress or help soothe common ailments such as back pain, headaches, or stiffness in the shoulders and neck. Practicing yoga in this way is unlikely to instill the inner calm of a more comprehensive approach, but at least it can help the situation at hand."

Before using a yoga posture to treat any condition, remember: "All movements should be slow, deliberate, and controlled, and performed only to the extent that is comfortable," Dr. Demers says.

For stress: Be a "Corpse." Don't let the name of this posture scare you. This posture is a rejuvenator that can defuse stress by reducing muscular tension throughout the entire body. Usually it's performed both at the beginning and end of a typical yoga session, but it can be used anytime life's ends just don't seem to meet. Take a few minutes to try it at work or at home whenever you're feeling about to boil.

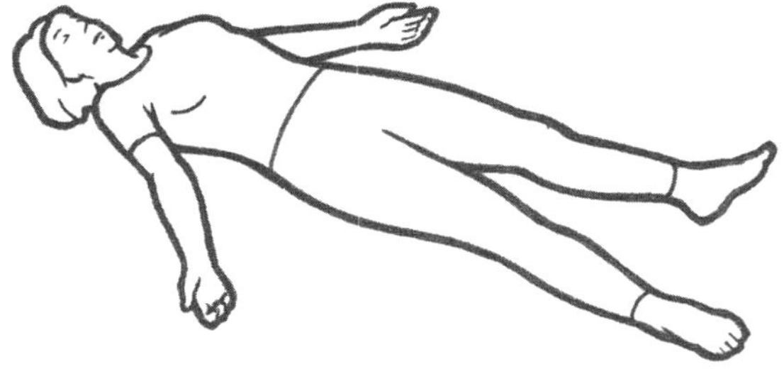

1. Close your eyes as you lie on your back with your arms spread slightly away from your body, palms up, and your legs slightly spread as well.

2. Relax as completely as possible while breathing slowly and deeply from your diaphragm, trying to clear your mind as much as possible of worldly concerns.

For low back pain: Become a "Cobra." With an estimated 80 percent of adults suffering from back pain at some point in their lives, this posture should be learned right along with the ABC's, Dr. Demers says. It can be particularly effective after long periods of sitting, which is a cause of low-back pain for many people.

1. Begin by lying stomach down and face down on the floor, with your palms pressed to the floor in close to your chest. Your legs should be together with your toes pointed.

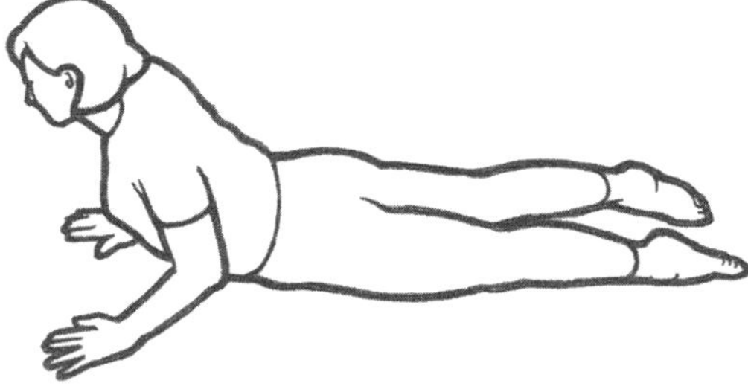

2. As you slowly inhale, gently begin to raise your head then your shoulders upward and backward, but always with your navel still in contact with the floor. Go slowly enough to get the feeling that you're moving each vertebra one at a time. It's critical to allow your arms to bear as little weight as possible to make sure the exercise works the muscles of the lower back.

3. Once you've gone as high as you can go, hold the position until the onset of fatigue—but not pain—and begin to lower your head slowly back to its starting position, again trying to go one vertebra at a time. Turn your head to the side when you've completed the maneuver and relax with deep, even breaths.

For the agony of a back attack: Use "Wall Power." Chronic back pain can be trouble enough, but an acute attack involving muscular spasms can be downright scary. Here's a posture that can help bring relief in such times of trauma:

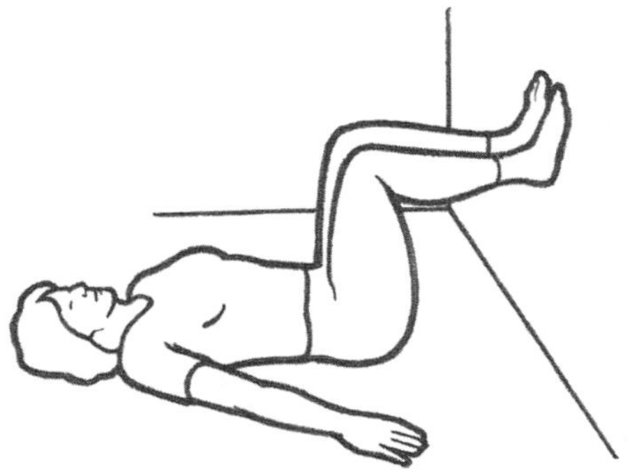

1. Lie down on your back and place your feet against the wall so that your thighs and shins form a right angle.

2. Now alternately press your feet gently against the wall and release, feeling your lower back press more tightly against the floor as you do. Several minutes of this should help your pain subside. If it doesn't, seek medical attention.

For varicose veins: Do some "High Fives." Logic alone supports the value of this posture, which employs gravity to help pooled blood drain from swollen veins of the legs. (Be sure to check first with your doctor before trying this one to be sure you're not at risk for dislodging a blood clot.)

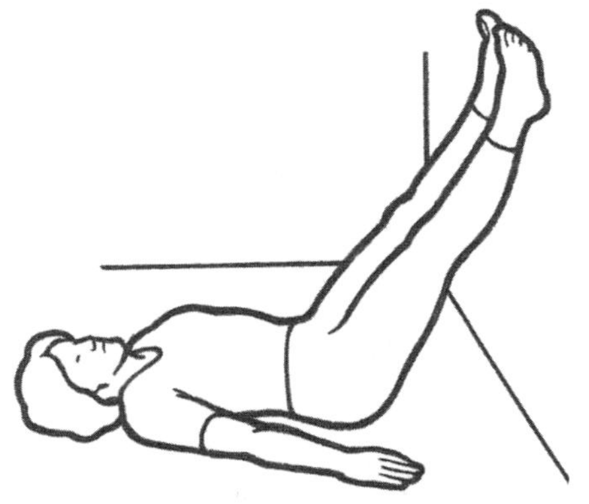

1. Lie close enough to a wall that you can rest your legs at approximately a 45-degree angle or higher. Breathe slowly and deeply, eyes closed. You may add a pillow beneath the buttocks for greater comfort.

For stiffness in the neck and shoulders: Do the "Twist." You can feel lousy and act grouchy when a bad day or a marathon car ride has put a crick in your neck or shoulders. Or you can do the Twist. Moreover, by giving a sideways twist to the spine in both directions this exercise can benefit the entire body by reducing pressure on spinal nerves, Dr. Demers says.

1. Begin by sitting on the floor with your legs stretched out in front of you. Slowly bend your right leg at the knee, pulling your heel in as close as you can to your crotch.

2. Bend your left leg and lift your left foot over your right thigh, placing it on the floor so the outside of your left ankle is now against the outside of your right knee.

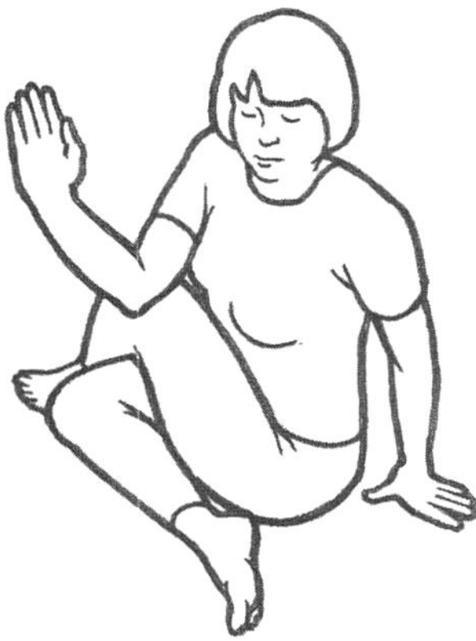

3. Inhale as you sit up as straight as you can. Exhale and turn your head and trunk to the left, raising your right arm over your left knee and bringing your chest against the inside of your left thigh. Turn as far as you comfortably can, hopefully to a point where the back of your right shoulder and upper arm will be pressing against your left knee and lower thigh. Your left hand should be placed on the floor behind your left hip to keep you steady.

4. Begin to breathe deeply once you've twisted as far as you can go. Hold this position for as long as you comfortably can (30 seconds or so), then slowly unwind and gently repeat the exercise in the opposite direction.

resources

Books

Light on Yoga by B.K.S. Iyengar (Schoken Books, 1995)

Yoga: The Iyengar Way by Mira Silva and Shyam Mehta (Knopf, 1995)

Back Care Basics by Mary Pullig Schatz, M.D. (Rodmell, 1992)

Living Yoga by Georg Feuerstein and Stephan Bodian (Jeremy Tarcher, 1993)

Magazines

Yoga Journal
Berkeley, California
800/I-DO-YOGA (800/436-9642)
www.yogajournal.com

Yoga International
Honesdale, Pennsylvania
(717) 253-4929
www.himalayaninstitute.org

appendix

USING ALTERNATIVE MEDICINES WISELY

Conventional medicine asks, "What disease does this patient have?" Alternative systems ask, "What disharmonies or imbalances disturb this person?"—*Leo Galland, M.D.*

Entering the brave new world of alternative medicine is like going to a bazaar in a foreign country and finding hundreds of food items on display. Your phrase book will tell you that arroz con pollo is rice with chicken or that le chou farci is stuffed cabbage, but it won't tell you which selection will make you feel better and which will send you back to your hotel room doubled over. For that, you need to proceed with caution, armed with expert guidance, research, and trustworthy instincts.

Alternatives Go Mainstream

No doubt the term "alternative" will soon be obsolete, as the practices we associate with it become as mainstream as blue jeans. In 1998 about 83 million Americans forked over $27 billion dollars to nontraditional health practitioners, exceeding the number of visits to primary-care physicians. The number of office visits to such practitioners increased by nearly 50 percent between 1990 and 1997. With demand like that, supply is sure to follow.

Sure enough, the number of chiropractors, acupuncturists, homeopaths, and other alternative therapists has mushroomed beyond what anyone could have predicted a decade ago, as has the quantity of natural remedies leaping off the shelves. This explosion is a boon in that it multiplies our choices and enhances quality in the long run, since competition keeps suppliers on their toes. But there is a downside to the colossal demand as well. Competition in a lucrative—and thus far pretty much unregulated—market also breeds false and exaggerated claims and brings all manner of quacks and charlatans out of the woodwork.

Fortunately, the potential for abuse has been a wake-up call for responsible experts. Information on alternative medicine is becoming as easy to obtain as a multiple vitamin, with a growing number of books, magazines, newsletters, websites, journals, and public speakers issuing guidelines, tips, and factual analysis. And, at long last, rigorous scientific studies are starting to ferret out exactly what works—and what does not—for whom and under what circumstances.

Research is underway at a number of prestigious medical institutions as well as the Office of Alternative Medicine (OMA) at the National Institutes of Health. This means you will enjoy ever-easier and more abundant access to knowledge—and so will your doctor.

The Good, the Bad, And the Ugly

Navigating the complex landscape of alternative medicine can be confusing, and the consequences of getting lost are far more significant than choosing the wrong long distance carrier or running shoe. There is an unfortunate tendency to assume that because something is "natural" it is, ipso facto, safe. While it is true that the potential for damage is far worse with drugs and surgery, at least we know about the side effects of drugs and surgery, and they're highly regulated.

Research on alternative medicine has barely scratched the surface, and, with a few exceptions, regulation is virtually nil. Take the widespread, and frequently haphazard, use of herbal supplements, for example. Just because something comes from a plant doesn't mean it's safe.

The product that helped your friend may be useless for your condition and may even do you harm. A remedy that proves beneficial won't necessarily do more good if you increase the dose; it might even make things worse. Something that's harmless or even beneficial on its own may interact with another herb or medicine to produce unexpected side effects.

And that's just looking at the myriad herbal products available over the counter. What about all the alternative practitioners vying for your medical dollar? We know that some M.D.s are more competent and more ethical than others; why shouldn't the same be true of naturopaths, homeopaths, massage therapists, and the rest? They too can be unscrupulous. They too can make mistakes. They too can be well-meaning but ill-informed.

On the whole, incompetence and fraud can wreak far less havoc in the alternative domain than with drugs and high-tech medicine. But there are fewer checks and balances on the fringes and less accountability.

Perhaps the greatest concern are acts of omission rather than commission. Critics cite the tendency of many consumers, disenchanted with conventional medicine, to rely on alternatives to the exclusion of conventional remedies that might help.

This may be inconsequential with a stiff neck, say, or indigestion, but with more serious conditions, it can lead to unnecessary suffering and even death. Take the case of a women we'll call Anna Russell. She's a San Francisco architect who believes strongly in alternative medicine.

Her back pain took her on a two-year odyssey of chiropractic, physical therapy, acupuncture, massage therapy, biofeedback, and hands-on healing, all of which provided temporary relief at best. Ultimately, the pain got so incessant and so severe that she yielded to the wishes of her family physician and had Xrays taken.

Sure enough, she had major damage to a vertebral disk. An orthopedist recommended surgery. Anna got a second opinion and a third. All concurred that surgery was needed. Another round of acupuncture and chiropractic failed to stem the tide. So, thousands of dollars later, she did what she swore she'd never do. The surgery was a success. Pain-free at last, Anna is happily jogging again—no small health benefit itself—and is now much more balanced in her attitude toward medicine.

Of course, for every story like Anna's there are dozens in which someone was healed by alternative therapies after years of frustration with mainstream medicine. But the potential danger of neglecting the conventional approach is real.

Samuel Benjamin, M.D., associate professor of pediatrics and family medicine at the State University of New York at Stony Brook School of Medicine and director of the University Center for Complementary and Alternative Medicine, cites this example: "I saw a young man who had been diagnosed at the very earliest stage of Hodgkin's lymphoma, a malignancy of the lymphatic system that can be easily cured by a well-known chemotherapy regimen.

"He was advised by an acupuncturist to stay away from standard medical care because natural medicine would be safer and would cure him. We saw him six months after his initial diagnosis. By then he had a very advanced stage of Hodgkins, which is quite difficult to treat and will, regrettably, result in his early demise."

The Best of Both Worlds

Most experts feel that the best and safest entry point to complementary medicine is through a primary-care physician who is both sympathetic and well informed. Such a doctor can serve as team captain, ensuring that one person knows everything you're doing for your health and can monitor your progress accordingly. He or she can also recommend alternative approaches that suit your condition, providing an element of consistency and quality control.

Another good reason for turning first to a knowledgeable M.D. is the diagnostic power of mainstream medicine. Western physicians are trained to use blood tests, imaging technology—Xrays, MRIs, CT scans, etc.—and other sophisticated methods to get precise, quantifiable diagnoses.

"If you have symptoms that have been persisting for some time and are accompanied by pain, fatigue, or problems with the immune system, you should definitely see an M.D.," says Cynthia Watson, M.D., a family practitioner in Santa Monica, California. "It's important to run tests to rule out the possibility that something serious is going on."

Once you have a diagnosis, you can make an informed decision about whether to see a holistic practitioner or use standard treatment—or both.

With a growing number of medical schools adding courses on alternative medicine, it won't be long before the average M.D. can advise patients knowledgeably about their options.

For now, most doctors are challenged when it comes to dealing with their patients' requests for alternative therapies, and many are downright hostile.

If that's the case with your doctor, you have two options. You might find a doctor who is more amenable to the use of alternative treatments. Or you could continue with your present physician and have a naturopath, nurse practitioner, or other health provider serve as gatekeeper for alternative care.

The Doctor as Partner

If you choose to stay with your current doctor, make sure you keep him or her well informed. Studies show that fewer than 40 percent of those using alternative modalities are disclosing that fact to their primary-care physicians. By keeping your physician in the dark, you risk using remedies that interact poorly with your conventional treatments.

"Let your regular doctor know what you are doing and encourage a dialogue between him or her and the alternative practitioner," advises Leo Galland, M.D., director of the Foundation for Integrated Medicine in New York City and author of *Power Healing: Use the New Integrated Medicine to Cure Yourself*. "There are certainly many doctors who just don't want to know, but there are also many who are interested in the fact that a patient has gotten benefit from some kind of therapy and will want to know about it."

By keeping your doctor informed, notes Dr. Galland, you not only improve the quality of your own treatment, you contribute to the much-needed integration of conventional and alternative medicines.

It's especially important to let your doctor know what medications and supplements you're taking. That means over-the-counter medications, vitamin supplements, herbs—any pills, capsules, herbal teas, whatever, that you're taking.

Your doctor wants to know about prescription medicines, too, but all these other therapies are also medications.

And if you're planning to try an alternative treatment method, broach the subject in a positive, declarative way. Volunteer to send your doctor information on the modality in question.

Foster communication between your doctor and your alternative practitioners. If you can't arrange for them to speak to each other directly, serve as a liaison, shuttling questions and answers between them.

The Integrated Approach

Experts are virtually unanimous in advising us not to think of conventional and alternative medicine as antagonists. That's why terms such as "integrative" and "complementary" are gaining favor. Says Dr. Galland, "Conventional medicine asks, 'What disease does this patient have?' Alternative systems ask, 'What disharmonies or imbalances disturb this person?'" In the first case, treatment naturally focuses on the disease; in the second, it is oriented toward restoring harmony and balance to the system as a whole. Both approaches have value.

"The process of integration is different depending on what the condition is," says James S. Gordon, M.D., director of the Center for Mind-Body Medicine in Washington, D.C., and author of *Manifesto for a New Medicine: Your Guide to Healing Partnerships and the Wise Use of Alternative Therapies*. "What's the diagnosis? What's the prognosis with conventional therapies? What do complementary and alternative therapies have to offer? How can you put them together in a way that makes sense to you?"

As a general rule for nonemergencies, he advises starting with treatments that have minimal side effects and are designed to enhance self-healing. "Only when those don't work would I look to drugs and surgery," he says.

In many instances, a simultaneous approach is called for. For example, many people with recurring headaches or chronic back pain turn to alternative practitioners to eliminate the underlying conditions that give rise to those symptoms. These individuals supplement that long-range plan with the judicious use of pain medication when their condition flares up.

Cancer patients, to cite another example, might undergo chemotherapy or radiation treatments to destroy malignant cells and at the same time take herbs to strengthen their immune system and reduce the side effects of treatment.

"Allopathic medicine has been lousy at dealing with things like chronic arthritis and the prevention of coronary artery disease, but we should acknowledge its incredible success in acute care," asserts Dr. Benjamin. "If you need a coronary artery bypass, you should have it, and you might consider acupuncture after the surgery to help with wound healing." (Allopathic medicine is the traditional, scientific medicine that your family physician practices.)

surfing the Net

If there is any correlation between information and wellness, the Internet might be the greatest blessing to public health since sanitation.

At the click of a mouse, you have access to cyberlibraries filled with facts, scientific data, and expert opinions. Unfortunately, it's not always easy to separate the experts from the cyberquacks who spread misinformation, whether to fleece eager customers or spread mischief.

Not only are there no regulations to protect us from false advertising, but chat rooms, newsgroups, and the like can be populated by "doctors" who in reality are no more qualified to give medical advice than your cable guy. All of which makes surfing the Net for health information as risky as body surfing off a rocky coastline.

Part of the problem is the proliferation of commercial websites. "If you did a search on coenzyme Q-10, of the first 20 hits, 10 would probably be someone selling supplements," says James Strohecker, executive editor of *Alternative Medicine: The Definitive Guide* and cofounder of HealthWorld Online, an Internet health network. "There are a lot of very aggressive people pushing the envelope of what they can legally get away with, and there are a lot of multilevel marketing schemes making all sorts of promises."

Ferreting out who is a reliable source of information and who is trying to sell you something is not always easy.

One safe bet is to favor the websites of well-known authorities such as Dr. Galland (www.mdheal.org) and Andrew Weil, M.D. (www.drweil.com). Also, a number of reputable institutions—universities, clinics, hospitals, etc.—have sites that include information on alternative medicine. These tend to be conservative, but at least they're not trying to fleece you or feed you flaky advice.

Medline, which can be reached through the National Library of Medicine's site as well as a number of others, is a treasure trove of journal articles on every conceivable medical subject, including alternative treatments. Then there's the website of NIH's Office of Alternative Medicine, perhaps the most prestigious institution devoted to the subject. HealthWorld Online (www.healthy.com) is a good starting point for investigating complementary medicine, with more than 30,000 pages of free content and 7,000 links, including the websites of various professional associations, a referral network, and Medline.

The opportunities for health education are virtually unlimited on the Net—but so is the potential for capriciousness and deception. Surfing effectively depends on common sense and technical know-how. In the meantime, if cyberspace seems as impenetrable as outer space, there are plenty of old-fashioned ways to get reliable information on alternative medicine. Knowledge, more than pills, is the most important ingredient in using alternative medicine wisely.

Finding an Alternative Practitioner

As in selecting any service provider, whether it be a plumber or lawyer, the best place to start is with a recommendation from someone you trust. Barring that, "you might inquire at local hospitals, clinics, medical schools, and professional organizations for the specialists you're looking for—or more unusual sources such as health food markets and phone directories where holistic clinics and individual practitioners might be listed," says Oscar Janiger, M.D., clinical professor at the California College of Medicine, University of California at Irvine.

State licensing boards and certification commissions are excellent sources; as a rule, those who have been licensed or certified have met basic standards of training and competence.

Locating a practitioner is one thing; choosing the right one is quite another. Here are some tips from a number of experts.

Beware of fanatics. "Just as there are doctors who are closed-minded when it comes to alternative modalities, there are others who are overzealous," Dr. Janiger points out. Be wary of practitioners who make what seem to be excessive claims. And watch out for ax grinding—such as overt hostility toward other systems.

"I'd look for someone who is not trying to push one treatment or another, but rather looks at you as a whole person and wants to help you figure out what you need to help yourself," says Dr. Gordon.

Make sure you can speak your mind. "When you talk with the person, you should feel free to ask all your questions," says Dr. Gordon. "And any concerns you raise should be handled in a respectful way. You should not feel that you're being coerced, seduced, or bullied."

If an unusual procedure is recommended, ask every question that comes to mind. Exactly why is it recommended? How does it work? What results can you expect? Are there potential side effects? "Once you are adequately informed, you can make an educated choice as to whether the approach is something you care to try," says Dr. Janiger. "If you don't feel comfortable with the answers you get, you are well advised to look elsewhere."

Choose someone who cares. "Evaluate whether this person really listens to you, encourages you to be an active participant in your own care, and shows concern for you as a person, " advises Dr. Galland. He describes the qualities he considers indicative of a caring health practitioner:

- Ability to explain
- Ability to listen
- Ability to show empathy
- Willingness to acknowledge your concerns
- Willingness to assess family and social support
- Willingness to offer encouragement, hope, and reassurance

Look for practitioners who know their limits. No one can be all things to all patients. "If a practitioner does not have the approach you need, he or she should recognize that and refer you to someone who can help you," says Dr. Galland.

- **Look for experience.** Make sure the practitioner has experience dealing with the kinds of problems you have. Don't be shy about asking, urges Dr. Galland. Find out what results they've had, and, if possible, speak to patients whom they've treated for similar conditions.
- **Examine your own expectations.** It's easy to get overly excited about a new and different treatment, especially if it resonates with your hopes for a perfect cure. Make sure you're not drawn to a person or practice because you are desperate to believe in something, advises Dr. Janiger, or because you're hoping for an effortless path to healing.

Complementary modalities tend to require some effort on the part of the patient, Dr. Watson points out. "You can put someone on lots of vitamins and herbs," she says, "but if they are not following healthy lifestyle practices—exercise, stress reduction, proper diet—then these things are not going to work as well." You have to be willing to make the effort and give the recommended procedures a chance to work.

- **Trust your instincts.** In the final analysis, your gut has to be satisfied that you're with the right practitioner. "Even if they have all the right credentials and somebody else thinks they're great, if you feel uncomfortable or you don't want to be there, leave," says Dr. Galland.

Safety and Warnings

Shopping in the bustling alternative marketplace can be confusing, given its newness, diversity, absence of regulation, and potential for abuse. Here are some red flags to watch for.

- **Lack of hygiene.** "If you enter a room and it looks dirty, trust your judgment and leave," says Dr. Benjamin. Same goes for the hygiene of the provider: "Somebody who is touching you or putting acupuncture needles in you should not have dirty nails."
- **Unwillingness to collaborate.** "Complementary medicine is not just physician based," says Dr. Benjamin. "It involves different people in the community who are involved in caring for individuals, and each one needs to understand the importance of collaboration." If your naturopath does not want to talk to your acupuncturist or neither one wants to know what your family physician has to say, that should be a warning sign.

"Patients should choose providers who are not so wrapped up in a philosophy or egotism that they don't want to share in the care of an individual," says Dr. Benjamin.

- **Arrogance.** "I would be concerned if somebody says, 'I've got all the answers, just do what I tell you,'" says Dr. Gordon. "You should feel like you are being encouraged to take care of yourself and not depend on yet another person."
- **Financial incentives.** Like everyone else, health-care providers can be seduced by the profit motive. It may be a good idea, for example, to be wary if someone insists on a

large number of visits in a brief period of time. Although it might be just what the doctor ordered, so to speak, it can also be financially motivated. "It's very hard to know in the beginning how much work it will take for somebody to do well," Dr. Gordon says.

- **Unwillingness to show you evidence.** If someone prescribes a treatment that does not make complete sense to you, ask to see proof. A good practitioner will make clear what is purely an opinion or hunch, what is an inference based on clinical experience, and what has been investigated scientifically. If evidence exists, he or she should be happy to show it to you or tell you how to look it up yourself. "You have every right to ask for evidence," says Dr. Gordon. "If they get irritated, then I would suggest it's time to move on."
- **Refusal to inform.** Part of a practitioner's role in complementary medicine is to serve as an educator. If he or she is impatient with your questions or refuses to explain procedures, proceed with caution.

"You should be careful about anyone who gives you products but won't tell you what's in them," warns Dr. Galland, "and also with anyone who won't share information freely."

- **Extravagant claims.** Dr. Benjamin's rule of thumb is: "If something sounds too good to be true, then most likely it is too good to be true."

Shopping for Herbs And Supplements

In a perfect world, you would be able to purchase any herb or nutritional supplement you cared to take and you would be sure you were getting an excellent product with exactly what its label said it contained. Unfortunately, this is not a perfect world. Supplements are regarded as food products, not medicines, so they are not regulated the way over-the-counter drugs are. This makes us vulnerable to unscrupulous manufacturers, clever wordsmiths, and careless vendors.

Even staunch supporters of alternative medicine feel we have to find a way to standardize products, ensure public safety, and guarantee truth in advertising without sacrificing consumer freedom.

"We think of herbs as being natural and therefore OK," says Dr. Watson, "but herbs are chemicals, and they can have a powerful effect on your system, so you have to be cautious about what you take and learn about possible side effects and contraindications."

For example, she says, a lot of people take a combination of echinacea and goldenseal every day. But, when taken over long periods of time, goldenseal can impair the absorption of B vitamins. Licorice root is another example of a health-enhancing herb that can have long-term side effects—in this case, high blood pressure.

But you can't rely on product labels to tell you any of that. Unlike the pharmaceutical industry, supplement manufacturers have no oversight agency to answer to. Where can you turn for reliable information? Probably not the health-food store clerk. "More often than not the person who is giving information in the health-food store does not have the education appropriate to advise an individual about what product to take or not take," says Dr. Benjamin.

A trusted health-care provider is one place to turn. The books and articles of reputable authors are another good source. A third option is to track down research data. As complementary medicine moves further into the mainstream, more and more information will be available from medical schools, teaching hospitals, and HMOs, institutions that can rigorously test the products they give their patients.

In addition to perusing the scientific literature, there are other steps you can take to help ensure your safety when taking supplements. Look to the source for one thing. "Be very cautious about products that come from foreign countries," says Dr. Galland. "There is a higher likelihood of contamination." Herbs from India and China, he says, are often contaminated with lead and heavy metals. If a product has been packaged in the United States, the odds are in your favor. But not all American manufacturers are equal. Unless you know the company is entirely reputable, you can't even be sure the package contains what the label says it does.

One way to know which products are dependable is to ask a health-care practitioner who recommends supplements to patients—assuming he or she can be counted on to have the patient's best interest at heart. It's your call: If someone sells a particular brand in his or her office, for example, it could mean that he or she has done the necessary homework and trusts that particular company. It could also simply mean that he or she is making a buck off your purchase.

Look for products whose ingredients have been assayed independently—meaning that an outside source has determined that the material inside is actually what the package says it is. If whoever sells you the product doesn't know if it's been assayed, call the manufacturer. Also, certain herbs—gingko biloba, ginseng, echinacea among them—are produced in standardized potencies. For example, a bottle of St. John's wort capsules should have a 3 percent standardized extract of hypericum, the active ingredient in depression treatment.

Dr. Watson also recommends products that use organic or wild-crafted (picked in the wild) herbs. "If a lot of the herbs in that particular line are wild-crafted or organic, you can be pretty sure they have good quality herbs," she says.

Perhaps the best way to safeguard your use of supplements is to have a trusted practitioner formulate a regimen, recommend specific products, and educate you as to what you can expect. "You can do a lot of the research yourself," says Dr. Gordon, "but it's much safer, at least in the beginning, to have someone help you put together a program."

One final precaution: If you are seeing several practitioners, it's very important that they all know what you are taking. "You need to communicate with all of them to make sure you are not being overprescribed," says Dr. Watson.

resources

These organizations can either help with referrals or supply helpful information:

Books

Power Healing: Use the New Integrated Medicine to Cure Yourself by Dr. Leo Galland, M.D. (Random House, 1998)

Manifesto for a New Medicine: Your Guide to Healing Partnerships and the Wise Use of Alternative Therapies by James S. Gordon, M.D. (Perseus, 1997)

Five Steps to Selecting the Best Alternative Medicine: A Guide to Complementary and Integrative Health Care by Mary and Michael Morton (New World Library, 1997)

Alternative Medicine: The Definitive Guide by the Burton Goldberg Group (Future Medicine, 1993)

Women's Bodies, Women's Wisdom by Christiane Northrup, M.D. (Bantam Doubleday, 1998)

Total Wellness: Improve Your Health by Understanding and Cooperating with Your Body's Natural Healing Systems by Joseph Pizzorno, N.D. (Prima, 1997)

Quantum Healing: Exploring the Frontiers of Mind/Body Medicine by Deepak Chopra, M.D. (Bantam, 1990)

Web sites

Alternative Medicine Center
www.alternativemedicine.net

Foundation for Integrated Medicine
www.mdheal.org

NIH's National Center for Complementary & Alternative Medicine
altmed.od.nih.gov/nccam

Andrew Weil, M.D., Internet Health Clinic (Ask Dr. Weil)
www.drweil.com

Newsletters

Dr. Andrew Weil's Self-Healing
P.O. Box 2057
Marion, OH 43305–2057
800/523-3296

Dr. Christiane Northrup's Health Wisdom for Women
P.O. Box 60042
7811 Montrose Rd.
Potomac, MD 20859–0042
800/211-8561

Dr. Julian Whitaker's Health and Healing
800/861-5967

home remedies

COMPLEMENTARY THERAPIES

I would be concerned if somebody says, "I've got all the answers." You should feel like you are being encouraged to take care of yourself and not depend on yet another person.—*James S. Gordon, M.D.*

The suggestions on the following pages are not a substitute for the advice of a qualified health-care practitioner. We encourage you to use the information in these pages to improve your health and vitality, but if you have a medical condition or symptoms that persist, be sure to seek appropriate medical guidance.

Acne

- **Cosmetics.** Among adults, women are more likely to have acne than men, primarily due to the use of oil-based cosmetics. Switch to cosmetics and creams that are water based.
- **Nutrition.** According to dermatologists, diet has nothing to do with acne. Many alternative practitioners, however, continue to insist that it does. What to do? It certainly can't hurt to cut back on excess sugar and fats, including fried foods. You should be minimizing these foods for your health in any case.

  Vasant D. Lad, BMS, MASc, author of *The Complete Book of Ayurvedic Home Remedies,* recommends cutting down on citrus fruits and spicy foods, as well as fats, meats, and sweets. (Dr. Lad's degrees are from India and indicate several years of training in ayurvedic medical school.)
- **Relax.** Stress is now regarded as a factor in acne, so take some time to unwind with long walks, soothing music, meditation, or any other stress-management method you find helpful.

Allergies

There are many types of allergies, including those caused by foods, pollens, chemicals, and environmental factors. The following recommendations are for

cautions

HERBS AND ESSENTIAL OILS:
During pregnancy, essential oils and herbs should not be used as home remedies without professional guidance. Some of these natural remedies are very potent, and their effects on the developing fetus are not fully understood. Some act as stimulants and could cause premature uterine contractions. Excessive exposure to others may possibly affect the cellular division of the fetus. It is best to be on the safe side and avoid taking herbs or oils if you are pregnant or intend to become pregnant.

MAGNETS:
According to Gary Null, Ph.D., author of *Healing with Magnets*, magnet therapy should not be used by pregnant women. Individuals using pacemakers should not place magnets near the chest or midback. People with cancer or any infection, including candida, viruses, or bacteria, should not use bipolar magnets.

HOME REMEDIES FOR CHILDREN:
Many alternative therapies are appropriate for children, but be aware that they must be adapted for children. Herbal and vitamin doses, for example, are smaller for children. Be on the safe side and coordinate all alternative therapies and home remedies with your child's pediatrician.

hay-fever-type allergies that affect the sinuses and have coldlike symptoms.

If you know you are allergic to something, stay away from it. This applies to foods, dust, mold, cat or dog hair, synthetic fabrics such as polyester, certain perfumes, and chemicals such as those in cleaning supplies. When the pollen count is high, stay indoors and use an air conditioner.

- **Acupressure.** Stimulate one or both of these acupressure points, recommended by Steve Shimer, L.Ac., coauthor of *Healing with Pressure Point Therapy.* (L.Ac. stands for Licensed Acupuncturist.)

1. With your left hand facing palm down, use your right hand (thumb on top, index finger underneath) to take hold of the webbing between your left thumb and index finger. Squeeze in the center of the webbing, pressing toward the bone of the index finger. Hold one minute, breathing deeply, then repeat with the other hand. This point helps to relieve symptoms such as headaches and congestion and balances the flow of energy in the body.

Warning: Pregnant women should *not* press on this point, as it may stimulate premature contractions in the uterus.

2. "At the inner end of your eye sockets, near the bridge of your nose, you will find a small indentation," says Shimer. Use the thumbs of both hands to press on this point for one minute. Close your eyes and breathe deeply as you press. You may also lean your head forward into your fingers.

- **Aromatherapy.** Essential oils for allergies include eucalyptus, pine, rosemary, mint, chamomile, and lavender. Tea tree oil is also effective. The best way to make aromatherapy home remedies for allergies is to use a diffuser. For more acute conditions, put a few drops in a pot of hot water, cover your head with a towel, and breathe the steam. (Be careful not to get your face too close to the hot water; you don't want to burn yourself.)
- **Herbs.** Herbalist David Crow, L.Ac., author of *In Search of the Medicine Flower*, recommends the following herbs for hay-fever: ginger, sage, mint, rosemary, eucalyptus, elder flowers, nettle, burdock, and green plantain leaf.

To use any of these herbs, make a tea infusion using about ½ teaspoon of the herb per cup of boiling water, steep about 10 minutes, and drink two or three times a day.

- **Homeopathy.** Dana Ullman, M.P.H., director of Homeopathic Educational Services in Berkeley, California, recommends using the homeopathic remedy *Euphrasia* when your allergies mostly affect the eyes, and *Allium cepa* if the nasal symptoms are more affected.

If there is copious nasal discharge, sneezing, itching in the nose, and red, runny eyes, try *Sabadilla*, he says. Ullman recommends using these medicines as often as once an hour, but only if the symptoms persist, reappear, or worsen.

Homeopathic remedies are available in many health food stores.

Angina

If you have angina, you should be under the care of a physician, so please seek medical attention. Angina is a warning sign of possible heart attacks and should not be ignored. The best "alternative" remedy comes out of mainstream medicine. Consider the therapy recommended by Dean Ornish, M.D. that is described in Vegetarianism on page 261. And because angina is such as serious condition, make sure you discuss all home remedies with your physician.

- **Acupressure.** An effective point for relief is on the palm side of your wrist, two thumb widths above the wrist crease and right in the center of the arm. Apply medium pressure; build up gradually, hold about a minute, and gradually release. Start with either hand but be sure to do both.

For acute pain, grasp the tip of the little finger of your left hand (the area above the first joint) with your right thumb and index finger, and hold it tightly.

- **Herbs.** The herbs most often recommended for this problem include hawthorn berry and ginkgo.

Look in natural food stores for an herbal circulatory formula that includes both these herbs. Garlic is also helpful.

• **Nutrition.** Favor a low-fat diet. Fat builds plaque in the arteries (atherosclerosis), narrowing the blood vessels and limiting the amount of blood that can reach the heart.

Increase your daily intake of fresh fruit and fresh vegetables, and eat more whole grains such as whole wheat, brown rice, and oats.

• **Relaxation.** Minimize stress. Spend at least 15 to 20 minutes every day practicing meditation or a relaxation technique. The "Relaxation Therapy" chapter on page 207 gives instruction in visualization, a meditation technique, and a sample of progressive muscle relaxation.

• **Yoga.** Try the yogic rest pose (the Corpse pose) described on page 307. This gentle version of the Spinal Twist will be beneficial: Lie on your back. Stretch your arms out wide, with the palms up. Bend your knees so your feet are flat on the floor, a few inches away from your buttocks. Keeping your feet and your arms on the floor, allow your legs to fall toward the left. As the legs go to the left, turn your head to the right. Hold for three or four breaths. Inhale and return your head and legs to the starting position. Repeat by turning head and legs in the opposite direction.

Anxiety

• **Acupressure.** For deep relaxation, press gently on the acupressure point known as the "third eye" point—between your eyebrows, just above the bridge of your nose. Use either your thumb or middle finger to press and use light to moderate pressure for up to two minutes. Close your eyes and take slow, deep breaths as you press.

• **Aromatherapy.** Helpful essential oils include lavender (the most beneficial), marjoram, rose, clary sage, ylang ylang, chamomile, orange, neroli, bergamot, geranium, and sandalwood. Aromatherapy for anxiety should be primarily in the form of massage with scented oil, but you can also use these essences in a diffuser.

• **Chinese medicine.** David Crow, L.Ac., recommends lavender, chamomile, skullcap, valerian, jatamansi, oat straw, passion flower, St. John's wort, and kava kava. "You can take most of these herbs as teas," he says. "They are all classified as 'relaxing nervines,' meaning that they calm the nervous system and at the same time are strengthening."

The most important of these herbs is kava kava. "I have found kava generally more effective, and more appropriate for most people, than medications for anxiety," says psychiatrist Harold H. Bloomfield, M.D., author of *Healing Anxiety Naturally.* "Whereas benzodiazepine tranquilizers can be addictive, impair memory, and worsen depression, kava improves mental functioning and mood and is not addictive."

Prepared kava products are readily available as tinctures or capsules. The standard dosage is 45 to 70 milligrams of kavalactones, three times a day.

Warning: Jean Carper, author of *Miracle Cures,* highly recommends kava for anxiety and stress but says, "Don't take kava if you are pregnant or nursing."

• **Exercise.** Regular daily exercise will also help you reduce your anxiety level, says psychiatrist James S. Brooks, M.D. Most people need only a daily walk for about half an hour, but if you like to play tennis, jog, swim, or dance, that's fine.

• **Homeopathy.** *Aconite* is an effective remedy for anxiety, according to Ullman. "Try aconite for intense fear or panic," he advises. *Argentum nitricum* is another homeopathic remedy for an agitated nervous system.

• **Meditation.** Dr. Bloomfield recommends the Transcendental Meditation program. "Deep relaxation is critical for anyone with anxiety," he says. "I've seen research indicating that TM may be twice as effective as other relaxation techniques for soothing anxiety."

• **Nutrition.** Cut out caffeine, says Dr. Brooks. "Coffee, tea, and colas are not what you need if you want to reduce your anxiety." Cut back gradually, because suddenly eliminating caffeine can cause headaches.

• **Yoga.** Yoga postures performed slowly offer great relief from tension and anxiety. If you only have a few minutes, try this simplified version of the Shoulder Stand: Lie on your back. Using your arms to support your torso, raise your legs and buttocks into the air and lean them back over your head. Your shoulders and arms will remain on the floor as your hands support your lower back. Keep your knees and ankles together, and your legs straight, but don't try to straighten your body out completely; keep your body bent at the hips.

Hold the posture for about 30 seconds at first. If you're comfortable, you can gradually increase the time up to three or four minutes over several weeks. To come down, bend your knees toward your chest; lower your arms and place your palms on the floor; slowly and gently lower your back and legs to the floor. Then lie still with your legs extended, arms by your sides, for a minute or two.

Arthritis

• **Bodywork.** A gentle massage with some warm oil for a few minutes once or twice a day over the affected areas can help relieve pain and reduce inflammation. Rub gently, mostly with your fingertips; don't use pressure directly on swollen or inflamed joints. You can use a little plain warmed up sesame oil or add a few drops of one of these essential oils: chamomile, eucalyptus, rosemary, juniper, lavender, lemon, or cypress.

• **Herbs.** The best Western herb for arthritis is called devil's claw, says David Crow, L.Ac. You will find it as a tincture or look for it as part of herbal arthritis formulas.

Other herbs, best taken as teas, include yarrow, black cohosh, honeysuckle flowers, dandelion, burdock, and nettle.

"Liniments are also good," says Crow. "They are usually based on camphor and menthol, and sometimes have spices such as wintergreen oil or cayenne added. These can be very soothing."

• **Hydrotherapy.** Swimming takes the weight off painful joints, reduces pain, and increases flexibility. Soaking in a warm bath may also relax muscles and stiff joints.

• **Nutrition.** Although there is little science to back this up, many alternative health practitioners have maintained for years that certain foods seem to aggravate arthritic conditions. You might try avoiding food in the nightshade family (tomatoes, white potatoes, eggplant, and sweet peppers). You might also greatly reduce or eliminate dairy products and stop eating red meat.

If your arthritis tends toward inflammation and is very painful, it may be helpful to avoid spicy foods and citrus fruits.

"Also, get yourself a juicer and make vegetable juices every day," says Crow. "Emphasize fresh green vegetables and also carrot juice. You can mix the veggies in with the carrot for a less intense flavor."

• **Relaxation.** Pain tends to worsen with tension. Sit with your eyes closed and take five slow, deep breaths. Keep your eyes closed and allow your breathing to return to normal, but follow it with your attention, observing the inhalation and exhalation. Sit quietly watching the breath for 10 to 20 minutes.

• **Supplements.** Try these only with your doctor's permission. Take 500 milligrams of vitamin C during the course of a day for a week or so (not on an empty stomach) and see if it helps.

Try glucosamine sulfate. Research is suggesting that this precursor building block for joint cartilage may be beneficial for osteoarthritis. Take 500 milligrams three times a day.

Asthma

Since most asthma attacks are related to allergens of one kind or another, "the first step in the natural approach to asthma is to reduce the allergic threshold by avoiding airborne and food allergens," according to Joseph Pizzorno, N.D., author of the *Encyclopedia of Natural Medicine.* Try to avoid dust, pollen, animal danders, mold, cigarette smoke, and other potential asthma triggers. "Removing dogs, cats, carpets, rugs, upholstered furniture, and other surfaces where allergens can collect is a great first step," says Dr. Pizzorno. He also recommends using an effective air purifier.

• **Acupressure.** Bend your head forward and locate the vertebra that sticks out on the back of your neck. With your elbows out in front of you, use your middle fingers (or if it's easier, use your index, middle, and ring fingers together) to press firmly on the points on either side of the protruding vertebra. Press for 30 seconds and repeat several times as needed. "This is the primary acupressure point for wheezing and asthma," says Steve Shimer, L.Ac.

• **Ayurveda.** Licorice tea helps provide relief. "Boil 1 teaspoon of licorice root in a cup of water for a couple of minutes to make a tea," suggests Vasant D. Lad, BAMS, MASs. "Just before drinking the tea, add ½ teaspoon of plain ghee (clarified butter). Take one sip of this tea every five to 10 minutes." You can use this tea regularly as a preventive measure, with one exception: People with high blood pressure can use it only for emergencies; it makes the body retain sodium, thus raising blood pressure.

• **Chinese medicine.** The most effective Chinese herbal formulas for asthma relief contain ephedra (ma huang), ginger, and/or pinellia. Look for them in Chinatown pharmacies or natural food stores. Ephedra is a powerful herb; do not take it without consulting with your physician.

• **Herbs.** Drink ginger tea several times a day to help reduce mucus congestion and relieve difficult breathing. Use ½ teaspoon of ginger powder or a few thin slices of fresh ginger per cup of boiling water.

• **Homeopathy.** Homeopathic medicines may help. Dana Ullman, M.P. H., recommends *Arsenicum* if you feel chilly or fearful during an attack, and the symptoms become aggravated between midnight and 3 a.m. Try *Spongia* if there is dry wheezing and little or no phlegm in the chest.

Homeopathic *Lobelia* is effective when there is wheezing, shortness of breath, and a feeling of constriction in the chest. *Ipecac* is the best choice when there is a great deal of phlegm and the person looks pale.

Take these homeopathic remedies up to once an hour for the first three doses, then repeat when the symptoms appear worse than before, up to every two hours, says Ullman.

• **Hydrotherapy.** Drink six to eight glasses of water a day. It should be room temperature, warm, or hot—never iced.

• **Nutrition.** A number of foods are known to aggravate or bring on asthmatic attacks in some people. These include dairy products such as milk, yogurt, ice cream, and all cheeses. Also avoid red meat and most fermented and salty foods. See if abstaining from wheat or minimizing wheat consumption (in the form of bread and pasta as well as cookies and cakes) helps you feel better.

Some people also need to avoid mushrooms, peanuts, walnuts and other nuts, and yeast.

Back Pain

• **Acupressure.** A point known as the "command point" for all low back problems is located behind your knee, in the crease that forms when you bend the knee, in the center between the two large tendons. Use your thumbs or middle fingers and press for 30 seconds to a minute. Be sure to press both legs.

• **Exercise.** Swimming, which takes pressure off the body, is an excellent exercise for low back pain.

• **Relaxation.** Tense shoulders can stretch all the muscles in your back. To relax them, pull your shoulders up toward your ears as you inhale, hold your breath for a few seconds as you tense your shoulders in that raised position, then exhale as you let your shoulders fall. Repeat at least three or four times, and do this several times a day.

You can also rotate your shoulders forward three times then backward three times. In general, remember the old rule: Lift with your knees, not with your back.

• **Yoga.** As a preventive measure, yoga stretching is an excellent way to increase strength and flexibility. One especially good posture is the Forward Bend, which stretches the lower back, legs, and hips. But be careful: Do not force the movements or stretch beyond your limits of comfort, or you may exacerbate your back pain.

To do this movement:

1. Sit on the floor (on a folded blanket or a fairly thick carpet) with your legs together and stretched in front of you. Keep your knees straight.

2. Extend your arms above your head, exhale, and slowly lean forward from the hips. Try not to curve your back. Depending on how stiff or flexible you are, take hold of your knees, calves, ankles, or big toes.

3. Hold for 15 to 30 seconds.

4. Inhale and slowly come back up to the starting position.

5. Repeat three times, then lie down and rest.

When your back hurts, do not do any yoga without expert guidance.

Bad Breath

- **Brush and floss..** Bad breath is often due to gum disease. Brush and floss your teeth regularly.
- **Exercise.** Be sure to get at least half an hour of exercise every day, either a good walk or something more strenuous if you are fit, to stimulate digestion and clear toxins from the body.
- **Nutrition.** Avoid foods that leave a strong taste in your mouth, such as onions, garlic, aged cheeses, and spicy meats like pepperoni or salami. On the positive side, eat more fruits and vegetables. These high-fiber foods help keep your intestinal tract clean. Fresh is best (rather than frozen or canned).

Include some fresh parsley. This little green leafy vegetable not only cleans your breath, but it also contains large amounts of vitamins and minerals. Drink plenty of plain water. Alcoholic beverages leave an aftertaste, as does coffee. As an alternative, try peppermint tea, which has a fresh taste and smell.

- **Yoga.** Some postures give the abdominal organs a good massage and may improve digestion and elimination. Try the Forward Bend, described under "Back Pain."

Burns

These recommendations are for minor burns. If you have a severe burn, you need medical attention immediately.

If possible, don't cover the burn with a bandage. It heals best in the open air. If you need to cover it, use some light gauze. The old advice to put something greasy on a burn is false; it just seals in the heat.

- **Aromatherapy.** Apply a few drops of pure, undiluted lavender oil directly on a smaller burn or make a lavender compress for larger burns. (See the "Aromatherapy" chapter on page 13 for directions on how to make a compress.)
- **Herbs.** Perhaps the best herbal remedy for burns is aloe vera. If you have an aloe plant, cut open one of the fleshy leaves and put some of the clear gel directly on your burn. Vasant Lad, BAMS, MASc, also suggests an ayurvedic remedy with aloe: Make a paste of sandalwood and turmeric powder (1/4 teaspoon each), mix with about 1 tablespoon of aloe vera gel, and apply it to the burn.
- **Hydrotherapy.** "The most effective way to treat a burn is with cold," says Dr. Lad. He recommends ice or cold water. "If you have no ice cubes, use a bag of frozen vegetables from the freezer," he says.

Colds

- **Aromatherapy.** Essential oils helpful for the common cold include eucalyptus, rosemary, thyme, mint, lavender, basil, and tea tree. Use these oils in a diffuser. Or place a few drops in hot water and make a compress by dipping a cloth or towel in the water; put the hot, wet cloth on your chest over a dry one.

You can also put a few drops of essential oil in a hot bath and soak for 15 or 20 minutes. Steam inhalation also is effective. Put a few drops of the aromatherapy oil in a pot of boiling water and remove it from the stove; place a towel over your head and stand over the pot inhaling the steam.

• **Ayurveda.** If you get repeated colds, David Crow suggests taking the Ayurvedic tonic, chyavanprash, to help build immunity. (Refer to the "Ayurveda" chapter on page 23 for sources.)

• **Herbs**. In both ayurvedic and traditional Chinese medicine, ginger is considered the best home remedy for colds. Vasant D. Lad, BAMS, MASc., recommends drinking a cup of ginger tea several times a day. Boil a few thin slices of fresh ginger or use ⅓ to ½ teaspoon of powdered ginger per cup.

Another useful herb is echinacea, which you can take either as a tea or in tincture form. You can also make an effective cold remedy tea out of common kitchen spices like sage, thyme, and rosemary, says Crow. These become even more beneficial with some added ginger, he says. Licorice root tea is also effective.

• **Homeopathy**. Many homeopathic remedies may be used for colds, depending on the individual's symptoms. Try *Aconite* for violent colds and coughs that come on suddenly, especially if there are chills, suggests Dana Ullman, M.P.H. He recommends *Spongia* for harsh coughs. *Belladonna* is called for if there is high fever and a headache. During the later stages of a cold, use *Kali bichromium*; it's also good for sinus headaches and blocked sinuses with nasal discharge.

When the cold has moved into the chest and has become largely a cough, says Ullman, use *Bryonia*. *Ipecac* is especially valuable in treating an infant's bronchitis. Adults can use it for a deep cough that has much accumulation of mucus in the chest.

• **Relaxation.** One of the most important healing factors when you have a cold is getting sufficient rest. Deep rest enhances the functioning of our immune systems.

"The value of sleep and rest during a cold cannot be overemphasized," says Joseph Pizzorno, N.D.

• **Supplements.** Vitamin C may help speed up recovery from a cold. Dr. Pizzorno recommends taking 500 to 1,000 milligrams every two hours, but take less if this dosage produces gas or diarrhea. (If you opt for this remedy, discuss it with your physician first. This is many times higher than the Daily Value for vitamin C.)

Dr. Pizzorno also recommends zinc lozenges supplying 15 to 25 milligrams of elemental zinc. It's best if the formula contains glycine as the sweetener. "Dissolve one in your mouth every two waking hours after an initial double dose," he says.

Do not continue taking this amount for longer than a few days.

Constipation

• **Ayurveda.** The best ayurvedic treatment for constipation is triphala, a combination of three herbs beneficial for all body types (doshas). One of the benefits of using triphala is that it doesn't develop dependency. (Refer to the "Ayurveda" chapter starting on page 23 for sources for these treatments.)

Before going to bed, steep the herbs in a cup of hot water for five to 10 minutes, then strain and drink. Start with ½ teaspoon and increase up to 1 teaspoon if the smaller dose is not effective.

Fresh aloe vera juice or gel is also effective. Take ½ teaspoon with water first thing in the morning.

If you are pregnant, you should avoid both triphala and aloe. Instead, try the bulking laxatives listed below or this remedy suggested by the ayurvedic physician Vasant D. Lad, BAMS, MASc.: add 1 or 2 teaspoons of ghee (clarified butter) to a cup of hot milk at bedtime. "This is an effective but gentle means of relieving constipation," Dr. Lad says.

Bulking laxatives include psyllium and flax seeds. "These laxatives are best for elderly people and pregnant women," says Crow, "because they don't overstimulate the system, but you have to drink a lot of water with them or they will cause gas and bloating."

- **Exercise.** All exercise is good for constipation. For most people, a brisk 30-minute walk is sufficient. Abdominal exercises from yoga, such as the Forward Bend (see instructions under "Back Pain" on page 327) and Spinal Twist (see "Angina" on page 323) may be quite helpful.
- **Hydrotherapy.** Make sure to drink enough. About 6 to 8 cups of water per day is recommended for most people. Coffee and tea don't count; they are diuretics and actually remove liquid from the body.
- **Nutrition.** Eat plenty of high-fiber food. Include whole grains, such as oatmeal, whole wheat bread, and brown rice, and serve yourself several portions of fresh fruits and vegetables every day. Some extra fiber, in the form of wheat or oat bran, will also help. Include bitter greens in your diet, such as dandelion and arugula.

A high-fiber, largely vegetarian diet is one of the best ways to stay free of constipation. Avoid processed foods and grains, such as white bread, as much as you can. Eating a lot of meat can also clog you up.

Cough

Most of the recommendations made under "Colds" on page 328 apply to coughs as well, so please check that section. If your cough persists longer than a week, it would be wise to see a physician.

- **Aromatherapy.** Good essential oils for cough include eucalyptus, rosemary, cedar, spruce, fir, and pine. Use them as steam, either by placing a few drops in a hot bath or by adding a few drops to a pot of just-boiled water and inhaling the steam. Remove from the stove, put a towel over your head, and lean over the steaming pot.
- **Herbs.** Ginger and licorice root are two of the most important herbs for coughs and can be easily prepared as teas. Or try a tea made from ½ teaspoon ginger powder plus a pinch of clove and a pinch of cinnamon steeped in a cup of boiled water.

Western herbalists say that mullein is also effective, as is horehound, one of the best herbs for lungs.

Horehound acts as an expectorant, thinning the mucus that causes the cough. Take it as a tea or tincture, or in capsules.

Vasant D. Lad, BAMS, MASc., says that for a productive cough (with mucus coming up) "the simplest home remedy is black pepper. Mix ¼ teaspoon with 1 teaspoon of honey, and eat it on a full stomach. The heating quality of black pepper helps to relieve congestion and drives out the cough. Take two or three times a day."

Depression

Clinical depression is a serious medical condition that requires the supervision of a medical doctor.

• **Aromatherapy.** Essential oils are helpful, both diffused in the environment and as part of a massage. For massage, add 10 to 20 drops of oil to an ounce of vegetable oil such as olive, avocado, or sunflower.

The best essential oils for depression include orange, tangerine, grapefruit, lemon, lime, and neroli. Several flowers are also good, including lavender, clary sage, geranium, and bergamot.

You can also use these oils as perfume. Jasmine, neroli, and rose are especially beneficial perfume oils for depression.

• **Chinese medicine.** Chinese herbal formulas for depression are mostly based on bupleurum and dong quai (angelica), says David Crow, L.Ac. "Ginseng can also be very effective for depression associated with fatigue and exhaustion, as can green tea and Siberian ginseng, which are both strengthening," he says.

• **Exercise.** Regular exercise serves as a powerful natural antidepressant, according to Joseph Pizzorno, N.D. Brisk outdoor walking is especially beneficial.

• **Herbs.** The best herbal remedy for depression is St. John's wort (*Hypericum perforatum*). "Research has shown that *Hypericum* can be at least as effective as prescription antidepressants for mild to moderate depression," according to Harold H. Bloomfield, M.D., author of *Hypericum (St. John's Wort) and Depression*. "In addition, it has far fewer side effects, and it costs much less," he says.

The usual dosage recommended is 300 milligrams of the standardized (0.3 percent hypericin content) herb three times a day with meals. "But be sure to give it time to work," says Dr. Bloomfield. "Four to six weeks of regular use are often required before results become significant."

Warning: If you are already taking antidepressant medication, do not use St. John's wort without consulting your physician.

• **Music therapy.** Prescribe some music therapy for yourself. Choose some music you really like and that will elicit some deeper feelings. Don Campbell, music educator and author of *The Mozart Effect*, suggests that music of the Romantic era (Brahms, Schubert, Schumann, Chopin) is good "to enhance sympathy, compassion, and love." Love songs, oldies, Beethoven's *Fifth*, the blues, salsa—it doesn't matter. Choose music that might cheer you up, or make you get up and dance, or make you cry. All have the power to help you heal.

• **Nutrition.** Diet is important. It's a good idea to eat a low-fat diet rich in fruits and vegetables. Avoid caffeine, other stimulants, and alcohol.

• **Supplements.** Michael Murray, N.D., author of the *Encyclopedia of Nutritional Supplements*, recommends a high-potency multiple vitamin and mineral formula, 500 to 1,000 milligrams of vitamin C three times a day, 200 to 400 international units (IU) of vitamin E, a daily tablespoon of flaxseed oil, and 800 micrograms of both folic acid and vitamin B12.

If you decide to take these supplements, discuss them with your physician.

Diarrhea

Diarrhea in infants and the elderly can be quite dangerous. Watch for symptoms of dehydration, such as sunken eyes, dry mouth and lips, light-headedness, or drowsiness. Dehydration is a serious medical problem that needs prompt attention.

- **Herbs.** Roasted carob powder has long been used for diarrhea in Mediterranean cultures. Mix it with warm water (not milk) the way you might make cocoa or coffee.
- **Hydrotherapy.** Drink plenty of water. Avoid milk products, alcohol, and anything with caffeine.
- **Nutrition.** Chinese medicine uses pearl barley for diarrhea. Eat it as a cooked grain (like oatmeal) or add to soups. If you have chronic diarrhea, adding a little barley and roasted carob powder to your diet on a regular basis will help prevent recurrences. Two other foods that may help are applesauce and a little cooked rice with one or two spoonfuls of fresh yogurt.

Earache

- **Acupressure.** Michael Reed Gach, author of *Acupressure's Potent Points*, recommends the following pressure points. In front of your ear, right where it attaches to your face, you will find a depression that deepens when you open your mouth. Holding the three middle fingers of your hand together, place your middle finger in the center of the indentation, your ring finger directly above it (at the top of the depression) and your index finger directly below it. "With your mouth partially open and your eyes closed, press all three points together on both sides of your face for three minutes," says Gach.
- **Ayurveda.** You might want to try this formula recommended by Vasant D. Lad, BAMS, MASc: "Mix together equal amounts of turmeric, goldenseal, and echinacea powders. Stir about ½ teaspoon of this mixture into hot water, steep a few minutes, and drink. Alternatively, simply swallow ½ teaspoon of the powder mixed in 1 teaspoon of honey."

  Dr. Lad recommends taking this three times a day, after meals, for one week. "This powerful antiseptic, antibiotic formula will help control the ear infection," he says.
- **Supplements.** These include vitamin C and the herbs echinacea and goldenseal, which aid the immune system in combating infection. You can take the herbs in capsule form.

Eyestrain

- **Acupressure.** A number of helpful points are located close to the eyes. Rub your thumbs and fingers all around your eye sockets or use a series of short presses. Be careful when pressing close to the eye.

  Warning: These points cannot be safely pressed with long fingernails.
- **Vision therapy.** Rub your hands together vigorously for about half a minute, then cup your palms and place them lightly over the eyes. (Don't press on the eyeballs.) Note the warm, healing energy flowing from your palms and soothing your eyes. Continue for one to three minutes. You can do this anytime, such as taking as a break from your work or when you stop during a long drive.

• **Yoga.** The inverted poses, including the Shoulder Stand (see "Anxiety" on page 324) and the Forward Bend (see "Back Pain" on page 327) help to increase circulation in the upper body and are said to soothe and nourish the eyes.

Fatigue and Chronic Fatigue

• **Aromatherapy.** Try an aromatherapy massage. Although you might think of massage as purely relaxing, it is extremely beneficial for fatigue, says David Crow, L.Ac. You can purchase an aromatherapy massage oil ready-made or make one yourself by adding 10 to 20 drops of essential oil to each ounce of a carrier oil such as almond, olive, avocado, sesame, or sunflower. Essential oils that have a stimulating, energizing effect include rosemary, eucalyptus, basil, peppermint, grapefruit, and lemon.

If you don't have someone to give you a massage, rub all the places you can reach yourself—head, arms, chest, abdomen, thighs, legs, feet, even your shoulders and part of your back.

• **Ayurveda.** Take chyavanprash, an ayurvedic rejuvenative tonic. Various brands are available at natural food stores or from suppliers of ayurvedic herbs.

• **Exercise.** Exercise increases vitality by pumping oxygen-rich blood to the cells. Excessive exercise, however, can be a cause of fatigue, so find the amount that energizes you and do it regularly. A brisk daily walk and some yoga stretching or tai chi is all most people need.

• **Herbs.** Green tea can help combat fatigue, as it has a strengthening effect. Try replacing coffee with green tea.

The herb gotu kola is also helpful for both physical and mental fatigue; try it in capsules or as a tea, using ½ teaspoon of the herb per cupful of hot water.

• **Music therapy.** A little music therapy can also get your energy going. Choose some lively music that you like, whether it's classical or rock, reggae or country-western. Instead of listening passively, as you would to relax, listen with lively attention, tap your feet, even get up and move around the room or dance.

• **Relaxation.** The main principle for building energy is to get more rest. In addition to sleeping more at night, brief naps can take the edge off fatigue and recharge your batteries.

Fever

• **Hydrotherapy.** Drink more to replenish the liquid lost by perspiring. Choose room temperature water or juices, or drink warm herb teas. Place cool compresses on the forehead. Each time the compress warms up to body temperature, dip it in cool water again. You can increase the cooling effect by also putting a compress over the navel area.

• **Herbs.** Make this herb tea from spices in your kitchen. Mix 2 parts coriander, 2 parts cinnamon, and 1 part ginger. Then steep 1 teaspoon of the mixture in a cup of hot water for 10 minutes before drinking. "Drink this every few hours until the fever breaks," says Vasant D. Lad, BAMS, MASc.

Try goldenseal. This herb, which is widely used as an herbal antibiotic, can help reduce fevers.

• **Homeopathy.** Dana Ullman, M.P.H., recommends *Belladonna* and *Aconite* during the first stages of a fever. Try *Belladonna* if the skin is hot and flushed, *Aconite* if you feel anxious, restless, or fearful.

Fasting for a day or two will help eliminate the accumulated toxins that are most likely causing the fever. But be sure to have enough to drink.

Headaches

Headaches may be caused by indigestion, constipation, poor posture, fatigue, eyestrain, or stress, so you might want to consult those sections also.

• **Acupressure.** Find the hollow areas on either side of the base of your skull. These points will be 2 to 3 inches apart and about an inch above your hairline. While pressing with your thumbs, lean your head slowly back, keeping your eyes closed. Press firmly for one to two minutes. Breathe deeply.

• **Aromatherapy.** Do a massage using essential oils of chamomile, lavender, elder flowers, or mint. You can make your own massage oil by adding 10 to 20 drops of one of these essential oils to an ounce of plain oil such as almond, sesame, sunflower, or olive. Using these in the form of herbs as a tea or in a hot bath or a diffuser will also help relieve your headache.

• **Bodywork.** Straighten up! Poor posture may put strain on your muscles and reduce oxygen flow to your brain.

• **Exercise.** Take a walk in the fresh air. Get some exercise every day. Aerobic exercise (even a brisk walk) increases the flow of oxygen to the brain.

• **Herbs.** The herb with the most science behind it for preventing migraines is feverfew. Take it in capsules or as a tincture.

• **Homeopathy.** The most common homeopathic remedy for headaches is *Belladonna*. Use it for intense, throbbing pain accompanied by sensitivity to light, noise, and touch, and when the headache is associated with a fever, says Dana Ullman, M.P.H. If your headache becomes worse when you move your head and seems to be centered over your left eye, try *Bryonia*, he says. For headaches brought on by prolonged mental work or by overeating, alcohol, or staying up too late, take *Nux vomica*.

• **Hydrotherapy.** Drink six to eight glasses of water every day.

• **Nutrition.** Eat a high-fiber diet. Many headaches are related to constipation. To prevent this problem, eat plenty of fruits, vegetables, and whole grains. Avoid clogging foods like red meat and refined (white) sugar and flour.

Other foods that commonly trigger headaches are red wine, chocolate, coffee, cheese, and bacon.

• **Relaxation.** Most headaches are caused by tense muscles in the face, skull, neck, shoulders, and upper back. Therefore, "learning how to relax and defuse tension goes a long way in the treatment and prevention of headaches," according to Joseph Pizzorno, N.D.

For daily prevention, or if a headache starts, use your favorite way to relax, such as a hot bath, a massage, listening to soothing music, yoga postures, meditation, or progressive relaxation.

One of the easiest relaxation techniques is simply to sit comfortably, close your eyes, and pay attention to your breathing for a few minutes.

• **Vision therapy.** Rest your tired eyes. Close your eyes for a minute, or, better still, rub your palms together vigorously for about 30 seconds, until they become warm; then close your eyes and place your palms lightly over the eyes. Don't press on the eyeballs. Hold your palms there for at least a full minute.

Heart Disease

• **Bodywork.** Straighten up! Poor posture may put strain on your muscles and reduce oxygen flow to your brain.

• **Exercise.** Get some exercise every day, but don't strain. It's true that regular daily exercise is essential for maintaining a healthy heart. But research suggests that vigorous aerobic exercise is not necessary; a 30-minute daily walk is sufficient.

"Moderate exercise is enough to provide you with almost all of the health and longevity benefits, without most of the risks of more intense exercise," according to Dean Ornish, M.D., author of *Dr. Dean Ornish's Program for Reversing Heart Disease.*

• **Nutrition.** Eat a low-fat diet. Cut down or eliminate red meat, whole milk, and full-fat dairy products. Eat more fresh fruit, vegetables, and whole grains.

• **Quit smoking.** Smoking puts an enormous amount of stress on the cardiovascular system, weakens the heart and lungs, raises cholesterol, and almost certainly shortens life span.

"If you are a smoker, quitting is the best thing you can do for your heart and your health," says cardiologist John Zamarra, M.D., assistant clinical professor of medicine at the University of California at Irvine.

Bookstores and libraries have books and tapes with programs designed to help you quit.

• **Relaxation.** "Stress has been identified as one of the major causes of heart disease," says Dr. Zamarra. To bust stress, spend 15 to 20 minutes twice a day practicing a relaxation technique.

Herpes

Treatment with antiviral medications effectively relieves symptoms and can prevent or at least lengthen the time between recurrences.

• **Herbs.** Steve Shimer, L.Ac., recommends an herbal tincture made from St. John's wort. Place a few drops directly on the affected area to help heal herpes lesions.

Applying some aloe vera gel directly on the affected area will help. If you have an aloe plant, slice open one of the long leaves and scoop out some fresh gel with a spoon; otherwise, purchase a gel.

• **Nutrition.** Favor peas, beans, lentils, fish, turkey, and chicken in your diet. These are good sources of lysine, as are most vegetables. Lysine is an amino acid that helps break the reproductive process of the herpes virus. Avoid chocolate and most nuts, especially peanuts and almonds. These foods contain arginine, an amino acid that facilitates the reproductive cycle of the herpes virus.

• **Relaxation.** Minimizing stress is important, as excess stress weakens the immune system and increases susceptibility to renewed herpes outbreaks. Try to get more rest and use relaxation techniques such as meditation, progressive relaxation, visualization, deep breathing, or listening to soothing music.

• **Supplements.** Michael Murray, N.D., recommends boosting your daily vitamin C intake to 2,000 milligrams during an outbreak. You might also take: bioflavonoid supplements of 1,000 milligrams per day; 30 to 50 milligrams of zinc; and 1,000 milligrams of lysine three times per day.

If you'd like to try these supplements, discuss them with your physician. The amounts of these nutrients are well above the Daily Values. Such high doses of zinc should not be taken on a regular basis.

High Blood Pressure (Hypertension)

If you have high blood pressure, you should be under the care of a physician. High blood pressure can do serious damage to the body if it's not kept under control.

"Most cases of high blood pressure can be brought under control through changes in diet and lifestyle," says Joseph Pizzorno, N.D. More than 80 percent of people with high blood pressure are in the borderline to moderate range, he says, and for these individuals "many nondrug therapies—such as diet, exercise, and relaxation—have proven superior to drugs."

• **Acupressure.** Steve Shimer, L.Ac, recommends pressing on a point known as the "source point" of the liver meridian. "It's on the top of your foot," he says, "between the big toe and second toe. Starting at the webbing between the two toes, slide your index finger slowly between the bones (up toward your ankle) until you feel a depression about ½ inch up. Still using your index finger, press between the bones (in the direction of the second toe). Start with light pressure, as this point can be sensitive, and increase until you are using moderate to firm pressure. Press for about one minute."

• **Aromatherapy.** Gentle massage with essential oils is beneficial, says David Crow, L.Ac. "A number of common oils, such as lavender, chamomile, bergamot, clary sage, and sandalwood are good," he says.

• **Exercise.** Get your body moving for half an hour, three to four times a week. A vigorous daily walk, yoga, tai chi, qigong, and other exercises that increase flexibility and improve circulation are all beneficial for cardiovascular health.

Be sure to consult with your physician before beginning any exercise program.

• **Herbs.** The best herb to treat high blood pressure is hawthorn berry, says Crow. You can use capsules or tincture, or make a tea using 1 teaspoon of the herb per cup of hot water. Crow also suggests taking relaxing herbs such as skullcap and valerian.

Warning: If you are currently taking antihypertensive medications, let your doctor know about any herbs you're taking. Cut down on prescribed medications only under the guidance of a qualified practitioner.

• **Music therapy.** For relaxation, music educator and author Don Campbell recommends Gregorian chant, slow movements of Baroque music (Bach, Handel, Vivaldi, Corelli), or New Age pieces—or anything you like that helps you feel settled and peaceful.

Sit or lie down with your eyes closed, take a few deep breaths, and let the music just wash over you.

- **Nutrition.** "Cut down on saturated fat," says John Zamarra, M.D., of the University of California at Irvine. "Foods high in animal fat and cholesterol clog the arteries, leading to atherosclerosis (hard fatty deposits on artery walls). The more clogged the arteries, the higher your blood pressure becomes, and the harder your heart has to work to pump the blood."

To cut down on saturated fat, avoid meat, especially beef and pork, dairy products (except for nonfat milk), heavy desserts, and all fried foods.

"A vegetarian diet is by far the healthiest for your heart and your blood pressure," says Dr. Zamarra. "If you choose to eat meat, limit yourself to fish and poultry."

Use natural diuretics. Watermelon, cucumber, and celery have a mild diuretic effect similar to medications prescribed for high blood pressure. If you have a juicer, make a fresh juice of cucumber and celery, with carrot added for flavor. Parsley is particularly helpful.

Eat less salt. Sodium increases the amount of fluid in your circulatory system and raises your blood pressure.

- **Relaxation.** "Stress can cause high blood pressure in many instances," says Dr. Pizzorno. "Using a stress-reduction technique is a necessary component in a natural blood-pressure-lowering program."
- **Yoga.** Vasant D. Lad, BAMS, MASc., suggests the yogic rest pose known as Corpse Pose. "Lie quietly, flat on your back with arms by your sides," he says. For deeper relaxation, "observe the flow of your breath. You will notice that after each exhalation there is a brief, natural stop and another natural pause after inhalation and before the next exhalation. In that stop, stay naturally quiet for just a few seconds. This practice will bring you deep relaxation, a natural antidote for hypertension."

High Cholesterol

- **Nutrition.** "The most important approach to lowering a high cholesterol level is a healthful diet and lifestyle," says Joseph Pizzorno, N.D. "Eat less fat and cholesterol by reducing or eliminating the amount of animal products in the diet." This includes red meat, eggs, and high-fat dairy products such as butter, ice cream, and whole milk. At the same time, eat more foods that contain fiber—fruits, grains, vegetables, and legumes. Also, reduce or eliminate coffee from your diet.

Specific foods that may be helpful in reducing cholesterol include pectin-rich choices such as apples, grapefruit, carrots, lettuce, spinach, cabbage, oranges, bananas, and grapes.

- **Supplements.** Michael Murray, N.D., recommends: a high-potency multiple vitamin and mineral formula; vitamin C (500 to 1,000 milligrams three times a day); vitamin E (400 to 800 IU per day); garlic (at least one fresh clove or 4,000 milligrams of allicin per day); and niacin (500 milligrams three times per day with meals).

Discuss these supplements with your physician before you decide to take them.

Incontinence

- **Chinese medicine.** According to Chinese medicine, "weakened kidney energy" is almost always involved in incontinence. The following exercise, recommended by Steve Shimer, L.Ac., is one of the best to cultivate that kind of energy. (For an explanation of the kind of philosophy behind this diagnosis, refer to the "Chinese Medicine" chapter starting on page 69.)

You may find this posture quite strenuous at first. If so, don't try to hold it for more than 20 to 30 seconds. Over time you can gradually build up to five minutes. Stand with your feet about shoulder width apart, feet pointing straight ahead (not angled outward, as they will tend to do). Hold your arms in front of you, elbows slightly lower than the hands. Your hands should be about 8 to 12 inches apart and roughly parallel (palms facing each other), but with the index fingers slightly closer to each other than the little fingers. Let your thumb and fingers relax.

Keeping your back straight, bend the knees. The more you bend your knees, the more difficult the exercise becomes, so start with just a slight bend. Over time, as you build strength, you can increase the amount of bend. If you can eventually sink 6 to 8 inches into the bend, that's enough. Don't strain. Holding your muscles tight will constrict the flow of energy.

When you start to get tired, relax into a more comfortable position for a few moments before resuming. See if you can feel the qi (energy) flowing, especially between your hands. It may feel like a soft breeze or a tingling in your hands.

• **Exercise.** Learn to do Kegel exercises. Many women have learned these exercises, which can be helpful in childbirth and are frequently recommended to improve sexual pleasure and the ability to experience orgasm. The first step is to tighten the sphincter (the ring of muscles) around the anus. These are the muscles you would use to hold back a bowel movement. Tighten them without tensing the muscles of your legs, belly, or buttocks.

Next, when you're urinating, practice stopping the flow about five times each time you go. This uses a different set of muscles, those in the front of the pelvis. Then combine these two sets of muscles. Work from back to front—tighten the anal sphincter muscles, then tighten the front muscles. Do this slowly, to a count of 4 or 5, and hold for a second or two before gradually releasing. Repeat five times. This is one "set." Do at least three sets every day, gradually increasing the number of repetitions in each set until you're doing a total of about 100 repetitions a day.

If you have an incontinence problem now, you may find it difficult to do even one set of five, because the muscles may be very weak. But with practice, they will gain strength.

Ask your physician for more specific instructions if you feel the need.

• **Nutrition.** Cut down or eliminate consumption of alcoholic beverages, caffeinated drinks (tea, coffee, soda), and grapefruit juice. These are all diuretics, which increase urine production and may increase the urgency of your need to go.

Drink a glass of cranberry juice every day. It is well known for its beneficial effects on the bladder and urinary system.

• **Quit smoking.** Nicotine adversely affects the bladder and urethra.

• Yoga. The posture known as the Forward Bend is said to help with bladder and incontinence problems. Instructions for this posture are in the section on "Back Pain" on page 327.

Indigestion

• Herbs. For excessive flatulence, California herbalist David Crow, L.Ac., suggests using common household spices such as cardamom, fennel seed, and ginger. Chewing a few fennel seeds after meals will help. Even better, grate or slice a little fresh ginger, mix with cardamom and fennel seeds, and chew after meals. Teas that will help alleviate excess gas include chamomile, peppermint, and sage.

• Homeopathy. If you have severe indigestion, with nausea, vomiting, diarrhea, or abdominal pain, try the homeopathic remedy *Arsenicum*, says Dana Ullman, M.P.H. For gas and heartburn, try *Nux vomica*; take *Ipecacuanha* for nausea and *Pulsatilla* for bloating.

• Nutrition. A commonsense rule to prevent indigestion is to avoid problematic foods. You may have food allergies or lactose intolerance. Or certain foods may not be good for your body type. For many people, eating spicy foods, pickles, hot peppers, and citrus fruits are a virtual guarantee of heartburn or stomach upset.

Other foods to avoid or minimize if you have chronic indigestion include anything with caffeine, alcohol, mints, milk, fatty meats, and all greasy, fried foods.

Eat less at a time. Consuming large meals is one of the main causes of indigestion. Also, an overly full belly tends to force acids back up into the esophagus, creating acid reflux or heartburn.

Ayurvedic tradition says a meal should consist of the amount of food you can hold in two cupped hands. Slow down. Eating too quickly is a main cause of upset stomachs. Take time to sit quietly and enjoy your food.

Insomnia

• Aromatherapy. Do a massage using essential oils of chamomile, lavender, clary sage, ylang ylang, rose, marjoram, orange, sandalwood, vetiver, or bergamot. To make your own massage oil, add 10 to 20 drops of essential oil to each ounce of a carrier oil such as sesame, olive, avocado, or sunflower. You might experiment by mixing two or three, using six to eight drops of each scent.

To treat yourself to a self-massage with these oils, gently rub your scalp and face (be careful not to get the oil in your eyes), then rub each arm, moving up from the fingers toward the heart. You can knead the muscles if you like or just rub over the surface. Spend some time on your shoulder and neck, where much tension tends to gather. Then give each foot a thorough treatment, working on each toe; proceed up the legs and thighs.

Massage your abdomen and chest (use a gentler pressure here) and reach behind to massage your lower back, above the kidneys.

Follow your massage with a relaxing bath. You can use a few drops of one of the same oils added to the tub water or choose another of these relaxing scents. Try sprinkling a few drops of lavender oil, or a mixture of lavender and marjoram, on your pillow.

• **Ayurveda.** "One of the simplest and most effective ways to induce sleep is to rub some oil on the scalp and the soles of the feet before going to bed," says Vasant D. Lad, BAMS, MASc. Use sesame oil, slightly warmed up, and massage gently. Remember to put on a pair of old socks after you finish or the oil will stain the bedsheets.

• **Herbs.** David Crow, L.Ac., recommends several herbs to help with difficulty sleeping. These include chamomile and lemon balm (milder herbs); vervaine and skullcap (medium strength); and California poppy, hops, passionflower, and valerian (strong). All or most of these are available in capsules, tinctures, or in various insomnia formulas at natural food stores or your local pharmacy.

Kava kava, a widely used herb for anxiety, is also effective for insomnia. Kava kava can be used during the day for general relaxation or just before bed. For insomnia, the standard dosage is 200 milligrams of kavalactones (the active ingredient) an hour before bed. (The information on how to get this amount will be on the label.)

A cup of chamomile tea before going to bed may be all you need to induce sleepiness. Or you may prefer a stronger herb such as valerian root.

Take capsules or up to 1 gram of the powdered herb 30 to 45 minutes before bedtime. (Some people find the odor of valerian root disagreeable, but the herb is effective.)

• **Homeopathy.** "We all know that coffee is a stimulant, but in homeopathic doses it can relax an overactive mind," says Dana Ullman, M.P.H. When sleep won't come because of a racing mind, try *Coffea*, a homeopathic remedy made from coffee.

Nux vomica can help if your insomnia is due to mental strain, or to abuse of coffee, alcohol, or other drugs. Ullman also recommends it if you tend to fall asleep at night, but wake up early and can't get back to sleep.

If you are sleepless because of anxiety and fear or you're overtired due to excessive exertion, try *Arsenicum*.

If you can't sleep because you're in pain, or if you've become dependent on sedatives, *Chamomilla* may be what you need, says Ullman.

• **Nutrition.** Eat lighter at night, and favor carbohydrates (pasta, hot cereal, potatoes) rather than protein (meat, fish, chicken). Reduce or eliminate your use of stimulants such as caffeine, whether in coffee, tea, soda, or chocolate.

• **Relaxation.** Take time every day for meditation, quiet listening to music, or another activity that helps you relax. Take a daily walk in nature, even in a local park. In bed, if you have trouble sleeping, try the Progressive Relaxation procedure described on page 213.

• **Supplements.** A magnesium supplement may help. If you have your physician's permission to do so, try taking 250 to 500 milligrams per day.

• **Yoga.** A helpful posture that you can do to help you fall asleep is the yogic rest pose, Savasana. Lie flat on your back, legs slightly apart, arms about 6 inches from your sides. This is very relaxing, even more so if you pay attention to your breathing.

Memory and Mental Clarity

• **Aromatherapy.** Essential oils that act as stimulants for the brain include rosemary, eucalyptus, grapefruit, and lemon. "They have a beneficial effect when diffused into the air and also when used to create an aromatherapy bath," says David Crow, L.Ac. Put about 5 drops in a tubful of hot water.

Vasant D. Lad, BAMS, MASc, recommends several foods helpful for improving memory. These include sweet potatoes, tapioca, okra, and spinach. Foods considered sattvic (pure) are traditionally said to be good for memory, including fresh fruits and vegetables, almonds, oranges, ghee (clarified butter), and milk.

"One food that is particularly bad for memory is heavy meat," says Dr. Lad. "This should be strictly avoided by anyone with memory problems."

• **Ayurveda.** An herbal tonic that is good for memory and the mind is chyavanprash, an ayurvedic formula available in natural food stores, Indian markets, and by mail order from suppliers of ayurvedic herbs. (Refer to the chapter on "Ayurveda," which starts on page 23 for more sources.)

You can also take triphala (an ayurvedic combination of three beneficial herbs) at night before bed. Steep ½ teaspoonful of triphala in a cup of hot water; let it cool 10 minutes, and drink.

• **Herbs.** According to Crow, the following herbs can be used as memory tonics: ginkgo, sage, ginseng (American, Chinese, or Korean), gotu kola, oatstraw, Siberian ginseng, rosemary, skullcap, St. John's wort, and vervaine. You can use any of these herbs alone, or purchase a formula that combines some of them.

• **Yoga.** The inverted poses (Shoulder Stand, Headstand) help increase circulation and bring more blood to the brain. If you don't know how to do these, instructions for a simple inverted posture are under "Anxiety" on page 324.

Menopause

• **Acupressure.** Steve Shimer, L.Ac., recommends a "master point" for healing and regulating the female organs. The point is a few inches above your ankle bone, on the inside of your leg. From the center of the ankle bone, measure up one palm width. The point is just off the shin bone, toward the back of your leg. When you find it (it is likely to be tender), press with your thumb or a knuckle. Increase pressure until you are pressing quite firmly, hold about a minute, and gradually release. Do both legs.

• **Aromatherapy.** Essential oils for female hormone regulation include lavender, clary sage, rose, geranium, bergamot, and ylang ylang, says David Crow, L.Ac. Use these as a massage oil (add 10 to 20 drops of the essential oil to each ounce of a carrier oil such as olive, sunflower, or avocado) and for a steam or herbal bath (add a few drops to a tub of hot water).

• **Ayurveda.** "Ayurveda has long recognized the value of female rejuvenative herbs at this stage of life," Vasant D. Lad, BAMS, MASc. These herbs "provide your body with natural food precursors of estrogen and progesterone."

He recommends making a mixture of equal parts of the ayurvedic herbs shatavari and vidari (you can substitute wild yam for vidari) and taking a spoonful of this mixture twice a day, after lunch and dinner, during the entire menopausal stage. Take it with a few sips of warm water or ½ cup of aloe vera juice.

• **Chinese medicine.** Chinese herbal formulas for menopause are typically made with dong quai (angelica), peony, and bupleurum, says Crow. Black cohosh is also used, as are blood-building tonics made with rhemania and shou wu (fo ti). These formulas are designed to relax the nervous system, balance hormones, and strengthen the uterus and the blood.

"The classic Chinese herbal formula for menopausal symptoms is called Zhi Bai di Huang Wan," says Shimer. "Any practicing acupuncturist should have it or be able to obtain it."

• **Herbs.** Crow recommends the herbs vitex (chasteberry), black cohosh, and alfalfa, all of which you may take as capsules, teas, or tinctures. St. John's wort is also helpful. You will also find combinations of these herbs in commercial formulas, available in your local natural food store.

• **Nutrition.** "Hot flashes and other menopausal symptoms rarely occur in cultures in which people consume a predominantly plant-based diet," says Joseph Pizzorno, N.D. Eat more fish and less red meat, very little dairy, and liberal amounts of fresh produce, whole grains, legumes, and soy products.

Research has demonstrated the benefits of soy products such as tofu, miso, and tempeh. Try substituting soy milk for cow's milk.

• **Relaxation.** To help maintain emotional equilibrium, spend some time every day in quiet meditation. If you've learned a technique that you like, practice it. If you haven't, try this: Sit comfortably, close your eyes, and mentally observe your breathing. Notice the cool air coming in through the nostrils and how your chest or belly expands. Notice during exhalation the warmer air against your nostrils and your chest and belly settling. For 10 to 15 minutes, just sit and maintain your awareness like this, bringing your attention quietly back to your breathing whenever you drift off. Twice a day is best.

• **Supplements.** Recommended supplements include a daily dose of 400 to 800 IU of vitamin E and 1,200 milligrams of vitamin C. Check with your doctor first.

• **Yoga.** For overall toning and to promote hormonal balance, yoga postures are outstanding.

Menstrual Difficulties
(See also, "Premenstrual Syndrome")

• **Aromatherapy.** Good oils include lavender, clary sage, rose, geranium, bergamot, and ylang ylang. Use these as a massage oil (buy them ready-made or add 10 to 20 drops of essential oil to each ounce of a carrier oil such as olive, sunflower, or avocado) and for a steam or herbal bath (add a few drops to a tub of hot water). Apply warm compresses. Dip a towel in warm water, wring it out, put on a few drops of one of these essential oils, and place it over your abdomen.

• **Bodywork.** Massage is helpful, especially localized massage of the abdomen (but just rub gently there, over the surface).

• **Exercise.** Some women say they feel better when they exercise during their periods. According to practitioners of ayurveda and ancient Chinese medicine, yoga postures, tai chi, and other forms of exercise are highly recommended all month—except during your period, when the basic prescription is to "rest, read, and relax" as much as you can. See which approach works best for you.

• **Herbs.** Ginger compresses generate a soothing, healing warmth. Pulverize some fresh gingerroot, spread it on the abdominal area, and cover with a piece of plastic and a hot towel. Drink ginger tea, using about ½ teaspoon of ginger powder or a few thin slices of fresh ginger per cup. Or try yarrow, mugwort, or chamomile as teas.

Other helpful herbs include dong quai, black cohosh, peony, and bupleurum. Many commercial formulas are available containing a combination of these herbs. Cramp bark (also called black haw) is particularly helpful for uterine pain.

• **Relaxation.** Exhaustion, unresolved emotions, overwork, and any form of excessive stress, anytime during the month, tend to affect your period. Take some time every day for meditation, a quiet walk, listening to music, dancing, or whatever you have found that works for you.

Nausea and Vomiting

• **Acupressure.** "Nausea is treated very effectively with acupressure," says Steve Shimer, L.Ac. "Recent research has confirmed this, both for morning sickness in pregnancy and chemotherapy-induced nausea. It can also be used for motion sickness."

The main point to use is on the palm side of your wrist, two thumb widths above the wrist crease and in the center of the arm. "This is the king of points to treat nausea," says Shimer. Use the thumb of the opposite hand to apply moderate to firm pressure for about one minute. Breathe deeply while pressing.

Acupressure bracelets (elastic wristbands with small plastic balls applied to acupuncture points on the wrist) are available in many drugstores and have been found helpful in combating morning sickness.

• **Herbs.** The best antinausea medicine is ginger. You can swallow powdered ginger as capsules or make a tea by simmering thin slices of fresh gingerroot or adding ½ teaspoon of powder to a cup of boiling water. Sip the tea as needed to settle your nausea. If you are traveling and have a problem with motion sickness, take some ginger capsules with you.

You can also chew a few raw or roasted fennel seeds, or one or two cardamom pods to dispel feelings of nausea.

• **Homeopathy.** Robin Hayfield, author of *Homeopathy: Simple Remedies for Natural Health*, suggests using *Arsenicum* for violent vomiting accompanied by pain in the stomach (also good for diarrhea). She recommends *Ipecac* for nausea that doesn't go away even with vomiting.

• **Nutrition.** Try fasting. Vomiting is your system's way of clearing out toxins, whether from illness or some food you've eaten. Fasting for 24 hours, longer if you are comfortable, gives your digestive system a chance to rest and heal. For an easy fast, drink just a little room temperature water or some juice, such as cranberry or sweet pineapple.

Neck and Shoulder Tension and Pain

• **Acupressure.** Steve Shimer, L.Ac., recommends trying one particular point: Hold out your left hand with the palm down and fingers out straight. Squeeze your thumb against the other fingers; the point to press is in the middle of the mound that pops up between the thumb and index finger. Squeeze in the center of the webbing, but toward the bone of the index finger. Hold one minute, breathing deeply, then repeat with the other hand.

Warning: Pregnant women should not press on this point, as it may stimulate contractions in the uterus.

• **Aromatherapy.** Massage your neck and shoulders with a few drops of warm oil. Plain sesame oil has a warming effect, or you can add a few drops of chamomile, cedarwood, lavender, or ylang ylang.

Rub your neck with your fingertips, then reach back over your right shoulder with your right hand and, starting close to the neck, squeeze, hold, and release the trapezius muscles (the large muscles at the top of your shoulders). Massage for a couple of minutes, moving outward, away from the spine. Repeat on the left side.

• **Bodywork.** Watch your posture. If your head is leaning forward so your ears are in front of your shoulders, tension builds up in the neck muscles.

Try to keep your head back and level, but with your chin tucked in. When you're working at a computer terminal, the screen should be at eye level. Try to keep your head up while you are reading or working at your desk. And don't tuck the telephone receiver between your neck and shoulder.

Sleep comfortably. Using a soft mattress or a pillow that is too thick or sleeping on your stomach, can all cause or aggravate stiff and sore necks and shoulders. Try sleeping on your back or curling up on your side.

• **Exercise.** Try neck exercises. Pull your shoulders up toward your ears, hold, then drop them down. Next, roll your shoulders forward, up, and back, forward, up, and back. Reverse, moving from back to front.

• **Herbs.** Chamomile and comfrey tea relax tense muscles.

Osteoporosis

• **Exercise.** The best thing people can do to strengthen their bones is physical activity, says Michael Murray, N.D. Regular weight-bearing exercise—walking, jogging, or any exercise (other than swimming) that puts weight on your bones—helps maintain bone density. But if you already have osteoporosis, be careful: a fall, or even a slight injury, may crack fragile bones.

• **Nutrition.** Coffee, alcohol, and smoking cause a negative calcium balance—more calcium being lost than taken in—and are associated with an increased risk of developing osteoporosis, says Dr. Murray.

According to a study published in the *American Journal of Epidemiology*, just 2 to 3 cups of coffee a day, whether regular or decaffeinated, increase the risk of osteoporosis-related fractures by nearly 70 percent. A vegetarian diet is associated with a lower risk of osteoporosis. On the other hand, researchers are finding that the high-protein diet typical of Americans increases the risk.

• **Supplements.** Experts recommend anywhere from 800 to 1,500 milligrams of calcium daily, preferably as calcium citrate, calcium lactate, or calcium gluconate. Talk to your doctor about the best dosage for meeting your needs.

• **Yoga.** Yoga postures are beneficial, but should be done with care by a person with osteoporosis.

Premenstrual Syndrome (PMS) (See also "Menstrual Difficulties")

If your PMS symptoms include headaches, depression, or anxiety, please refer to those sections for extra help.

• **Acupressure.** Steve Shimer, L.Ac., recommends a point on top of the foot. Between the big toe and second toe about ½ inch up from the webbing, you will feel a depression. Using your index finger, press between the bones in the direction of the root of the second toe. Start with light pressure, as this point can be sensitive, and increase as much as you can until you are using moderate to firm pressure.

Press for about 1 minute. Press both feet simultaneously if you can. If you have trouble bending down or reaching your feet, try rubbing the area on your left foot with your right heel and vice versa.

• **Aromatherapy.** Essential oils you might use for a massage include rose, geranium, clary sage, bergamot, chamomile, grapefruit, jasmine, neroli, orange, sandalwood, and ylang ylang. Use a few drops in a carrier oil, such as sesame or olive. You might also prepare yourself an aromatherapy bath by putting a few drops of one or more of these oils in a tub of warm water.

• **Exercise.** Be sure to get regular aerobic exercise (walking, jogging, swimming, whatever you enjoy) during the entire month, up until your period.

• **Herbs.** The most helpful herbs for PMS are vitex, black cohosh, chamomile, lemon balm, vervaine, skullcap, passionflower, and valerian, says David Crow. L.Ac. You can obtain them in capsules, tinctures, or in various formulas at natural food stores or your local pharmacy. Another beneficial herb is kava kava, he says. Chinese herbal formulas typically include dong quai, peony, and bupleurum.

• **Homeopathy.** Homeopathic remedies recommended by homeopathic author Robin Hayfield include *Pulsatilla*, a remedy for when you feel emotional and "weeping and the feeling of neediness is prominent;" *Sepia* "where there is anger and exhaustion;" and *Lachesis* "for the more extreme symptoms of violent anger, jealousy, and suspicion."

• **Nutrition.** Your diet is important. Try to base your diet around whole grains and cooked vegetables, fruits, legumes, nuts, and seeds. If you can follow a mostly vegetarian diet, that might prove helpful.

"Reduce your intake of fat," suggests Joseph Pizzorno, N.D. "Eliminate sugar and caffeine, keep salt intake low, consume small to moderate quantities of meat and dairy products, and increase your intake of soy foods."

Watch out for chocolate cravings (high in fat and sugar) and cut down on spicy foods and alcohol.

• **Relaxation.** Stress may be unavoidable in life, but you need a program to help you deal with it. Learn progressive relaxation, meditation, yoga, tai chi, or qi gong. Make the time to practice daily, even if you think you're too busy. Even 10 to 15 minutes a day of deep relaxation will make an enormous difference.

• **Supplements.** "Nutritional deficiency is relatively common among women with PMS," says Dr. Pizzorno. He recommends taking a high-quality multiple vitamin and mineral supplement that provides adequate levels of vitamin B6 and magnesium. He also suggests taking vitamin E (400 IU), zinc (15 to 20 milligrams), and a tablespoon of flaxseed oil every day.

Discuss these supplements with your doctor to determine whether they are appropriate for you.

Prostate Problems

More than 50 percent of American men will develop prostate problems, including enlarged prostate (benign prostatic hyperplasia or BPH) and prostate cancer.

• **Exercise.** As for virtually any health condition, exercise is helpful. Research verifies that men who are physically fit have less prostate trouble than those who are not. "I recommend that everyone get 30 minutes of aerobic exercise (such as walking, swimming, or bicycling) at least five days a week," says Andrew Weil, M.D., author of the best-selling *8 Weeks to Optimum Health* and director of the Program in Integrative Medicine of the College of Medicine at the University of Arizona in Tucson.

Sitting exerts pressure on the prostate. If you sit a lot—and that includes driving as well as sitting at a desk—get up and walk around regularly.

• **Herbs.** Men have reported good results using herbal products to relieve symptoms of BPH. The most widely used and documented is extract of saw palmetto (*Serenoa repens*).

"Roughly 90 percent of men with mild-to-moderate BPH experience some improvement in symptoms during the first four to six weeks after beginning to take saw palmetto extract," says Joseph Pizzorno, N.D., who recommends taking 160 milligrams of standardized saw palmetto extract twice a day.

Another effective herb is *Pygeum africanum*. Many formulas are on the market combining these two herbs, sometimes with added zinc. You may also have good results from stinging nettle extract (take 300 to 600 milligrams a day). Additional beneficial herbs for prostate, according to herbalist David Crow, L.Ac., are corn silk and uva ursi. If your problem is prostatitis (inflammation of the prostate), try goldenseal.

• **Nutrition.** "The best strategy is prevention," according to Dr. Weil. "Dietary and lifestyle measures—from eating soy foods to getting regular exercise to taking specific supplements—may significantly reduce your odds."

Eat less saturated fat. Many studies confirm that the men who eat the most animal fat (from meat and dairy products) are the most likely to die of prostate cancer.

"Focus on whole, unprocessed foods," suggests Dr. Pizzorno. Eat more soy products (tofu, tempeh, soy milk), which may help to prevent both prostate cancer and BPH.

Eat your veggies. "I advise eating five to nine servings of fruits and vegetables a day," says Dr. Weil. Dr. Pizzorno suggests eating "a quarter-cup of raw sunflower seeds or pumpkin seeds each day" and eliminating alcohol (especially beer), caffeine, and sugar from your diet.

• **Supplements.** Michael Murray, N.D., recommends a daily supplement of: zinc (45 to 60 milligams); flaxseed oil (1 tablespoon); and an amino acid mixture of glycine, glutamic acid, and alanine (200 milligrams each). Dr. Weil recommends selenium (200 micrograms daily), vitamin E (400 to 800 IU), and vitamin C (1,000 milligrams twice a day). Talk to your physician about which of these supplements might be appropriate for you.

Sinus Problems
(See also "Allergies" and "Colds")

• **Acupressure.** Use the following sequence of pressure points around your nose, eyes, and forehead to relieve sinus headaches, pressure, and congestion.

- Press at various points around the eye sockets, using your thumbs for the upper points and your middle fingers for the lower points. Do not press hard around the eyes. You will find several natural depressions that help locate the points for you. Press both sides simultaneously for three to five seconds, release, and repeat twice.
- Press along the bottom edge of the cheekbones. Press with three-finger pressure on both sides. Again, press for three to five seconds, release, and repeat twice.
- Use three fingers to press on the temples, in a straight line from the corner of the eye toward the ear. Use medium pressure at most, pressing and releasing.

• **Aromatherapy.** Boil a pan of water with a few drops of eucalyptus oil or a little powdered ginger in it. Turn off the heat, cover your head with a towel, lean over the pot, and inhale the steam.

• **Hydrotherapy.** One of the best ways to help clear up sinus congestion is to wash your nasal passages with a mild saline solution. Add ¼ teaspoon salt to ¼ cup warm water. Pour a little in a small cup (an eye cup or a small paper cup works well) or in the palm of your hand, and sniff it up, one nostril at a time. Tilt your head back and let the salt water slip partway down into your throat, then spit it out.

If you find this uncomfortable, just sniff it in, then gently blow your nose. Or use an eye dropper and put 5 or 6 drops into each nostril. Repeat this several times a day.

Just standing a while in a hot shower is also effective.

Skin Problems
(See also "Acne")

• **Aromatherapy.** Steam your face with essential oils. Put a few drops of essential oil in a pot of hot water (after you remove it from the stove), cover your head with a towel, and let the steam rise onto your face. Use bergamot, tea tree, or chamomile. If you don't have the essential oil you could put a chamomile tea bag in the water.

• **Ayurveda.** The main factors in clear, healthy skin are a clean colon and healthy liver, says David Crow, L.Ac. To accomplish this, take triphala at night. Add ½ teaspoon of the powder to 1 cup of hot water, steep 10 minutes, and drink.

• **Exercise.** Exercise keeps the organs healthy and promotes healthy digestion and elimination. Try to get half an hour of aerobic exercise at least four or five times a week. Try walking, bicycling, jogging, aerobic dancing, swimming, or whatever you enjoy and are in shape for.

• **Herbs.** "Burdock root is a very helpful herbal blood purifier," says Crow. "It also works as a liver decongestant." Make burdock tea by adding ½ teaspoon of the herb per cup of water; drink it two or three times a day.

"In addition," says Crow, "buy yourself a juicer and make lots of green drinks: parsley, fresh burdock root (if you can get it), celery, cucumber. Bitter greens, like dandelion and arugula, are best."

Other beneficial herbs for the skin are milk thistle seed (in capsules or tincture); turmeric (capsules), and yellow dock. A standard commercial formula for skin care might contain a mixture of these herbs, plus red clover and perhaps echinacea.

For an anti-inflammatory skin wash, make a tea of any of the following herbs, then make a compress by dipping a washcloth in the tea and placing it over your face. Or simply rinse your face with the tea (once it cools). Effective herbs include calendula, chamomile, and St. John's wort. A compress or rinse with witch hazel is also effective. Mix some comfrey, slippery elm, and aloe to make a slippery paste; and apply topically as a mask.

Taking goldenseal is helpful for the infectious stage of skin problems. This herb is effective both internally (in capsules) and externally as a paste or wash.

• **Nutrition.** Alternative health practitioners point to a number of foods they say can aggravate skin conditions: fried foods, chocolate, salty and greasy foods such as potato chips, dairy products, and spicy food.

Especially avoid saturated fats found in meat and dairy. Also avoid alcohol, white sugar, and refined flour. Instead, eat fresh, healthy foods, rich in fiber, which help keep the colon clean and elimination regular.

Fresh fruits and vegetables are vital. Everyone should eat five to nine servings each day.

Water helps your kidneys eliminate toxins, which otherwise might be released through the skin. Drink six to eight glasses per day.

Sore Throat

• **Acupressure.** Use the following point to help relieve your sore throat. It is located on the thumb, at the bottom corner of the nail—the corner farthest away from your little finger. Stimulate the point by holding your right thumb between the thumb and first two fingers of your left hand; press with the thumb.

You want the pressure to be right where the cuticle meets the nail corner. To properly stimulate this point, you need to press hard. Slowly rock the thumb that you're pressing back and forth as you press. Remember to build up pressure, hold about a minute, then gradually release. Repeat with the other hand.

• **Aromatherapy.** Boil a pint of water in a pot, remove from the heat, put a towel over your head, and breathe normally through your nose as you lean over the pot and inhale the steam. Add a few drops of aromatherapy oil to the water if you wish; eucalyptus, clary sage, rosemary, or lemon oil would be beneficial.
• **Chinese medicine.** Dairy products such as yogurt, milk, and cheese tend to aggravate sore throats. It's best to avoid them.
• **Herbs.** A soothing and healing herbal tea, recommended by Vasant D. Lad, BAMS, MASc, is a mixture of ginger, cinnamon, and licorice root. Mix the herbs in equal proportion and use ½ teaspoon of the mixture per cup of hot water. Plain ginger tea is also effective. You may add a spoonful of honey after the tea starts to cool a little.

David Crow, L.Ac., recommends the following herbal remedies. If the sore throat is infectious (not just from irritation), use goldenseal and echinacea. Licorice root and slippery elm (made as teas) are soothing for sore throats and also help relieve hoarseness. If you have laryngitis, try raspberry, yarrow, or white oak bark prepared as teas.
• **Hydrotherapy.** The simplest and least expensive home remedy for sore throats, and one that is quite effective, is gargling. Use 1 cup of warm water (as hot as you can comfortably handle) with ½ teaspoon of salt added.

Toothache

The following home remedies can relieve pain, but they cannot cure a toothache caused by infection or inflammation. For that, you need to see a dentist.
• **Acupressure.** For immediate pain relief, press the following point. With your left hand facing palm down, use your right hand (thumb on top, index finger underneath) to take hold of the webbing between your left thumb and index finger. Squeeze in the center of the webbing, pressing toward the bone of the index finger. Hold one minute, breathing deeply, then press the other hand. You can repeat this procedure as needed for pain relief.

Warning: Pregnant women should not press on this point, as it may stimulate premature contractions in the uterus.
• **Herbs.** Vasant D. Lad, BAMS, MASc, suggests placing a clove next to the aching tooth (between the cheek and tooth) to help alleviate the pain. Chew the clove for a few minutes to release the juice, then just let it stay there.

You can also use clove oil or tea tree oil; use a cotton swab to place a little on the surrounding gums.

Weight Gain

To lose weight and keep it off, you need to make a commitment to two things: a healthier, lighter, low-fat diet and regular exercise.
• **Acupressure.** Press the "appetite control" point. It is located on the ear and is easiest to find while looking in a mirror. Place your fingers on your jaw, in front of your ears. Open and close your mouth a few times until you feel your jaw bone moving underneath your fingers. Now try putting one finger where you feel the most movement of the jaw. Your finger should be right next to a little fleshy protrusion of the ear (not the ear lobe). Grab this part of the

ear with your thumb and index finger and press with steady pressure for at least a minute. Remember to press both ears.

• **Exercise.** The bottom line: "You need to use up more calories than you take in—spend more than you earn—not just today or this week, but for the rest of your life," according to Leonard Doberne, M.D., an endocrinologist in the San Francisco Bay area. "That's why you need long-term strategies, like riding a bicycle to work instead of driving."

"For most people, trimming some fat from the diet and getting a sensible amount of exercise three or four times a week will be enough to help you lose weight," says cardiologist John Zamarra, M.D.

First, get some regular aerobic exercise. Jogging, swimming, bicycling, skiing, or action sports like basketball or tennis help you lose weight by increasing the rate at which your body burns fuel. You don't need to buy expensive equipment, special clothing, or health club memberships. Just increase your physical activity.

Take a half-hour walk at your lunch break or to unwind when you get home. Park a mile from work and walk the rest of the way. Instead of hiring someone to do them for you, use household chores like raking, sweeping, scrubbing floors, shoveling snow, or moving furniture—even carrying bags of groceries—to increase your metabolism and tone your muscles.

• **Nutrition.** Along with regular exercise, eating less fat is crucial to your weight-loss program. Say goodbye to packaged foods, sweets, and meats. Fill up your shopping cart with vegetables, fruits, legumes, and whole grain breads and cereals.

Follow these guidelines:

- **Eat more salads, cooked vegetables, and legumes,** such as lentils and kidney, pinto, and navy beans.
- **Use whole grain bread** rather than white bread.
- **Eat more potatoes,** baked or boiled.
- **Choose whole grain cereals** such as oatmeal.

• **Relaxation.** Many health experts advise a more relaxed pace of eating to foster better digestion, but taking your time also helps you consume less food. Six additional tips for healthy eating:

1. Eat in a calm, settled atmosphere. Eating in a noisy environment makes you pick up your pace and get out of touch with how much food you really need.

2. At the start of the meal, take a moment to relax. Sit quietly and close your eyes. Take a few deep breaths and let the tension melt away. If you know how to meditate, practice your method for a few minutes. Quiet and centered, you'll be less likely to eat too much.

3. Use a little music therapy to help you slow down. Play soft, relaxing music while you eat.

4. Cut your food into smaller pieces.

5. Put down your fork after each mouthful.

6. Take time to savor the taste and texture.

index

a

d-e

i-m

W–Z